Dyslexia and Counselling

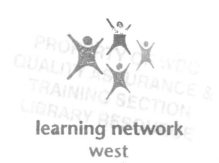

learning network
west

This book is dedicated, with all my love, to my sons
Jamie and Jonathan

Dyslexia and Counselling

ROSEMARY SCOTT

East Court School for Dyslexic Children, Ramsgate

Consultant in Dyslexia

MARGARET SNOWLING

University of York

W

WHURR PUBLISHERS
LONDON AND PHILADELPHIA

© 2004 Whurr Publishers Ltd
First published 2004
by Whurr Publishers Ltd
19b Compton Terrace
London N1 2UN England and
325 Chestnut Street, Philadelphia PA 19106 USA

British Library Cataloguing in Publication Data

A catalogue record for this book
is available from the British Library.

ISBN 1 86156 395 7

Typeset by Adrian McLaughlin, a@microguides.net
Printed and bound in the UK by Athenæum Press Ltd, Gateshead, Tyne & Wear.

Contents

Ackowledgments   xiv

About the author   xv

SECTION ONE: DYSLEXIA   **1**

Chapter 1   Dyslexia as an individual difference   **3**

Summary

Social and historical perspective   **3**

Does dyslexia exist? • How many people are dyslexic? • Is dyslexia a modern problem? • Is there a history of writing? • What is the history of dyslexia? • What is 'specific learning difficulty'? • Is dyslexia just part of a general decline in reading ability? • Is dyslexia an international problem? • Do attitudes to dyslexia vary between countries? • Do some languages favour the dyslexic person?

The physical differences associated with dyslexia   **8**

Is dyslexia a medical disorder? • Is dyslexia a single condition like colour blindness? • Is dyslexia inherited? • Is reading difficulty inherited? • What is the genetic evidence for the heritability of dyslexia? • What is the genetic point of dyslexia? • Are there brain differences in dyslexics? • Are dyslexic brains wired differently?• Do dyslexics have memory problems?

Literacy   **14**

Is there a single defining feature of dyslexia? • What is the phonological deficit? • How important is the phonological deficit? • What does a phonological deficit look like to a dyslexic? • How does the phonological deficit affect the process of reading? • Can a dyslexic ignore the phonological deficit? • Does dyslexia vary in severity? • Is there a single, best help for dyslexic people? • What happens if help is not given early? • What is the 'Matthew Effect'? • How are dyslexic children taught? • Is dyslexia teaching a specialist skill? • Do dyslexics have problems with reading comprehension? • Do dyslexics have an inherent problem with grammar? • What about spelling? • Does speech therapy help? • Do unhelped adult dyslexics ever learn to read? • Do adult dyslexics ever learn to write?

Diagnosis of dyslexia   **23**

What are the main signs of dyslexia? • Is dyslexia linked to intelligence? •

Is reading linked to intelligence? • Are there any early identifiers for dyslexic children before difficulties start? • How is dyslexia diagnosed? • Do people always know that they are dyslexic? • Is dyslexia a fixed problem through life? • Are other conditions linked to dyslexia? • Is there a gender difference in dyslexia?

Chapter 2   The social landscape of dyslexia   31

Summary • How do dyslexics feel about being labelled with a disability? • Can dyslexics be good at sport? • Do dyslexics get lost easily? • Do foreign dyslexics have problems with English as a foreign language? • Does dyslexia affect other cultural and ethnic groups in British society? • Is it hard for a dyslexic to learn a foreign language? • Are dyslexics at risk while driving a car? • Is chess a particular skill for dyslexics? • Does music present a problem for dyslexics? • Do dyslexics get confused? • Are there more left-handed dyslexics than non-dyslexics? • Do dyslexic people work harder than non-dyslexic people? • What single daily activity do dyslexic people find difficult? • Are dyslexics naturally isolates? • Do dyslexic people just reverse b's and d's? • Do dyslexics have problems with pronunciation and vocabulary? • Is there a distinctive dyslexic cognitive and learning style? • Do dyslexic people have a creative gift? • Is there a link between creativity and the severity of the dyslexia? • Why do dyslexics enter the creative professions? • Can dyslexics excel at written imagery? • Are there many famous dyslexics? • Are difference and eccentricity linked to dyslexia? • Is dyslexia linked to giftedness and high intelligence? • Do dyslexics reverse left and right and east and west? • Do dyslexics confuse time and dates? • Are dyslexic people a political group?

SECTION TWO: SCHOOL   51

Chapter 3   The effects of school   53

Summary
School   53
How important is school? • What are the general effects of school on dyslexics? • Is this an overreaction? • How do dyslexic children fail at school?
Transition   58
Does it help to go to a new school or a new class? • What are the problems with school and class transition? • Is the transition to secondary school any easier? • Do things improve when dyslexic children leave school?
Reaction   59
Are dyslexics hypersensitive to criticism? • Does anxiety affect the work of dyslexics? • Is dyslexic self-esteem linked to academic failure? • Do dyslexics idealize academic ability? • Do dyslexics feel out of control at school? • What maladaptive behaviours do dyslexic children learn at school? • Do dyslexic children have the means to express their anger about school? • Do dyslexic academic problems develop over time at school? • Is isolation an enduring feature of school life for dyslexic children?

School organization   **64**
What about the education authorities? • Are special classes in mainstream
school helpful for dyslexic children? • Are special schools better for dyslexic children than mainstream schools?
School phobia   **67**
Do dyslexic children experience school phobia? • What is school phobia? •
Who and how many are affected by school phobia? • Is separation anxiety
an important factor in school phobia among dyslexics? • How important to
school phobia are fear and anxiety about school? • Is school refusal a rational learning response? • What is the best treatment for school phobia?

Chapter 4   The effects of teachers and peers   72

Summary
Teachers   **72**
How important is an individual teacher to a dyslexic child? • How do teachers have such power to influence a dyslexic child? • Can the personality of
the teacher have a negative effect on a dyslexic child? • Why can the relationship between the teacher and dyslexic child be so intense and difficult?
• How does this transference occur? • Does it compare to counsellor transference? • Do teachers acknowledge this transferential aspect of the dyslexic child's education? • What types of transference and counter-transference
can occur in the teacher-dyslexic-child relationship? • How do teachers act
out these feelings towards dyslexic children? • How have teachers been
helpful to dyslexic children?
Peers   **86**
Are peer relationships important to children? • Do dyslexics have good
relationships with their peers? • What is the effect of peer-relationship
problems for dyslexic children?
Bullying   **88**
Background
Are dyslexic children more likely to be bullied than non-dyslexics? • Do
dyslexic children bully others? • Does bullying occur more in mainstream
schools than special schools for dyslexic children? • How are dyslexics bul-
lied? • Does their dyslexia feature in the bullying? • What effect does bullying have on dyslexic children?
Help against bullying
Who do dyslexic children go to for help? • Do teachers help? • Do friends
help? • Does anyone help a bullied, dyslexic child?
The context of bullying
What is the main personality difference between bullies and victims? • Is
bullying a social activity? • Are there different types of bullying?
Action against bullying
What can be done about bullying and dyslexia? • What does the literature
on bullying suggest? • Is there any evidence on what actually works to stop
bullying? • Can a counsellor do anything at all to help a client who is being
bullied? • How can a counsellor use the counselling process to help a
victim?

SECTION THREE: FAMILY   101

Chapter 5   In the home of the dyslexic child   103

Summary
The arrival of dyslexia: changes in the home   103
Will family relationships change when a child is diagnosed as dyslexic? • Are
the family influences on dyslexic clients unusual? • How does the family first
realize a child is dyslexic? • Does a home have to be organized for dyslexia?
• Does a rigid or relaxed family structure help the dyslexic child? • Do the
family and school unite to help the dyslexic child? • Is it a good idea to teach
a dyslexic child to read at home? • Are there particular problems with hyperactivity (ADHD)?
Siblings   109
How are siblings important in understanding a dyslexic child? • How do
siblings cope with the dyslexic child's disability? • What is the normal reaction of siblings to each other? • Do dyslexic children attract violent and
aggressive sibling behaviour? • Is there a pattern to sibling conflicts with
dyslexic children? • Do the effects of sibling relationships outlive childhood?
• What happens if a dyslexic child is not favoured over siblings?
Disability   114
How do parents react when they realize that dyslexia is a disability? • Does
parental reaction determine how a dyslexic child copes with their disability? • Do parents determine a dyslexic's self-image? • Can helping the mother to cope help the dyslexic child to cope? • Does it help if parents are
informed? • Are disability feelings transferred from the child to the parent?
• Do parents give up play? • Do dyslexic children cause problems in public? • Are parents of dyslexic children isolated? • Does the disability of
dyslexia harm the home? • Does the dyslexic child's disability affect the sex
life of his parents? • Does family life ever return to normal? • Do parents
of a dyslexic child rediscover normality? • Do family members want to
make the dyslexic child 'better'? • What are the parents' most difficult feelings about dyslexia as a disability? • Are there feelings that a counsellor
might find hard to acknowledge? • Does counselling help with the notion
of disability?
Bereavement   123
What is lost when one gains a dyslexic child? • Does the grief for a 'normal'
child ever end? • Which family member needs bereavement counselling? •
What are the signs and stages of bereavement? • Does pathological mourning occur?

Chapter 6   The parents of dyslexic children   127

Summary
Parental reaction to their child's diagnosis of dyslexia   128
Do parents feel guilty? • What is the main response of dyslexic parents?
• What has happened? The bewildered response of non-dyslexic parents •
Do dyslexic parents have to 'come out' about their dyslexia?
Parental reaction to their dyslexic child?   130
What is the initial reaction? • Do parents defend their dyslexic child against
school? • Does dyslexia cause marital difficulty? • What about the genetic
inheritance of the dyslexic gene? • What is the role of parental anxiety?
• Are parents emotionally abusive to their dyslexic child? • What about

ambitious parents? • What about unambitious parents? • Are there problems with damaged dyslexic parents? • Do dyslexic children have to parent
a dyslexic mother or father?

Mothers and the dyslexic child   136

Who is the main carer of the dyslexic child? • Who picks up the child's
dyslexia first? • Who acts to solve the dyslexia? • How does the child's
dyslexia affect his mother? • Does she give practical support to her child?
• What about emotional support? • What positive effects does all this have
on her child? • What is the most helpful maternal quality? • What are the
problems faced by dyslexic mothers of dyslexic children?

Fathers and the dyslexic child   139

Is the father as relevant and present as the mother? • Is it useful to reintegrate the absent father? • Can the father become usefully engaged with his
dyslexic child? • How useful is spouse support of the father to the mother?
• Do fathers provide useful role models? • What about critical fathers? •
What about paternal horseplay with dyslexic children? • Do fathers protect
their dyslexic children?

Overprotective parenting of dyslexic children   142

How is overprotective parenting relevant to dyslexia? • Is overprotection
common with dyslexic children? • Is there a repressed and denied dislike
of the dyslexic child? • Does the mother have a problem in separating from
her child? • What is the role of the mother's own separation anxiety? • Is
the mother's mother important? • Is overprotection the embodiment of
the female 'tiger' role? • Can overprotection be a valid action against a hostile, jealous father? • Are there simpler reasons for overprotection, such as
fear or transference? • What happens in a parent-child alliance? • What are
the effects of overprotection on the child? • What particular counselling
issues arise because of parental overprotection?

Positive family support for a dyslexic child   150

How important is family support? • What family characteristics are helpful
to a dyslexic child?

SECTION FOUR: EFFECT   153

Chapter 7   The psychological and social effects of dyslexia   155

Summary
Research on reading problems   155

What do we know of the effects of *general* reading disability? • What do we
know of the effects of *specific* reading disability in dyslexia? • Do the social
and emotional effects of dyslexia vary over time? • What do we know about
the effects of dyslexia on girls? • What are the broad indications of existing
research on the effects of dyslexia?

The inner-directed effects of dyslexia   158

Stress

Is dyslexia linked to stress? • How do dyslexics acquire PTSD? • What are
the behavioural effects of PTSD? • What are the psychological effects of
PTSD? • What is 'Complex' (or Type II) PTSD? • What are the physical
effects of PTSD? • Are dyslexics especially vulnerable to PTSD? • Is PTSD
ever cured? • What are the protective factors against PTSD? • What is the
counselling response to PTSD? • What is the theory of 'daily hassle' stress?

• Do daily hassles cause stress to dyslexics? • Are daily hassles general or particular? • What common causes of daily stress are also associated with dyslexia? • Is there a 'final straw' with daily hassles?
Depression
What is the evidence of depression among dyslexics?
Anxiety and fear
Is there more evidence of anxiety in dyslexics? • What is normal anxiety? • What are the common causes of anxiety in childhood? • What is excessive anxiety? • Is there a link in dyslexia between levels of anxiety and intelligence? • Do physical and psychosomatic symptoms of anxiety affect dyslexics? • Do dyslexic children suffer from bed-wetting (enuresis)? • Do dyslexics experience obsessive–compulsive disorder (OCD)? • Is anxiety a protective factor for dyslexic children?

The externalizing effects of dyslexia   174
Conduct disorder
Are there higher incidences of conduct disorder in dyslexic children?
Dyslexia and crime
Is there a link between general reading disability and crime? • Is there a link between dyslexia and criminal behaviour? • Is there help for dyslexic prisoners? • Why is dyslexia linked with crime?
ADHD
Does ADHD increase the chances of a dyslexic having conduct disorder? • Are dyslexics with ADHD more likely to commit crime? • Is it possible to counsel dyslexic children with ADHD?
Suicide
Is dyslexia a cause of suicide? • What are the signs of suicidal tendency? • What are the facts about suicide? • How do counsellors work with dyslexics and suicide?

Chapter 8   Isolation   183

Summary
Isolation and dyslexia   183
How do dyslexics become isolated? • Do dyslexic isolation problems start with parents? • Do dyslexic isolation problems start with siblings? • Do dyslexic isolation problems start in peer relationships? • What is the main vehicle for relationship problems in dyslexic people?
Isolation through non-verbal skills   187
Are non-verbal skills important in communication? • How do dyslexics demonstrate poor non-verbal skills? • Why do other people not look beyond this dyslexic demeanour? • Specifically, how do dyslexics create problems in non-verbal communication?
Isolation through language problems   193
What are the dyslexic's language problems? • Why do dyslexics have problems in conversation and information processing? • What sort of problems with articulacy, speech and delivery do dyslexics have?
Isolation through kinaesthetics   196
How do dyslexics manage space (kinaesthetics)?
Isolation through lack of social cognition   197
What is social cognition? • Do dyslexics have good social cognition? • Is social-cognitive-skills training effective?

Isolation through victim behaviour 198
Is victim behaviour common in dyslexics? • Why does the dyslexic adopt victim behaviour? • What is learned helplessness?
Isolation through the latency stage 200
How is the latency stage relevant to relationship problems? • How is the latency stage important in social relationships? • What are the effects of problems in the latency stage?
Misinterpreting dyslexic isolation 202
Can dyslexic isolation be cloaked? • Is isolation the same as 'lonely' or 'alone'?

Chapter 9 Survival strategies and dyslexia 204

Summary
Self-esteem and dyslexia 204
How does self-esteem feature in dyslexia? • Do dyslexics have lower self-esteem than non-dyslexics? • Are there associated bodies of evidence? • Do special schools enhance dyslexic self-esteem? • Is dyslexic self-esteem a single unity? • Is dyslexic self-esteem judged fairly? • Does poor self-esteem in literacy contaminate everything else? • Is 'poor self-esteem' a strategic psychological choice by a dyslexic client? • What improves self-esteem in dyslexics? • Would getting rid of dyslexia itself help?
The infantilized dyslexic 208
Are dyslexics generally mature or immature for their age? • How do dyslexics internalize the notion that they should not grow up?
Coping strategies: balancing out the negative 214
Can dyslexics survive their negative experiences? • Is there acknowledgement of the dyslexic's ability to cope? • Do dyslexics develop coping strategies? • What coping strategies do dyslexics commonly use? • Do dyslexic's find ways of coping with academic work? • Do dyslexics benefit from their experiences? • What is post-traumatic growth? • How can a counsellor use the theory of post-traumatic growth?
Research on the social and psychological effects of dyslexia: a critique 220

SECTION FIVE: COUNSELLING 223

Chapter 10 Counselling practice with dyslexic clients 225

Summary
Effective counselling systems for dyslexics 225
How do effective counselling systems work? • What systems have used combined assessment and counselling to help dyslexics? • Are there voluntary projects? • Are there any counsellors who have dyslexia?
Counselling for dyslexics in primary care 227
Is dyslexia understood in primary care? • Do dyslexics use primary care for help? • Are GPs a useful area for dyslexic referrals? • Is there counselling provision for dyslexics in GP surgeries?

Counselling adults with dyslexia   229
Are there specific issues to consider in counselling adult dyslexic clients? •
Do dyslexic adults have problems at work? • Does literacy continue to cause
problems in employment? • Should a dyslexic employee disclose their
dyslexia or not? • Is there practical support for dyslexics a work? • How do
dyslexics make the right career choice? • Do dyslexics make unwise career
choices? • Are dyslexic employees bullied at work?

Counselling students with dyslexia   234
What provision is available for dyslexic students? • What are the recommendations of the *Singleton Report*? • How many students are dyslexic? •
What problems do dyslexic students face that are different from those
faced by non-dyslexic students? • Do dyslexic students benefit from counselling services? • What about disclosure at university? • What help is available for study skills?

Counselling dyslexic children at school   238
Is there counselling help for dyslexic children at school? • Are school-based
counsellors useful to dyslexics? • Is outside referral a good option?

Assessment of dyslexia: a counselling tool   240
What are the practicalities of assessment for a dyslexic client? • When
should a dyslexic be assessed? • Is counselling useful before or after diagnosis? • What are the effects of assessment?

Chapter 11 The counselling process with dyslexic clients   244

Summary
The counselling relationship   244
What is the single most important aspect of counselling for a dyslexic
client? • Do dyslexic clients disclose their dyslexia to a counsellor?

Counselling communication with dyslexic clients   246
Verbal communication
Do dyslexics have poor vocabulary? • Why does my dyslexic client always
sound depressed even when he says that he is not? • Are there problems in
expressing language? • Will a dyslexic client and counsellor understand
each other? • Do I need to build a time lag into my responses? • Why do
we keep talking over each other? • Will my dyslexic client be happy to do
CBT homework and keep a diary? • Why do some dyslexic clients talk in a
stop-start way? • Do dyslexic clients prefer vague or concrete responses? •
Should I avoid counselling jargon? • Why do dyslexic clients often waffle?
• Why do dyslexic clients just seem to seize up sometimes? • Are words as
important to dyslexics as to counsellors? • How do dyslexics play for time?
• Do dyslexic and non-dyslexic clients use 'intention' words in the same
way? • Are words, images and metaphors better for counselling with dyslexics? • Are dyslexics creative in counselling? • How will a dyslexic's sequencing difficulty affect counselling with them? • How do short-term memory
problems affect dyslexics in counselling?
Physical factors
Why do my dyslexic clients arrive late, early or sometimes forget to come?
• Are dyslexic clients always fidgety and restless? • Why are dyslexic
clients so languid? • Why are dyslexic non-verbal skills so strange? • Do
dyslexic clients use a lot of comfort and transitional objects? • Would it be

considered tactless to give a dyslexic client forms to fill in? • Are dyslexics easily distracted during counselling? • Do dyslexic clients get bored?
Defences   257
Are dyslexic clients good at defences? • What defences are common in dyslexic clients?
Boundaries   262
Are boundaries important in dyslexic counselling? • What types of boundaries are most important?
Challenge and change   263
How do dyslexic clients respond to challenge? • Do dyslexic clients like change?

Chapter 12 Specialist counselling approaches   265

Summary
Contributions from the 'inner critic'   265
What is the 'inner critic'? • Does the dyslexic child take in more negative introjects than other children? • What is the effect of the inner critic?
Contributions from cognitive behavioural therapies (CBT)   267
Why is CBT so useful for dyslexic problems? • Can CBT techniques be integrated into other therapeutic practices? • Do I work with cognitive skills or cognitive processes? • What negative thoughts and beliefs are particularly common withdyslexic clients? • Which CBT statements and challenges work well with dyslexic clients? • What other CBT approaches can be used?
Contributions from Transactional Analysis   276
How can I use the theory of strokes? • Is the notion of PAC (parent-adult-child) useful? • What TA drivers and injunctions are relevant to dyslexic clients? • Are notions of 'scripts' unwise for dyslexic clients? • What is the main OK/not-OK position for dyslexic clients?
Contributions from Ecosystemic Therapy   278
What is Ecosystemic Therapy? • How does it work?
Contributions from Psychodynamic Theory (transference)   279
How important is transference in working with a dyslexic client? • What aspects of transference are particularly relevant when working with dyslexic clients?
Contributions from humanistic therapies: empathy and congruence   283
What problems are there in communicating empathy to a dyslexic client? • Are words or images more important in communicating empathy to a dyslexic client? • How important is congruence to a dyslexic client?

Conclusion The individuality of dyslexia   287

Appendices   289
References   313
Index   333

Acknowledgements

Since writing this book, I have come to appreciate, more than ever, the value of two things: simple human encouragement and practical support. They are like oxygen.

Throughout the entire preparation of this book, Nick Dermott gave me both these things generously and imaginatively. I give him my love and warmest thanks. He also makes a cracking cup of tea.

I also want to thank the other people who helped me.

These are Michael Thomson, Principal of East Court School, for his natural kindness, and for enthusiastically promoting the original idea for this book; my big, beautiful sons Jamie and Jonathan, who were a bit perplexed by it all but correctly read the importance of random hugs; Polly Klinefelter, a gifted therapist and easy, natural teacher, for her inspiring combination of really clear thinking, common sense and irrepressible warmth; my best counselling mates Bridget, Judi and Veronica who know me rather too well and, consequently, gave great advice; Tim Bettsworth, a very good publishing editor, who made a hellish job fun, and Colin Whurr, for his impressive mad-author management; my Mum, Irene, whose life philosophies of 'have fun', 'never give up' and 'so – what's stopping you?' have always inspired her four daughters; my three lovely sisters Diane, Trisha and Jillie, who usefully insulted me in the way sisters do; my late Dad, Bill, my late cats Bean, Sam and Mabel, and our late dog Lili, who always rest quietly underneath my thoughts.

I also want to acknowledge those many dyslexic people – adults and children – whom I have known over my twenty years at East Court School. They have given me some extraordinary, happy memories, and the most exuberant and satisfying counselling ever.

They have my respect. I hope they like my book.

About the author

Dr Rosemary Scott is co-owner, with Dr Michael Thomson, of East Court School for Dyslexic Children in Ramsgate, Kent. East Court holds 'Approved' status from the Department for Education and Skills (DfES) for the education and care of children with Special Educational Needs, and is registered for 'Special Provision' with CReSTeD (the Council for the Registration of Schools Teaching Dyslexic Pupils).

Dr Scott is also Director of the East Court Dyslexia Support Service, an integrated facility to provide psychological assessment, specialist counselling and teaching for dyslexic adults, as well as psychological assessments for children.

Dr Scott has a PhD in Applied Psychology from the University of Aston in Birmingham and is an Accredited Counsellor with the British Association for Counselling and Psychotherapy. Before co-founding East Court School in 1983, she worked in business management and, for twelve years, as a university lecturer and freelance journalist.

For over twenty years, she has worked at East Court School as a counsellor with dyslexic children and their families and, in private practice, with dyslexic adults. She has also worked with dyslexic students in her capacity as a Visiting Counsellor in the Student Counselling Department at the University of Kent. Dr Scott lectures and writes on the subjects of 'Dyslexia and Counselling' and 'The Social Psychology of Dyslexia' and is the author of a module on these subjects for the distance-learning course for specialist dyslexia teachers at the Hornsby International Dyslexia Centre.

Dr Scott is currently researching material on dyslexic counsellors, and case study material on the different therapeutic approaches to dyslexic clients.

Contact details:
Dr Rosemary Scott
East Court School for Dyslexic Children
Victoria Parade
Ramsgate
Kent CT11 8ED
Tel: 01843 592077
Email: rscott@eastcourtschool.co.uk

For information about the school, visit www.eastcourtschool.co.uk
For information about the East Court Dyslexic Support Service, visit www.dyslexiadiscovered.co.uk

Author's note

Of the individual members of the British Association for Counselling and Psychotherapy, 83% are female and 17% are male. For this reason, the counsellor/therapist in this book is taken to be female. It was once believed that dyslexia was predominantly a male problem. Recent research, as we shall see, has shown this to be wrong. However, to differentiate between the therapist/counsellor and their client in this book, the dyslexic client is taken to be male.

SECTION ONE
DYSLEXIA

Introduction

There are 250,000 people working with counselling skills in the United Kingdom. Of these, 20,000 are individual members of the British Association for Counselling and Psychotherapy (BACP) and 4000 are accredited counsellors (Couchman 2003).

Statistically, up to 10% of the population is dyslexic. Applying this percentage to the number of counsellors in the United Kingdom, there must be about 25,000 dyslexic people working with counselling skills, and just 400 accredited dyslexic counsellors. There are, however, over 6 million dyslexic adults and children in the UK.

Whichever way we look at it, it is evident that matching a dyslexic client to a dyslexic counsellor is considerably less likely than a dyslexic client being matched with a non-dyslexic counsellor.

It is, therefore, important that a non-dyslexic counsellor has some understanding of the dyslexic experience. This must include not only the biology of dyslexia that leads to literacy problems but also the secondary effects of dyslexia, whose poisonous roots reach far more widely, dig more deeply and cause more insidious destruction than the simple literacy difficulties with which dyslexia is stereotypically associated.

This book is designed to fill some of these information gaps for non-dyslexic counsellors. I hope that it will facilitate a deeper empathic response to the millions of dyslexic clients who need their help.

This first section is designed to paint a broad picture of what it is like to be dyslexic. Like the rest of the book, it is based on four sources: current research in the dyslexia field; anecdotal evidence from dyslexic adults and children, including dyslexic counsellors; a straw poll of non-dyslexic counsellors, who told me what they would like to know about dyslexia; and my experience of working with dyslexic clients.

The first chapter in this section looks at dyslexia as an individual differ-ence, and draws the outline of dyslexic people in physical and biological terms. The second chapter adds the detail and colour of what it is like to live with dyslexia.

The rest of the book will be built on the basic facts outlined in this section.

CHAPTER 1

Dyslexia as an individual difference

Summary

A constellation of specific physical characteristics makes dyslexic people different from non-dyslexic people. These are physical differences. These are not problems. It is the educational and social effects of living with dyslexia that convert these differences into problems, and it these problems that lead dyslexic people to create adaptive behaviours – some useful and some not at all useful. Specifically, it is these problems and adaptive behaviours with which this book is concerned since they will be the principal reasons why a dyslexic person seeks the help of a counsellor or therapist. It is essential that we know how to separate the physical aspects of dyslexia so that we do not misread what presents to us.

Social and historical perspective

Does dyslexia exist?
Yes.

I refer to one of the major reviews of dyslexia by Grigorenko (2001). She says, 'the existence of developmental dyslexia as a complex cognitive and behavioral syndrome is at this point beyond doubt' (p. 91).

How many people are dyslexic?
It depends on your definition, but most sources quote figures of between 4% and 10% of the population.

In Britain, the population in July 1991 was around 60 million, which would give an estimated dyslexic population of between 2.4 million and 6 million people, including half a million school children. Compared to other significant minority groups, this would put the number of dyslexic people in this country (adults and children) as greater than the numbers in the main ethnic groups combined (West Indian, Indian, Pakistani, Welsh and Irish). There are also more dyslexics in the United Kingdom than some of its main religious minorities combined (Presbyterians, Methodists, Jews, Sikhs and Muslims) and only slightly fewer than its entire Catholic population (The World Factbook 2002).

Furthermore, the world's population is 6 billion. So, on these estimates, between 240 and 600 million people worldwide are dyslexic. This would translate, even at the lower estimate, to half the population of India or China, a little less than the whole population of the USA and twice the population of Russia.

Is dyslexia a modern problem?
No. Dyslexia is as old as the human race.

Dyslexia, as a problem, however, can only exist in literate societies. This is when just one aspect of the dyslexic syndrome, the phonological deficit (see below), moves into focus. Before the advent of literacy, all the other aspects of dyslexia – for example outstanding three-dimensional and visuospatial skills and the ability to see things from many complex perspectives at once – would have made dyslexic people desirable and successful. These skills would have been much in demand when it came to developing military strategy, designing buildings, engineering and weaving political webs.

It was the advent of universal literacy that led to universal misery for the individuals who were born with the cluster of biological features now known as 'dyslexia'.

Is there a history of writing?
Written language and literacy are evolutionary newcomers. They evolved to save spoken words in a lasting format, in a time when history was fundamental to the identity of a culture.

Literacy can only develop with the evolution of biologically based mental faculties that enable this skill to be acquired (Russell 1982). Writing appeared around 3500 BC in ancient Egypt and Mesopotamia and has been available to humanity for around 5500 years, but it took 3000 or more years before the 23-letter alphabet was devised by the Romans in the first century BC.

The first stage of writing was picture script or ideograms, which are symbols of pictures. They do not require language. Dyslexics would have found them easy and would have been adept at both creating and reading them. Ideograms have no connection with the spoken word and do not require phonemic awareness – which is where all the problems with dyslexia arise.

Phonetic writing and phonography arose later to carry the more subtle aspects of language. This process went – via hieroglyphs and cuneiform – to the alphabetic system that was based on speech sounds. The development of perfected script over the centuries has 'depended on it becoming increasingly phonetic. This process is likely to have been generally adaptive to human cognitive and linguistic faculties and facilitatory for the encoding of spoken language directly onto the written cypher' (Russell 1982, p. 398).

This evolution of an alphabet was only maladaptive for the minority of readers who had poor phonological processing skills, that is dyslexia. This group has been left behind by the demise of pictograms and has still not caught up.

What is the history of dyslexia?
A hundred years ago, an article in the *British Medical Journal* described a boy, Percy, who, in spite of normal intelligence, could not read. Percy's writing reveals many of the signs characteristic of dyslexia.

Early research in 1877 referred to children who were congenitally 'word blind', and the term 'dyslexia' appeared early last century. It was derived from the medical custom of using Greek terms: *dys* (difficulty) and *lexis* (word). Most of the early research into the neuropsychological and emotional effects of their handicap on dyslexics originated in Germany in the 1930s, and influential remediation research was spearheaded in the USA in the 1940s. Russia was one of the first countries to remediate dyslexia and was well advanced in research in the 1920s. At that time, the Russian government ordered all teachers to bring dyslexic children to the expected level or risk being sent literally to Siberia. This educational strategy succeeded in virtually eliminating literacy problems associated with dyslexia. By contrast, awareness of dyslexia in India only originated in the 1980s and in Hong Kong in the last ten years. Japan still denies it exists.

In the UK, in the 1940s and 1950s, dyslexic symptoms were still considered a psychiatric disorder, but, in 1962, the Invalid Children's Aid Association established that some people had innate difficulties in learning to read. In 1970, the Chronically Sick and Disabled Persons Act was passed, and, in 1972, the British Dyslexia Association (BDA) was founded. In 1972, the seminal *Tizard Report*, which coined the term 'specific learning difficulty', was published.

What is 'specific learning difficulty'?
It is the official term for 'dyslexia'.

It is used most by professionals in this field and used least by sufferers and their families, who universally use and prefer the term 'dyslexia' (Riddick 1996; McLoughlin 2002). It is derived from the *Tizard Report* that was based on the Isle of Wight study of Rutter, Tizard and Whitemore (1970).

This study found that children could be divided into those with a 'general reading difficulty' (for example a ten-year-old with an IQ of 80 who read at the eight-year-old level and may be considered a slow reader) and those with a 'specific learning difficulty (for example a ten-year-old with an IQ of 120 who would be expected to read at the 11- to 12-year-old level but who was reading at the eight-year-old level).

Children whose reading age is well below their age level but not out of line with expectation because their IQ is low are known as generally 'backward readers' or, in the USA, as 'garden variety readers'.

The *Tizard Report* finally laid to rest the medical model of dyslexia and placed it firmly in the educational arena. From then on, 'a child is deemed to have a specific problem with reading if their reading attainment is significantly below that predicted from their general ability; in other words, if they show a *discrepancy* between expected and actual attainment' (Snowling 2000, p. 16).

Is dyslexia just part of a general decline in reading ability?

No. There is an argument that dyslexia *represents* most of the general decline in reading ability. To explain this, you need some comparison over time.

Hurry (1999) examined reading records from 1840 to the present day. She found that, up to 1964, there was a steady rise in literacy standards, particularly in the 20 post-war years. Between 1971 and 1988, literacy standards remained largely unchanged, with the greatest improvement in the 11-year age group. Between the 1980s and early 1990s, there was some evidence of a drop in standards but, on closer analysis, it was only the worst readers who were getting worse. 'The significant overall decline was entirely explained by an increase in the "hump" at the lower end of the distribution' (Hurry 1999, p. 99), that is, the poorest attainers.

Turner (1990) makes a similar point. Comparing literacy in the United Kingdom with that of other countries, he found that general literacy in the United Kingdom had, in fact, improved by the end of the last century and was better than that in the USA, Sweden and Italy, and was comparable to that in Spain, East Germany, Canada and Cyprus. The best readers read better than all but five of the 27 countries, but all the worst United Kingdom readers had got worse, having a lower reading ability than all but three of the 27 countries.

Importantly, this decline in the literacy of the worst readers matched the decline in the early teaching of phonics. The worst readers, in effect, lost their best method of learning to read. Of these, dyslexics would have been a significant majority.

Is dyslexia an international problem?

Where there are human beings and written language, there is dyslexia.

It is a human phenomenon throughout every country, race, culture and language of the world.

The universal nature of the problem is indicated by the fact that the International Dyslexia Association (IDA) grew from 28 members in 1949 to 12,000 in 50 countries by 1997. A multilingual/dyslexia conference in June 2000 summarized work in Russia, Japan, South Africa, Chile and India.

Magiste (1986) notes: 'we are faced with a condition that affects countless numbers of people worldwide [and] a substantial loss of skills to society which neither developed nor underdeveloped countries can afford' (p. 54).

Grigorenko (2001), in noting the existence of dyslexia across many cultures and continents, concludes that the majority of research results 'support a consistent pattern in specific dyslexia which does not depend on any one writing system or geographic location' (p. 96).

Do attitudes to dyslexia vary between countries?

Yes – but the effects of dyslexia are largely mediated through a culture and how much dyslexia is disabled through that culture (Frith 1999), and the most surprising countries have the best policies towards dyslexia.

In Russia, for example, children are evaluated soon after oral language appears. They are then assessed by psychologists, speech therapists, neuropsychologists, pedagogic specialists and medical doctors. Specialists aim to remediate dyslexia by the age of ten (Malofeev and Kukushkina 2000).

Chile also makes good provision for dyslexia. Every school has special-education classes, and all suspected learning-disabled children have evaluations at private centres with access to specialist tutors (Shaw 2000).

In India, the intention is positive but the scale of the problem is immense. There are 100 million children at school at any one time, and there is a policy to increase literacy from 50% to 90% by the end of this century. Taking an estimate of dyslexia at 10% of the population, there must be up to 10 million dyslexic children in India alone and at least a further 30 million dyslexic adults. Unsurprisingly, 'The professionals and policy makers are alarmed by the prevalence figures' (Ramaa and Kurian 2000, p. 16), especially as any child can be dyslexic in every one of up to three languages, and there exist hundreds of different languages and dialects throughout the subcontinent.

In the USA, the full extent of national dyslexia only emerged in 1986 with evidence to Congress from the Office of Special Education Programs that the percentage of the school population classified as learning-disabled had doubled from 2% in 1978 to 4% in 1983. Students with learning disabilities now represented about 40% of the handicapped students receiving special education. Millions of secondary students were found to be functioning at reading levels significantly below grade placement so that most 17 year olds had a reading age of nine to ten years, and only 5% could read at the advanced levels needed in many technical and professional jobs. One observer concluded: 'Learning disabilities is now recognized as one of the leading causes of school failure in the United States' (McKinney and

Feagans 1987, p. 104). Since this time, research on learning disabilities, including dyslexia, has received increased federal support.

In cultures where disability is considered shameful, dyslexia is either not recognized or actively kept hidden. In Japan, for example, less than 1% of the population is said, officially, to be dyslexic, whereas research puts the figure at over 6% (Yamada 2000). South Africa is still in the early stages of identifying dyslexia, and 46% of adults are illiterate. There is a '40-year educational backlog' (Freinkel 2000, p. 24).

Some countries see dyslexia as a language problem with associated behavioural problems, such as England. Other countries see it as a behavioural problem in which language is central, such as Norway.

Do some languages favour the dyslexic person?
Very much so.

The English language, for example, is the very worst for a dyslexic that could possibly be imagined. It is a highly irregular language with an irregular 'deep' orthography, and, not surprisingly, the highest frequency of reading disability is observed in English-speaking countries. The recent International Adult Literacy Survey (1996), for example, showed that 'the UK has more severe problems than most other countries' (Fawcett 2003, p. 119). Other 'deep' irregular orthographies are French and Danish. The more regular, or 'shallow', orthographies are Finnish, Greek, Italian, Spanish, German and Norwegian. The intermediate languages are Dutch, Swedish and Portuguese. These are all much easier for a dyslexic. On this basis, learning to read in Czech, Polish, Hungarian or Hebrew is relatively easy compared to English (Goulandris 2003).

Two things about a language cause problems for a dyslexic: its phonological structure, and the differences between its spoken and written form. Character-based languages cause some different problems, but the Japanese child using Kanji makes precisely the same kinds of reading errors as the dyslexic English-speaking child who is seeing his words as line drawings instead of representations of sounds (Miles 2000).

The physical differences associated with dyslexia

Is dyslexia a medical disorder?
No. It is not a disease to be cured, nor do people 'grow out of it'.

Dyslexia originates from organic quirks – some right down at the genetic level – that represent human difference, not human illness. Frith (1999), in her observation of the three components of dyslexia, suggests that one must seek explanations of dyslexia at three different levels: the biological, the cognitive and the behavioural. Only then will we have some under-standing of reading failure in dyslexics.

Is dyslexia a single condition like colour blindness?

No. It is not a binary thing – either on or off. It is a complex matter that is best seen as a constellation of difficulties, or a syndrome.

It has a complicated basis. Grigorenko (2001), reviewing the latest find-ings on dyslexia in an enormous review of its cognitive, developmental, educational, psychological, behavioural, genetic, molecular-genetic and neuroscience research traditions, concludes that all disciplines 'stress the complexity of dyslexia, and, therefore, the likely complexity of the under-lying etiological mechanisms' (p. 91).

In fact, Snowling (2000), in her elegant review of the current state of dyslexia, suggests that, in future, the use of the term dyslexia 'may be replaced, at least clinically, by the concept of a dyslexia spectrum' (p. 216).

Is dyslexia inherited?

Yes.

Evidence from twin, family and molecular-genetic studies suggests that developmental dyslexia is hereditary. Consequently, it is the norm rather than the exception to work with dyslexic people who have several dyslexic family members. Counsellors, in fact, need to devise methods of commu-nicating safely with the parents of dyslexic children who, being dyslexic themselves, will forget information, give telephone numbers out of sequence or addresses with chunks missing. It is not unusual to find that a client has as many as six or seven close family members, male and female, who have some form of reading difficulty.

It has been known for many years that dyslexia runs in families (Orton 1937), and more recent work has confirmed that reading and its related skills are heritable (Grigorenko 2001). Thus, there is a good chance that a child will be dyslexic if one or both parents are. There is a 50% probability of a boy becoming dyslexic if his father is dyslexic and about 40% if his mother is. The odds increase to 80% if both parents are dyslexic.

The research on the family component of dyslexia also shows that there are many individuals who are dyslexic in any one family. Scarborough (1984) reports that 65% of children whose families had a history of dyslex-ia could be classified as reading-disabled at eight years old. Riddick (1996) found that 50% of the children in her study were brought up in families in which one parent was thought to have dyslexia. In some cases, several members had reading and spelling difficulties, including uncles, aunts, cousins and grandparents. In some cases, several siblings in the same fam-ily were affected, with the degree of severity varying between them.

Is reading difficulty inherited?

Strictly speaking, no.

What is inherited is not reading disability – which is a social, not a bio-logical, phenomenon – but aspects of language processing. Results of studies on twins have found that there is a greater chance of inheriting the phonological, as opposed to the visual, aspects of reading. Also, there is a heritable variance linking phonological reading skills and phonological awareness; that is, the ability to reflect on the sound structure of spoken words. Gallagher et al. (2000) found that a high proportion of children selected to be at genetic risk of dyslexia scored with significantly lower lit-eracy skills than a control group.

What is the genetic evidence for the heritability of dyslexia?

Considerable.

Grigorenko (2001), in an influential review of developmental dyslexia, concludes:

'Today, the field of developmental dyslexia is the only area of genetic studies of human abilities and disabilities in which linkages to the genome have been robustly replicated in independent laboratories' (Grigorenko 2001, p. 91).

Different chromosomes may be responsible for different underlying dif-ficulties in the reading process: specifically, a region on the short arm of chromosome 6 has the most significant and replicated evidence for linkage to dyslexia; there are also reported linkages for dyslexia on chromosomes 1, 2, 15 and 18 (Olson 2002).

Molecular geneticists have also found evidence that dyslexia is not a product of a single gene but involves the effects of many different, interact-ing genes, each of which will account for only a portion of the average genetic influence on the group deficit in reading. One gene might limit development of phonological skills, while another might spoil higher-level language skills. There is 'accumulating evidence for more than one region of the genome that is linked to dyslexia, and we are likely to find that dif-ferent individuals have different specific genetic etiologies for their reading disabilities' (Olson 2002, p. 155).

What is the genetic point of dyslexia?

This is open to much speculation.

The genetic inheritance of dyslexia has evolved through millennia of human reproduction. Dyslexic people are one of the largest generic sub-groups of humanity. There is, therefore, a species advantage to dyslexia. It is not a mistake, and it is not an accident. It is certainly not a human trait that is suited to a literate society, but, for it to have remained in our genetic inheritance, there must be some importance to dyslexia for human survival (Galaburda 1983).

Much of the writing on the dyslexic 'gift' (see Chapter 2) relates to visuospatial skills, and there is a view that humanity needed such spatial awareness when we were nomadic hunter-gatherers. Visuospatial skill is an aspect of human intelligence that has mostly dropped out of use, but has been reactivated recently in computer graphic design and military field technology. Notably, in all these areas, dyslexics are much in demand.

The broad consensus is that the idiosyncratic talents associated with dyslexia are not an anomaly but rather 'a normal variation of human intelligence, which is important for the survival of the species' (Dummer-Smoch 1998, p. 65).

Are there brain differences in dyslexics?

Yes, but the extent of these differences is still unfolding.

Importantly for the counsellor, brain research on dyslexia is developing in the context of two new strands of neuropsychological research. These demonstrate that behaviour, psychology and brain structure are intimately linked. There is evidence, first, that experience directly affects brain structure; for example, that regular exercise can set up new neural pathways in the brain and that early abuse destroys brain tissue (Grossman et al. 2003, Glaser 2000).

Second, there is also evidence that differences in brain structure will define behaviour (Grigorenko 2001, Nicholson 2000, Snowling 2000). This second area of research has shown that it is the brain differences between dyslexics and non-dyslexics that account for dyslexics' problems not only in literacy but also in all areas of behaviour. For example, brain scans show that adult dyslexics and non-dyslexics use different parts of their brains for tasks – hence the dyslexics' unusual way of doing things. There are also structural differences in areas relevant to verbal short-term memory deficits, and reduced activity in the insula, a region of the brain known to be involved in the transmission of language.

There are, however, three significantly distinctive aspects to the dyslexic brain. First, there is evidence of *cerebellar dysfunction* in the dyslexic brain that might cause problems with coordinating movements of limbs, eyes and voice, and lead to clumsiness.

Second, there are *magnocellular deficits* that hinder rapid processing, including that of speech sounds. Time estimation – on which dyslexics are far weaker than controls – is also implicated in cerebellar function. Dyslexics are less sensitive to temporal frequency, so they are often late. Magnocellular deficit also leads to poor automaticity – the ability for skills to move from the 'think about every action' stage to the automatic. This explains why dyslexics can be slow at doing certain things, including reading, and why they need more practice before tasks can be performed easily. The magnocellular system is also a flicker-motion detecting system that transmits information about stimuli change and general shape. Deficits in this will inhibit the ability to pick up information when a person is reading.

Third, dyslexics have *symmetrical brain hemispheres*. The normal pattern for non-dyslexics is asymmetry, with a large planum in the left hemisphere. The degree of symmetry has been correlated to the phonological coding difficulties found in dyslexics which are principally linked to their reading problems. Lundberg (1995) found that symmetry in the plana temporale was especially marked in dyslexics with pronounced phonological problems.

Are dyslexic brains wired differently?
Yes – in the sense that the electrical activity in the dyslexic brain is different from that found in non-dyslexics.

Results of childhood electrophysiological studies using EEG show 'a clear physiological deficit in children with reading disability' (Grigorenko 2001, p. 98). These aberrant brain signals are not found in a single area but are 'spread throughout much of the cortical region ordinarily involved in reading and speech' (op. cit., p. 98).

The net effect of this is that the dyslexic brain makes the same electrical response to nonsense words as it does to real words. Furthermore, 'dyslexic EEG responses to words hardly differ from dyslexic response to meaningless flashes' (op. cit., p. 98).

Non-dyslexic readers, on the other hand, respond to the two types of stimuli very differently.

This eccentric wiring may account for the dyslexic ability to read text as easily upside down as the right way up (Miles 1993), and also explains why dyslexics can rapidly reconfigure letters into a range of symbols, as shown in Figure 1.1 with the word 'cat'.

Do dyslexics have memory problems?
Yes, but in short-term, or 'working', memory not in long-term memory.

This is a major factor in day-to-day problems for a dyslexic. Short-term memory is the term used to refer to the mental workplace in which information can get temporarily stored while we are using complicated daily activities, such as talking, listening and mental arithmetic. Dyslexics have problems retaining visual information, but problems with short-term memory are most marked when retaining verbal items. For dyslexics, taking messages or remembering instructions are like holding a handful of fine sand. This has important consequences for a child's ability to pick up knowledge in the classroom.

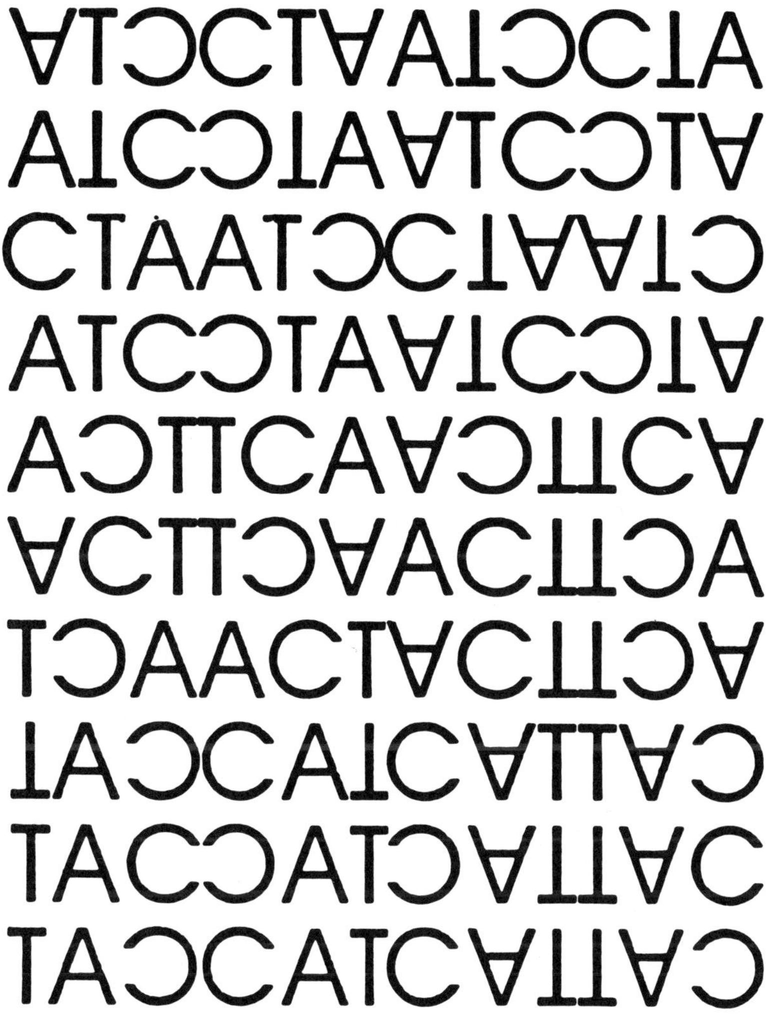

Figure 1.1 Davis's Visual Combinations for the word 'CAT'

'Dyslexic learners may be described as "quick forgetters" as they often seem quick to grasp something but fail to retain it, as opposed to slow learners who may only learn in small painstaking steps' (Morgan and Klein 2000, p. 14).

Gathercole and Pickering (2001) found that the very poor working-memory capacities of dyslexics largely affect their ability to process and sort different, incoming categories of information simultaneously. Like the old Space Invader game, as fast as they are attending to one piece of information another is arriving.

Dyslexics also have problems remembering dates, number strings, information and where they left keys, laptop, gloves, watch, cigarettes, essay, coat and shoes. They rely on long-term memory, which is based more on association, context and understanding – all of which are dyslexic strengths.

Literacy

Is there a single defining feature of dyslexia?
Yes.

The genetic and brain differences of dyslexics lead to one, significant, life-defining fact: the *phonological deficit*.

What is the phonological deficit?
It represents an inability to link the written and spoken form of a word. Normally, we build up our reading by recognizing that certain alphabetic letters represent certain sounds, known as 'phonemes'. This is known as *phonological awareness*. Good phonological awareness makes a good reader. 'Extensive research evidence has demonstrated the central role of phonological processing skill as a determinant of success in literacy learning' (Rack and Hatcher 2001, p.11).

The link between the written and spoken word seems utterly straightforward to a non-dyslexic, but to a dyslexic this link can be incomprehensible. A dyslexic cannot associate the letter with the sound and 'the images of the sounds of words stored in a dyslexic brain are fuzzy or blurred' (Snowling 2000). Dyslexics cannot make that cognitive jump from the word *looking* like something to *sounding* like something. 'Put simply, the way in which the dyslexic person encodes phonology is different from that of the normal reader' (Snowling 2000, p. 60).

How important is the phonological deficit?
No other aspect is as important in understanding dyslexia, nor its development through the dyslexic's life.

Snowling (2000) considers the phonological deficit to be the 'key characteristic' of dyslexia (p. 215). Stanovich (1986) proposed that dyslexia could be defined entirely through the 'core phonological deficit'. Other writers and researchers give the same emphasis:

> 'the main weakness of a person with dyslexia will be with phonological processing abilities' (Thomson 2001, p. 125)

> 'we have consistently found that most children with dyslexia have clear deficits in phonological language processes that are largely independent of any differences in IQ' (Olson 2002, p. 146)

'Many researchers consider phonological impairment to be the major deficit [in dyslexia] and a few theorize it may be the only proximal cause of reading failure' (Ackerman and Dykman 1996, p. 1)

Phonological deficit is considered to be the nuclear pile that fuels most dyslexic problems.

The most recent research on this – a multiple-case study conducted in order to assess three leading theories of developmental dyslexia: the phonological, the magnocellular (auditory and visual) and the cerebellar theories – found that 'a phonological deficit can appear in the absence of any other sensory or motor disorder, and is sufficient to cause literacy impairment. Overall, the present data supports the phonological theory of dyslexia, while acknowledging the presence of additional sensory and motor disorders in certain individuals' (Ramus et al. 2002, p.1).

What does a phonological deficit look like to a dyslexic?
The word on the page remains a symbol to dyslexics, no matter how hard they look at it.

It does not convert into anything – sound or otherwise – any more than you can convert a piano into an orange by looking hard at it. To dyslexics, symbols do not mean sounds. You might as well expect a painting to growl at you. When a dyslexic sees the word 'dog' and is told what it is, he wonders why everyone is lying to him. Those black shapes are not wagging their tail. The incongruence that makes dyslexics so anxious has its roots, I believe, in this first clear perception that adults are either mad or liars, but if you don't humour them, you get into big trouble.

Davis (1997), writing as a dyslexic about learning to read, observes that dyslexics often see the letters three-dimensionally, as if they were floating in space. He explains, for example, that there are at least 40 different possible visual combinations of the three letters evoked by 'cat', if you see the letters as letter shapes rather than symbols. Only six of these are correct in writing terms and only three in spelling terms (see Figure 1.1).

Dyslexics can eventually get to grip with words because they can bypass the phonological bit and create a mental picture in their head. 'Horse' and 'table' are easy. Even abstract concepts such as 'goodness' and 'happiness' can be converted into images (a halo and a new pair of football boots).

Words such as 'and' and 'because' are not easy. Davis calls these 'trigger' words, of which he estimates there are more than 200, since they trigger confusion, disorientation and intense concentration in most dyslexics. All dyslexics have problems with abstract concepts and are far more at ease with concrete, visual images.

How does the phonological deficit affect the process of reading?
It makes it a torment.

It disorientates the dyslexic, forces superhuman concentration, makes him anxious and, ultimately, turns him off the whole nasty, frightening, discouraging process.

Davis (1997) illustrates beautifully how this can happen in his example of how a dyslexic child will read the sentence: 'The brown horse jumped over the stone wall and ran through the pasture' (see Figure 1.2). A dyslexic himself, Davis shows how comprehension starts to disappear as the disorientated child, concentrating intensely, loses his grip on the meaning of the words in front of him. Then, exacerbated by anxiety, his short-term memory problems intensify and extinguish earlier words in the sentence, like waves rubbing out words in the sand. What the dyslexic is left with is not what was written down.

'When asked what he has just read, he is likely to answer with something like *a place where grass grows*. He has a picture of a horse in the air, a stone wall, himself playing ball and a grassy place, but cannot relate the separate elements in the sentence to form a mental image of the scene described' (op. cit., p. 25). By the time he reaches the end of the sentence, the dyslexic reader has not understood any of what he has just read but 'he doesn't care that he didn't understand it. He's just thankful that he survived the ordeal of reading aloud' (op. cit., p. 27).

He is also exhausted, and his disorientation and performance anxiety have rattled him so much that he will underperform on other tasks for quite some while (see Chapter 3).

Can a dyslexic ignore the phonological deficit?
No. In modern society, the dyslexic's phonological deficit is fundamentally and tragically central to his future.

Being phonologically aware and, therefore, being able to make the link between the written word and the sound it represents is the foundation of all literacy and, thereby, success in modern society. A phonological deficit is, by the same token, the foundation of all illiteracy and leads – through the resultant academic failure – to a whole quilt of social and emotional problems. The dyslexic phonological deficit is a physical and permanent difference, so it will never go. It is a life-long problem.

Does dyslexia vary in severity?
Yes – both in the types of dyslexic difficulties and the extent to which an individual experiences it.

A dyslexic reads one sentence:

The brown horse jumped over the stone wall and ran through the pasture

Word	Reaction	The dyslexic sees/thinks	Says
The	picturing process stops concentration begins	blank picture	'the'
brown	concentration continues	brown colour	'brown'
horse	concentration continues	brown horse	'horse'
jumped	concentration continues	front of the horse rises	'jumped'
over	concentration continues	back of the horse rises	'over'
the	picturing process stops concentration doubles	blank picture	'the'
stone	doubled concentration	rock	'stone'
wall	doubled concentration	rock wall	'wall'
and	picturing process stops disorientation occurs concentration triples	blank picture	OMITS WORD

Short-term memory is now starting to struggle. Anxiety starts to rise.

ran	disorientation continues tripled concentration	running	'runs'
through	disorientation continues tripled concentration	throwing a ball	'throws'

Panic is added to anxiety. Like acid, it starts to dissolve what memory remains. The first part of the sentence starts to disappear.

the	picturing process stops disorientation continues concentration quadruples	blank picture	OMITS WORD

Short-term memory gives up. Sentence now looks like Chinese. A jumble of visual images remains. Anxiety and panic are uncontrollable. The child, looking like a rabbit in headlights, is overwhelmed with stress chemicals. His heart rate is elevated and his palms are wet.

pasture	disorientation continues quadrupled concentration	a grassy place	'pasture'

A mystified and frozen child stares at the page.
'He has acquired the emotional distress needed to become a fully-fledged dyslexic.' (Davis 1997, p. 89)

Figure 1.2 Adapted from Davis (1997, p. 26)

According to Snowling (2000), the extent of variation in dyslexia 'can be attributed to variations in the severity of the underlying phonological deficit, modified by other language and cognitive skills intrinsic to the child, in interaction with environmental factors' (p. 212). Dyslexia can just be an annoyance to some but a life-threatening and life-wasting, severe disability in others. The difference is not one of perception but of glaring actuality. It is the difference between arthritis in one knee or in every joint: the same affliction, different degree: the same disability, different quality of life. In absolute terms, one walks with some pain, while the other does not walk at all.

Is there a single, best help for dyslexic people?

Yes – early assessment followed by intervention, the earlier, the better.

If this is done, the virus of phonological deficit has not had time to proliferate and produce increasingly disabling literacy problems. Once the dyslexia is confirmed, early phonological training – the very best course for dyslexic children – can start. It is the 'neglect of phonological skills training, especially in the early years of reading instruction' that so disadvantages children at risk for literacy problems (Waring et al. 1996, p. 166). Indeed, it was the specific conclusion of the *Ofsted Report* (1999) that dyslexic children are helped most of all when their condition is identified early and is known to all their teachers.

Dozens and dozens of sources point to the overwhelming need for early help for dyslexics. For example:

'early and appropriate intervention [is] the best chance for people with dyslexia to achieve their maximum level of literacy' (Viall 2000, p. 3)

'early screening needs to be carried out ... whether by teachers, psychologists, SENCOs or whoever' (Cooke 2001, p. 49)

'early intervention for children at risk of specific learning difficulties should be high priority for educationalists, and health professionals' (Prior 1996, p. 164)

'early intervention [can] circumvent what otherwise can be a downward spiral of literacy impairment and educational achievement' (Snowling 2000, p. 214)

It is not as if the message is in any way ambiguous.

Yet, 60% of dyslexics are still undiagnosed in adulthood, and most children will be lucky to obtain a diagnosis before they are teenagers.

What happens if help is not given early?

If help does not come early, the main result is insidious and accelerating failure.

This is not only cruel but 'the cost of failure in terms of reduced self-esteem and in terms of wasted time and resources is inordinate' (Cooke 2001, p. 48). She adds that the practice of some Local Education Authorities to wish to see clear evidence of failure through reading retardation before a child receives special help is 'thoroughly objectionable' (p. 48).

The longer the wait for remediation, the further behind a child falls. This is known as the 'Matthew Effect'.

What is the 'Matthew Effect'?

Things get slowly worse when you're dyslexic. The Matthew Effect is a New Testament reference to the rich getting richer and the poor getting poorer (Stanovich 1986).

In other words, without the firm base of phonological skill, dyslexics cannot build the further skills required to learn to read. They get further and further behind, and everyone else gets further and further ahead. With less access to print, other benefits gleaned from reading, such as general knowledge, also remain out of reach.

Thomson (1990) showed how dyslexic children who do not receive help make an average of five months' progress per year in reading and three months' in spelling. Thus, they drop behind their peers in both skills. Without intensive remediation, the children remain stuck and do not show any progress.

This is the critical moment when a dyslexic embarks on a lifetime of significant difficulty: '[of the] few longitudinal studies of outcome for children with reading problems, ... those that exist are generally quite pessimistic in their findings, with poor educational, social and employment outcomes highly likely for a substantial proportion of children with early reading difficulties' (Waring et al. 1996, p. 160). This is also known as the 'learning disabilities loop' where poor school performance leads to lowered school-related success, followed by the rejection of the values of school and learning to read and, ultimately, the rejection of education in its entirety.

How are dyslexic children taught?

A specialized approach to teaching is required for children with dyslexic difficulties. This is known as 'structured phonics' and also involves elements of 'multisensory' learning and 'over learning'.

Structured phonics involves teaching the relationship between letter combinations and their sounds specifically, and relating them to spelling patterns. This builds up the pupil's vocabulary gradually and in a very systematic way. It also involves starting at a level just below the child's reading and spelling attainments. For example, the child who is having difficulty identifying simple words and letters would start with CVC (consonant-vowel-consonant) words. The next stage would be consonant blends and large letter clusters. The teaching process moves through two-syllable regular words, vowel combinations (e.g. 'ai' saying 'a') and spelling rules such as how to add suffixes to words, e.g. *hop* into *hopping*, as well as attention to more difficult orthographic units, e.g. *tion* spelling *shun*.

The important thing is that a child should receive a systematic programme geared towards writing sounds and symbols, spelling patterns, rules and regulations of the written language in a way that is geared to their particular level of reading and spelling and their learning difficulty.

There are other multisensory techniques that can be used, involving whole-word tracing, using plastic or wooden letters or tracing over sandpaper. These are all additional aids to the child's weak auditory memory and help to combat the sound-coding difficulties that many dyslexic children have. As well as these, there might be a programme specifically on phonological awareness and sound coding. Examples of this include 'Sound Linkage' by Peter Hatcher and taped programmes such as 'Units of Sound'. Sometimes, these programmes can be used as an adjunct to other teaching methods, with individual parts picked out to suit the child. With other children, they can be used as a complete programme. Another important aspect of these programmes is the relating of the articulation of letter and word formation in speech to its written form; that is, showing a child relating whereabouts in his mouth sounds are produced and the consequent representation of those in letter formation. It is not the particular programme that is important so much as the general approach.

Teaching a dyslexic involves much 'over learning' (approaching a subject from many different angles, over and over again) and a great deal of patience.

Thomson (2001) observes that the path of reading ability in dyslexics follows a certain growth curve. There is an initial improvement followed by a plateau or slower rate, and then another surge, reflecting the initial learning of 'phonics', i.e. basic alphabetic, regular word teaching, based on phonological weaknesses. The rest of more complex phonology, e.g. vowel combinations as well as irregular words and more complex orthography, takes longer to remediate. Nonetheless, this specialized teaching is very effective. It eliminates the 'Matthew effect' and 'the widening gap between a dyslexic's chronological age and his/her attainments can be closed' (Thomson 2003, p 3).

Is dyslexia teaching a specialist skill?

Yes – and it requires training from diploma to degree level.

There are many different courses available, but the specific skills to teach dyslexics are not integral to general teacher training courses.

Different accredited courses are available through the British Dyslexic Association and the Dyslexia Institute, including a variety by distance learning. (Appendix C provides a number of useful websites and lists some relevant publications.)

Do dyslexics have problems with reading comprehension?

Yes. Good comprehenders can decode words accurately and quickly, have a good vocabulary and can summarize, predict and clarify as they read. They also have good short-term memory. In other words, they are not dyslexic.

The main difference between good comprehenders and dyslexic readers is in the amount of recall after reading a passage of prose. Lack of automaticity means that acute concentration on the mechanism of reading takes place to the detriment of understanding. It is like driving a car. It is hard to enjoy the scenery if you are focusing on working the pedals and gear stick: 'word identification processes are still too resource-demanding at the cost of the amount of attention available for comprehension' (Hummel 2000, p. 23).

Dyslexics also have deficits in the verbal reasoning ability that allows reading between the lines, and a lack of knowledge about different writing conventions, vocabulary and syntax. They also have a poor understanding of certain words – mainly owing to a lack of experience with books. Hummel concludes: 'students with specific learning difficulties are often identified as poor comprehenders' (p. 23).

Do dyslexics have an inherent problem with grammar?

No. Their talent in understanding context means that dyslexics are, intuitively, better at grammar and in using it correctly than non-dyslexics. Their problems with grammar are intricately related to their phonological problems. The initial advantage that dyslexic children have in the understanding and use of grammar will, however, be lost within a year. Their phonological problems affect their spelling. This, in turn, leads to the loss of advantage in grammatical awareness and, finally, all grammatically based spelling sequences – such as 'there' instead of 'their' – as well. Their use of context and intuition will not help them so, although dyslexic children have 'a linguistic strength as well as a linguistic weakness' (Bryant et al. 1998, p. 509), it is the weakness that prevails and, ultimately, disables them.

What about spelling?

Dyslexics will have spelling problems all their lives.

It may improve, but it will never be secure and, on a bad day, it will be the first skill to desert them. 'This spelling deficit often remains when the child's reading disability has improved, and indeed frequently remains a life-long handicap' (Stevenson et al. 1993, p. 1137).

Dyslexics cannot decode unfamiliar words or reflect on the sound structure of words to try and work out how to spell them. This spelling problem is directly linked with the phonological deficit, and one of the most significant and persisting consequences of a phonological deficit is a difficulty with spelling. Dyslexics see a written word as a symbol composed of several alphabet symbols. Dyslexics do not pick up that the letters on the page are representations of what we say. Spelling mistakes are, thus, the outer manifestation of dyslexia.

Does speech therapy help?

Very much so.

It is the case that children with literacy problems often have difficulties with speech and language problems, so speech therapy helps with verbal and oral dyspraxia, the processing of information and difficulties with articulation.

Speech therapists are excellent at 'unplugging phonology' (McCormick 2003, p. 1). They help the dyslexic to grow the connection between letters and sounds like a skilled surgeon can grow a tube of skin graft from one part of the body to another. Speech therapy can coax sound and symbol together in the dyslexic child's cognitions establishing, it has even been suggested, new neural pathways to phonological processing. In fact, speech therapists can also help with the difficult problem of poor eating habits by helping those dyspraxic dyslexics whose mouth sensitivity has turned them into fussy or messy eaters.

Do unhelped adult dyslexics ever learn to read?

Yes.

Adult dyslexics use various compensatory, context-based strategies to learn to read, just as they find ways to compensate for their emotional difficulties: 'there is no question that dyslexic children change and can compensate' (Snowling and Nation 1997, pp. 9). This means that although 'reading problems tend to be the key behavioural symptom of dyslexia in the early years, many adults with a childhood history of dyslexia are fluent readers' (Snowling 1998, p. 7). Not all adult dyslexics manage to do this, however, but they can compensate in other ways (Snowling 2000). The issue of compensation in the guise of coping strategies will be a continuing theme throughout this book, and the subject of more detailed discussion in later chapters because it forms an essential plank in counselling dyslexic adults and children.

Do adult dyslexics ever learn to write?
Often – but it will rarely be a secure skill.

Sterling et al. (1998), in a study on adult student dyslexics, found that they wrote more slowly, produced shorter essays, used more monosyllabic and fewer polysyllabic words and their spelling-error rate was much greater than non-dyslexic students. These differences were not markedly different from those found in dyslexic children, who also wrote fewer words and scored significantly lower on measures of story construction in comparison to their non-dyslexic peers (Thomson and Snow 2002).

Diagnosis of dyslexia

What are the main signs of dyslexia?
The presenting symptoms of dyslexia will vary, depending on whether the dyslexic is an adult or a child.

- The main sign of dyslexia in every age group is a puzzling discrepancy between intellectual ability and the achievement of literacy. Dyslexic adults and children cannot read and write easily. Spelling in dyslexics is particularly poor and will always remain a major weakness. Some dyslexics can learn to read and write, but those who are severely dyslexic will remain illiterate all their lives.
- Dyslexia is associated with disorganization, awkwardness, and with forgetting things. Handwriting is poor and often very untidy. Dyslexics can be clumsy, and many have poor communication and social skills. A significant number of dyslexics have problems with language. They find it difficult to express themselves, and many have a lack of verbal fluency, including problems in pronunciation and word finding. They can be untidy in their appearance.
- Dyslexics have problems with sequencing, so they often cannot tell left from right and east from west. Days, months, years, letters – any type of symbols – get mixed up. Since dyslexics confuse number order, mathematics and arithmetic become difficult, if not impossible.
- Dyslexics find abstract concepts very difficult, and prefer a more visual, concrete and kinaesthetic way of learning. They have a poor sense of time and are often late.
- The brain structure of dyslexics means that automatic actions in certain tasks are not mastered, so some skills, such as golf, handwriting and driving, may never become fluent.
- Dyslexics can have profound problems in concentrating and may 'disappear' psychologically in the middle of a sentence and during a lesson.

They can forget what to say mid-sentence or in the middle of carrying out instructions. By contrast, they can find it difficult to sit still and may be restless.

More details of dyslexic symptoms are given in Appendices A and B.

Is dyslexia linked to intelligence?
No. Dyslexia is independent of intelligence.

It used to be thought that being dyslexic was associated only with high intelligence. The reality is that dyslexia is spread normally over the full range of IQ levels and occurs at all levels of intellectual ability.

Where it does link with intelligence is in the 'discrepancy theory' that is used extensively in the diagnosis of dyslexia. Dyslexia is suspected if there is a puzzling and significant discrepancy between a person's performance on literacy and their intelligence. This is a significant feature of assessment.

It works like this. If you would expect a child with a certain IQ to be reading at, say, the 12-year-old level, and testing discovers the level to be at the nine-year-old level – which is a reading age of 18 months below expectation (this is usually the minimum discrepancy) – then dyslexia is indicated. If a low IQ links with a low reading age, then other problems – such as being a slow reader – might be suspected. With a very intelligent child, it would be expected that their reading age would be up to five years higher than their chronological age. As children's written language performance improves with teaching, their discrepancy between ability and IQ lessens. This is also a good measure of improvement.

Is reading linked to intelligence?
Yes. There is a strong relationship between reading and intelligence.

The seminal Isle of Wight Study (Rutter et al. 1970) established this association for all children and, since then, many researchers have also demonstrated that bright dyslexic children make the most progress in reading. A recent study, for example, found that there were 'high and significant correlations between intelligence and written language skills' in a wide sample of dyslexic school children (Thomson 2003, p.10).

Are there any early identifiers for dyslexic children before difficulties start?
Yes. There are some clues that point to a good possibility that a child is dyslexic. Phonological impairment, including early language and speech difficulties, is considered a particularly powerful subclinical marker for dyslexia, and there is 'converging evidence of phonological difficulties as early signs of dyslexia at school entry from children learning to read in

different school systems (the United States, Australia and Denmark)' (Gallagher et al. 2000, p. 204).

Adding to this, Mardell-Czudnowski (2001), in her report for the American government, identified the following as the top-ten predictors for children at risk of learning difficulties. In order of strength of research evidence, she cites:

1. phonological awareness tasks and difficulty rhyming words
2. difficulty naming known objects quickly
3. pronunciation problems
4. trouble learning the alphabet and numbers
5. being extremely restless and easily distracted
6. slow vocabulary growth
7. late talking compared to peers
8. trouble interacting with peers
9. clumsiness (gross and/or fine motor)
10. poor ability to follow directions or routines

Another indicator is the presence of dyslexic siblings and parents and, in this context, it will soon be the case that gene markers for dyslexia will be identified for affected families leading to early help for dyslexics in the preschool years.

How is dyslexia diagnosed?
Dyslexia must be diagnosed properly with specialist psychometric tests and trained psychologists. It must not be confused with other reading problems, and any overlap of other conditions needs to be established. Without a proper diagnosis, the right help cannot be given. Details on diagnosis are given in Appendices A and B.

Do people always know that they are dyslexic?
No. In fact there is a huge, untapped, undiagnosed core of dyslexia in the population. This is why assessment is so important (see Chapter 10). Grant (2002), for example, found that 60% of the university students referred to him for diagnosis had not been identified as dyslexic at school.

Is dyslexia a fixed problem through life?
Dyslexia is a developmental problem.

This means that it is a problem that changes as the sufferer develops and matures. Consequently, it is defined differently at different stages of development, even within one individual. This development is mainly defined by the changing nature of the presenting symptoms of dyslexia. These will involve four changing components.

First, there is the hierarchical system of reading, involving layers of cognitive semantic processes building one on the other. Second, there are maturational developments in the individual. Third, there are the situational and individual features such as the type of school, peer response, social/behavioural difficulties that change and develop with age, and how the individual copes with their dyslexia. Fourth, there are teaching advances, which mean that a bad reader may make single-word errors when young but, with remediation, have fewer in middle school.

The dyslexic will never be bored with the range of his problems during his lifetime.

Are other conditions linked to dyslexia?
There are several. The most common are *dysphasia* (a speech and language delay/deficit), *dyspraxia* (motor and coordination difficulties), *attention deficit disorder* with or without hyperactivity (ADD/ADHD) and *dyscalculia* (difficulty with numbers).

New data suggest that there is an unexpectedly high co-morbidity (overlap) between dyslexia and ADHD, dyslexia and specific language impairment, and dyslexia and dyspraxia. When there is co-morbidity with other conditions, the presenting features of the dyslexia will be different with different associated behaviours. Like in a recipe, one basic ingredient will give a different flavour with the addition of different ingredients. A counsellor does need to be aware of these overlap conditions, since they are very common in dyslexia and will lead to differences not only in how the dyslexic person lives but also in how they will present in counselling.

Dysphasia and language difficulties

There are many links between literacy and language difficulties amongst dyslexics. McArthur et al. (2000) observe that there are two striking similarities between these two conditions: both refer to failures in communication, one written and one oral, and both occur in children who are normal in every other obvious way. Their review and research show that a large percentage of children could be equally classified as having reading or language difficulties.

Snowling et al. (2000) have reviewed the considerable evidence for a developmental link between language and literacy. They conclude: 'delays and difficulties in language development are more common in children with dyslexia than control samples' and, looking at children with language disability, 'studies of children with speech–language impairments frequently report a high incidence of reading difficulties' (p. 587).

Dockrell (2001) reviewed studies on the effects of language difficulties and observed that this was a risk factor for a number of other difficulties, including numeracy and social skills. Communication difficulties in childhood can affect the fluency of children's expressive language and social interaction between friends: 'even minor problems can affect a child's ability to access and contribute to daily experiences' (p. 75).

Dyspraxia

All dyslexic children can be slow and clumsy to some extent. This is a particular problem when they are distracted by other tasks that can impede automaticity and overload their already poor, short-term memory.

Nonetheless, for a child with dyspraxia – a physical coordination disorder – everything is difficult because attention has to be given over to body control of every sort. This disorder comes from an immaturity in the way the brain processes information, resulting in messages not being properly transmitted. It is also known that many dyspraxic children are impeded in their physical development by retained, primitive reflexes. These are 'automatic, stereotyped movements directed from the brain stem with no involvement of the cortex' (Flory 2003, p. 71). These reflexes are neural blockages that prevent the development of more sophisticated and mature movements and are best extinguished by certain specialist exercises.

Dyspraxic children, or 'clumsy children', will be affected on many different levels – in feeding and eating, speech, dressing, gross and fine motor skills, handwriting, drawing, body image, language, play, and organization of themselves and their belongings. They also have poor balance and poor awareness of body position in space so that they bump into people and knock things over, have poor social skills, poor posture and are very excitable. They do not know right from left and find copying and writing difficult. Just as the core problem with dyslexic children is reading, the core problem for dyspraxic children is motor coordination.

Between 2% and 10% of the population are thought to have some degree of dyspraxia, and it affects boys four times more than girls. 'The stress levels for the dyspraxic pupil who has trouble spatially, can't remember a long sequence of instructions and lacks an awareness of time can be very high indeed' (Underdown 1999, p. 16).

The large amount of physical effort required for tasks means that dyspraxic people tire very quickly. Unfortunately, fast moving, coordinated people find them irritating, so they are rarely popular. Although dyspraxic and dyslexic difficulties often occur in the same person, there is some disagreement over whether they are linked genetically. Many dyslexics, for example, are very clumsy, while it is possible for a dyspraxic child to have normal reading and spelling skills.

Attention deficit hyperactivity disorder and attention deficit disorder (ADHD/ADD)

Children with dyslexia often have attention control problems and are very wriggly, often because they are bored and distractible. This inattentiveness has been observed in 15.6% of dyslexic children (Snowling 2000), but it is not ADHD. Overlap of dyslexia with ADHD is something else altogether and a much more serious problem. 'When a child is affected by both dyslexia and ADHD, the impairments are likely to influence almost every area of development' (Knivsberg et al. 1999, p. 43).

What complicates matters is that there is a clear overlap between ADHD and *general reading disability*, as opposed to the *specific learning disability* of dyslexia. Rucklidge and Tannock (2002), in a review of the literature, conclude: 'The overlap between ADHD and Reading Disability is substantial and important' (p. 988) with a co-occurrence of 15% to 40%.

Chadwick et al. (1999) reported on a genetic link: one chromosome seems to influence reading and ADHD symptoms: '[About] 75% of the observed covariance between spelling and hyperactivity can be explained in terms of shared genetic factors, [and] research points to the likelihood that genetic factors constitute an important common causal influence' (p. 1049).

Other studies do report a more specific link between dyslexia and ADHD, but it is hard to interpret why the frequency of ADHD in children with dyslexia is significantly higher than normal, but the frequency of dyslexia in children with ADHD is not. A great deal of research tries to disentangle the effects of these two conditions, but the default position seems to be that both ADHD and dyslexia contribute to reading problems but by different routes and need different types of help. The more hyperactivity, the more adverse will be the outcome (McGee et al. 2002).

Overall, if a child has ADHD and dyslexia, they are more likely to resemble a child with dyslexia alone than one with ADHD alone (Chadwick et al. 1999). In terms of reading remediation, dyslexic children with ADHD will not benefit from medication or other treatment for ADHD alone. Similarly, they will not benefit from motor control exercises alone if there is a dyspraxic link with dyslexia.

Dyscalculia

Dyscalculia is a specific learning difficulty in mathematics, and there is such a considerable overlap between it and dyslexia that it is now generally recognized that difficulty with some aspects of mathematics is a feature of dyslexia (Milton 2000). It can even emerge as a difference in studies where it is not expected. Rack and Hatcher (2001), for example, found, in a study on literacy: 'Perhaps surprisingly, given that the pupils were selected for literacy difficulties, 70% were below the expected standard in Maths' (p. 12).

The British Dyslexia Association estimates that about 60% of dyslexics have problems with mathematics (BDA 2003). Of the 40% of dyslexics who don't have maths problems, about 11% excel in the subject (Einstein was dyslexic). The rest do as well as children of the same age who have no learning difficulties. Some dyslexics just have problems with tables, while others are troubled by even the simplest of numerical tasks, such as selecting the larger of two numbers or counting the number of objects in a display (Chinn et al. 2001, Milton 2000).

Number difficulty in dyslexics takes two forms. The first, assumed to be 'true' dyscalculia, is an independent condition that features profound difficulty with number concept. The second, and more common, type is linked to the same literacy problems as dyslexia: they 'may understand the mathematics and be able to solve the question but may use the wrong operator or record digits inaccurately' (Clayton 2001, p. 19.).

It is not surprising that those who have difficulty in deciphering written words and symbols should also have difficulty in learning the various notations and symbols that are used in mathematics: 'the underlying cognitive difficulties that affect a child with dyslexia will also be the core factor affecting their progress in mathematics' (Weavers 2003, p. 33).

Thus, dyslexics with sequencing difficulties may give the correct answer but with the digits in the wrong order. Short-term memory weakness also makes it hard to learn basic numerical relationships, number bonds and – most fiendish of all – multiplication tables. Speed of processing may also be slow. Often dyslexic children are placed in a lower-ability group than their real mathematical skills warrant. On the other hand, some dyslexics do well at this subject because they can visualize the solution as a mathematical pattern.

Is there a gender difference in dyslexia?
Yes, but the gap is closing.

Dyslexia was once considered a predominantly male condition – about four out of five diagnosed dyslexics were male – on the basis that the female bias to greater verbal dexterity protected them from dyslexia. Recent research now disputes this (Prior et al. 1995, Wagner and Garon 1999).

Shaywitz et al. (1990), for example, uncovered a more even distribution of 1.3 to 1.5 boys for every girl affected by dyslexia, with no significant differences in the prevalence rate between the sexes. Furthermore, there is no evidence that boys and girls experience a different type of dyslexia. On the contrary, 'the evidence suggests that dyslexia in girls is of exactly the same kind – based in a linguistic, and especially phonological, deficit – as in boys' (Turner 1997, p. 190). This suggests that the male skew in dyslexia may have been the result of referral bias and assessment rates (Anderson 1997). Also, fewer females are diagnosed early, and more are diagnosed later. One study found, for example, that, for 68% of female students, this was their first diagnosis (48 out of 71). The comparable figure for male diagnoses was 31% (11 out of 35) (Grant 2001).

This may be because teachers more readily identify boys than girls as having learning difficulties, and previous reports of differential sex ratios reflect a reliance on school-identified, as opposed to research-identified, samples (Lewis et al. 1994).

At school, for example, girls have to show far worse difficulties than boys before they are referred. Also, boys who have reading problems are much more likely to have troublesome and visible behavioural problems than girls, who tend to become more withdrawn, anxious and, thus, less visible or problematic (Vogel 1990, Snowling 1998). There is also an argument that sexism still exists in education.

The lack of identification of girls with dyslexia has led to hardly any data on female dyslexics. Most research is predominantly concerned with male dyslexics.

CHAPTER 2
The social landscape of dyslexia

Summary

A dyslexic person does not live with his equal plana temporale, his poor magnocellular processing or his core phonological deficit. He lives with the effects: disorganization, forgetfulness, confusion, the endless pressure of having to do so many things in a series of bits – usually in the right order – instead of fluently and automatically. His problems with reading and writing, which permeate every little, last detail of modern society, constantly circle overhead, and will continue to do so for the dyslexic person's entire life.

This chapter looks at a few selected details of life as a dyslexic. They are gleaned from questions that I am commonly asked.

How do dyslexics feel about being labelled with a disability?
This does not come up with dyslexic people.

To be honest, most dyslexics are so relieved to have a label for their perplexing problems that the label itself becomes fondly associated with relief from stress. It is seen as a magical and wonderful explanation, so dyslexics do tend to have quite a positive view of the term 'dyslexia'. McLoughlin et al. (2002) also observe that the commonly preferred term among dyslexic adults is 'dyslexic(s)' or 'dyslexic people'.

What is much more important is that dyslexics loathe the adjectives, such as 'stupid', 'thick' and 'spastic', which were so much part of their childhood. When I interviewed dyslexic clients and counsellors for this book, this was the aspect of dyslexia that made them the most angry. Other labels for dyslexics such as 'maladjusted', 'retarded', 'disturbed', 'brain injured', 'handicapped' and 'backward' are part of recent educational culture.

In 1985, for example, one study was referring to children with dyslexic difficulties as 'the dull group', and noting that 'the distinction between dull and retarded children has little impact on educational practice' (Van der

Wissel and Zegas 1985 pp. 3–8). Undoubtedly, many dyslexics who were failing at school in 1985 – and who would now (in 2003) be between 25 and 36 years old – would, therefore, have been referred to by their teachers as 'specifically retarded' or 'dull'. Older dyslexic clients would certainly have grown up with the 'spastic', 'backward', 'brain-damaged' or 'mentally retarded' labels that have been commonly used in schools for failing readers in the last 50 years.

Can dyslexics be good at sport?

Yes – although those dyslexics who do well at sport – and there are many – tend to excel in those sports requiring individual skill and dogged determination, such as swimming (Duncan Goodhew) and rowing (Steve Redgrave). Sports requiring hand-eye coordination present more of a difficulty.

In cricket, for example, dyslexics make a much better bowling than batting side. 'There is something about the information processing required in detecting the line of a ball and moving a bat in such a way as to intercept that line and making contact' (Thomson 1995a, p. 54) which dyslexics find very hard. It calls for quick and accurate processing within microseconds of the output response and, for a dyslexic, too many things are happening at once. Rugby, however, seems to suit dyslexics. The contextual and visual imaging of the pack, combined with a collective, eccentric creativity and outstanding visuospatial skills, can disorientate a non-dyslexic side, many of whom start to look quite thoughtful at half-time, and alarmed thereafter.

Dyslexics who are clumsy or dyspraxic are not good at sport and usually avoid it. Their problem is often less to do with their poor sporting ability than the articulate scorn of others who tend to exclude them.

Do dyslexics get lost easily?

Some do and some don't.

Most dyslexics seem to have good visuospatial skills and seem to just know where they are, even in a strange city. Some 'have a superb memory for landmarks, a kind of visuospatial map in their heads' (Morgan and Klein 2000, p. 16). Such dyslexics hate to use a map and are not good with verbal instructions. Personally, I have never known a dyslexic get lost. Yet, I have heard of some dyslexics whose directional problems, confusion of right and left, and sequencing difficulties lead them to get lost easily. 'I can get lost in a square room' observed one dyslexic woman (op. cit., p. 16).

Do foreign dyslexics have problems with English as a foreign language?

Yes. Furthermore, the problem is that the English language may be one of the worst for dyslexics worldwide, but it is extremely desirable, in economic and academic terms, to learn English.

In Germany and Israel, students who fail to learn English adequately prior to high-school graduation will not have access to higher education. In India, because of the many different languages and dialects, 'English is the medium of education at universities and of communication in large businesses. Learning the English language is a high priority and of great advantage' (Ramaa and Kurian 2000, p. 17).

Soon, in a world 'where language contact across state borders is expanding rapidly ... increasing numbers of children and adults will be required to learn to read in their second (or third) language' (Cline et al. 2000, p. 1). Unfortunately, it is not just across borders. There are also Sylheti English speakers in Scotland and German/English speakers in Austria. Japanese children learn two writing systems, and Indian schools have a three-language education policy. Welsh and English are taught to children in Wales, and Dutch secondary schools are coping with serious spelling problems in English and Dutch. Sometimes a dyslexic will have to deal with 'dual literacies, that may be presented in different scripts, printed in different media, based on different orthographies and taught by different means for different purposes' (Cline 2000, p. 8).

Does dyslexia affect other cultural and ethnic groups in British society?
Yes – and the problem can become complex.

Morgan and Klein (2000), for example, refer to a dyslexic woman who is fluent in spoken English, Portuguese and French but cannot read or write fluently in any language. Culturally, too, it is not always appropriate to admit there is a dyslexic problem. Some families attach great shame to having a learning problem, however well it may be explained. The Chinese, Japanese and African cultures, for example, can see diagnosis of dyslexia as a stigma.

The problem is that members of these groups are rarely assessed for dyslexia so their incidence is unknown.

Morgan and Klein (op. cit.) found 'very few non-white, working-class or bilingual speakers from non-European countries who were diagnosed at school' (p. 54). This was because low expectations surrounding black and Asian children, along with the effects of second-language difficulties, concealed their dyslexia.

Importantly, all ethnic-group dyslexics felt that their learning problems, rather than class or race, were most significant in setting them apart.

Is it hard for a dyslexic to learn a foreign language?
It is not only hard but also extremely unwise.

It is not the same as learning a native language. The first language is learnt orally and at home, and the second is learnt using writing and at school. Additionally, learning another language involves auditory sequencing and discrimination, syntax, speed of processing information, good attention span, automaticity – all of which are stunningly difficult for dyslexics in one language, let alone another.

Good language learners normally have good phonological processing skills, while phonological impairment is the main feature of dyslexia. Crombie (2000) notes that dyslexics are likely to encounter fairly serious difficulties in foreign language learning. This is borne out worldwide (Ganschow et al. 1995). The physiological or biological limitations that block the learning of a first language will similarly block the learning of a second language.

Miles (1993), after speaking to many dyslexics who had tried a foreign language, observes: 'I think it likely that only a very bright dyslexic subject would be able to achieve [GCSE] standard in written (opposed to oral) French, and my experience was that those who had struggled with it were usually very relieved at the thought of giving it up' (p. 140).

Are dyslexics at risk while driving a car?

It depends. Dyslexics, for example, confuse right and left. This is not a helpful skill when driving a car – either in negotiating the controls or in finding directions.

Miles (1993), however, makes the point that confusion over the concept of left and right is not the same as acting on this confusion by, say, cutting across traffic. He asserts that a dyslexic's three-dimensional skills would help to locate them in relation to other traffic. Failing to wait or take care are not problems for dyslexics. Miles knew of no dyslexic adult who had been involved in a serious car accident, and he saw no distinctive risk in a dyslexic driving a car. There is also an argument that the dyslexic's intuitive and three-dimensional skills would make them better instinctive drivers. Certainly, the dyslexic Jackie Stewart would bear out this opinion.

The other view is that dyslexics are not good drivers. Kirkby (1995), who runs his own driving school and has taught dyslexic drivers, describes their biggest problem as being unable to process traffic information in real time. They can be 'overwhelmed by unimportant facets of the scene before them, and fail to recognise where real danger lies' (p. 130). Some dyslexics had problems extrapolating what happens next, others mixed up sequences, such as the order of clutch and gear change. Kirkby observes that the worst dyslexics were graphic artists and technical draughtsmen. This is probably because these would be the most severely dyslexic and, therefore, think most visually and contextually rather than sequentially. They would also have more information processing delays.

Morgan and Klein (2000) also observe how miscopying directions, mis-spelling and not being able to read road signs are hazards for the dyslexic driver.

Is chess a particular skill for dyslexics?
It seems so, and I often hear this assertion.

I have known a number of dyslexic children who have become outstanding chess players with very little training, and who easily and quickly learn to beat competent, adult, non-dyslexic players. The chess skill of dyslexic players is conceivably based on their ability to think visually, conceive of an object from many positions at the same time and mentally move objects through three-dimensional space. Miles (1993) supports this view, and many of his subjects were good chess players. Chess does not depend on memory of past moves so much as visualizing successive moves in the future. Miles saw no reason why dyslexics should not make first-class chess players and, from his evidence, 'it is plain that some of them are' (p. 144).

Does music present a problem for dyslexics?
Yes – but it does not have to be a handicap.

The British Dyslexia Association (BDA 2003) has published one of their helpful factsheets on this issue. This details how dyslexic symptoms impede, but do not prevent, the acquisition of musical ability in dyslexics. Violet Brand, Chair of the Music and Dyslexia Committee of the BDA (Brand 2000), observes that dyslexics all have problems with musical notation – even though they may have a good musical ear and a good sense of melody. This is because written music has to be decoded; spatially adjacent marks on paper have to be converted into sounds that form a temporal sequence. In addition, it is necessary to learn the function of many different symbols, assign correct names (e.g. minim, clef, largo) and associate them with the complicated motor behaviour which is involved in playing a musical instrument.

Learning to play an instrument is an occupation that also demands a high degree of physical coordination, and a dyslexic who has motor problems, poor spatial ability or directional confusion is not going to find this easy. It is for these reasons that music examination bodies give dyslexics more time.

It is a credit to dyslexic musicians that they do go on to achieve so well, and Miles and Westcombe (2001) show how dyslexics can be gifted musicians, if they are not put off from studying the subject early on. There are also committed music teachers who use the same techniques as specialist dyslexia literacy teachers since the phonological problems are similar. In literacy, the match is between letter and phoneme; in music it is between a written note and a sound note (Oglethorpe 1996).

Music also seems to attract dyslexics and I think that there are three reasons for this. First, the music profession attracts the type of iconoclastic and creative personality with whom dyslexics feel at home. Second, the enormous effort put into learning and playing music has a more satisfying and immediate reward. A dyslexic quickly hears the music he creates, whereas, in order to appreciate a story he is writing, a dyslexic has to push through another disability – reading. The logjams of literacy create an impediment to writing that does not exist in music. Third, there are a number of role models in music who demonstrate that disability is not a hindrance to success – such as the one-armed drummer, Rick Allen, in Def Leppard, the blind Stevie Wonder and Jose Feliciano, and the deaf percussionist Evelyn Glennie.

Do dyslexics get confused?
Yes – and disorientated.

Many dyslexics, in fact, have a disconcerting way of tuning out at almost any time, and their intense curiosity and visual acuity mean that they can be transfixed by visual stimuli that a non-dyslexic does not notice. Davis (1997), a dyslexic writing on dyslexia, argues that confusion is an essential part of the dyslexic way of relating to the outside world – what he calls a process of positive disorientation. Dyslexics use this distorted perception to shift their view of events – like the turn of a kaleidoscope.

Are there more left-handed dyslexics than non-dyslexics?
Yes.

Among dyslexic children, 13% are left-handed, and 20% are right-handed compared to 4% and 68% respectively among non-dyslexic children (Thomson 2001). This is because the dyslexic right hemisphere is considered to be dominant and, since brain hemispheres and lateralities are crossed, favours the left hand. (One opinion suggests that this accounts for dyslexic creativity, since the right side of the brain is considered to be the artistic, creative side.) Nonetheless, the difference in dyslexics' handedness is interesting, but it is not significant.

What is more interesting is the ambidexterity of some dyslexics. Only 28% of non-dyslexics are ambidextrous compared to 67% of dyslexics. This enables many of them to do mirror writing. They can also use both hands to write, including changing the pen in the middle of the page and coming back in the opposite direction, like the tracer on a heart monitor. Dyslexics are also mixed lateral – in that they can favour a dominant hand for different activities such as writing, playing tennis and crossing their arms. This mixed laterality is part of the dyslexic diagnosis.

Do dyslexic people work harder than non-dyslexic people?
My experience is that they do.

There is generous evidence that dyslexic people work much harder than others and are more persistent. Also, when I have asked dyslexic counsellors and clients what they consider to be the most useful thing that dyslexia has given them, almost all of them have responded with some reference to their capacity for hard work and the ability to keep going.

Grant (2001) observed this factor when doing psychological assessments with dyslexic students. 'I have been struck by the number of times they have told me they have to work harder than others at school and university in order to achieve the same mark as their peers. It is the case that many dyslexic children have to spend more time than others completing educational tasks' (p. 4).

Parsonage (2002), a dyslexic writing about the views of other dyslexics, also observed that all his subjects' childhoods were typified by 'working harder than others' (p. 12).

Olson (2002) comments on the extra effort put into work by dyslexic children who 'may reach normal or even above-normal levels of reading fluency only through extraordinary amounts of reading practice and support' (p. 156).

Fawcett (1995) supports this: 'children with dyslexia actually input considerably greater resources in all skills, not just literacy skills, to achieve the same level of performance as other children' (p. 14).

Dyslexia, it seems, can create its own solutions by inspiring those who suffer from it to succeed against the odds. Dyslexic people need to work harder than others to maintain their position, like sharks swimming constantly to stay afloat. In doing this, they acquire impressive inner resources, particularly when – as is often the case with dyslexics – there are no others available.

Some dyslexics, of course, do not manage this. They can succumb to learned helplessness and a victim persona (see Chapter 12). My experience, however, is that even these dyslexics do have resources and coping abilities, but they have either forgotten that they are there or have learned useful reasons for ignoring them.

What single daily activity do dyslexic people find difficult?

Writing cheques. In fact, this is used as a criterion for software self-assessment of dyslexia (Quick Scan, see Appendix B). All of the dyslexic subjects in the study by Riddick et al. (1999), for example, found writing cheques stressful. 'Cheque writing is the ultimate real world literacy task. It requires complete accuracy under a close time constraint with no rehearsal while being observed by another person' (p. 243). Performance anxiety makes a difficult task harder (see Chapter 3).

Are dyslexics naturally isolates?

Dyslexics are not easily understood, and many suffer such a degree of exclusion during their life – especially at school – that they learn to stand alone.

They are also isolated by their problems in processing language, under-standing others and poor social skills (see Chapter 8.). On the other hand, I think that dyslexics can choose isolation and self-sufficiency as a coping tactic and then learn that it has advantages. One therapeutic view is that dyslexics both experience and resolve anxiety about isolation earlier and more effectively than other people, and it is this that contributes to their tough, compassionate character.

Do dyslexic people just reverse b's and d's?

Not really – despite this being a stereotype of the condition. In fact, dyslex-ics do not make reversal errors that often, and they account for only a small proportion of reading errors made by disabled readers. Dyslexics are more likely, in fact, to reverse 'p' and 'q' and confuse letter sounds such as 'k' and 'g', although the reason for this is not fully understood (Miles 1993).

Jumbling the order of letters is, however, common, and this can give rise to striking, metaphysical ambiguity. One dyslexic boy, confusing the letter order of 'how', once wrote to his parents 'Dear Mum and Dad, who are you?'

Do dyslexics have problems with pronunciation and vocabulary?

Yes.

Dyslexics have difficulty in pronouncing certain words, particularly poly-syllabic ones. Pronunciations such as 'preriminary', 'statstistical' or 'amenome' are more frequent in dyslexics than in controls. Dyslexics will also make word reversals such as 'dikkifult', 'par cark' and 'Jackercrack' (Miles 1993).

A particular problem for a counsellor who is reflecting back to a dyslex-ic client is whether to use the client's incorrect mispronunciations or not. Using the correct word and ignoring a dyslexic client's incorrect one does have a 'teacher' resonance. I avoid the whole issue by scrabbling rapidly in my head for euphemisms. This rapid scrabbling is an important counsellor skill when working with dyslexic clients. Their poor vocabulary, because of limited literacy access, and problems with abstract concepts, because of their cognitive style (see below), mean that they prefer concrete and plain language rather than vague, abstract and multisyllabic words.

Is there a distinctive dyslexic cognitive and learning style?

Yes – very much so. The evidence points to a specific visuospatial and con-textual style.

Visual and three-dimensional style

Dyslexics are highly sensitive, visual thinkers, and some dyslexics can circumvent learning blocks by translating verbal into visual information. They also have an ability to turn things around in three-dimensional space in their mind, often at great speed. I have met some architects who do this – going into a sort of trance while they do so. This skill is also useful in some branches of medicine. One dyslexic orthopaedic surgeon, who could not easily process written material, nonetheless found that his three-dimensional talent made him superb at piecing together fractures and other multidimensional human puzzles.

Many chiropractors are dyslexic, and think nothing of mentally rotating skeletal frames and the manipulation required to recalibrate them. Hiscock (1995), observing how this dyslexic style can infuriate non-dyslexic people, counters with the fact that dyslexics can become equally frustrated that non-dyslexic people cannot just feel how something should work. 'I say "feel" because the solution exists as some form of whole three-dimensional entity in my brain; it's not visual and it's not written, but it's there all the same' (p. 129).

Contextual style

Dyslexics have a way of pulling out embedded patterns and seeing the context of problems in very complex, fast-thinking and intuitive ways. It is this contextual style that enables both adult dyslexics to teach themselves to read and dyslexic children to find a mathematical answer by visualizing the pattern of the numbers and intuitively going to the correct answer. It is also through this route that many dyslexics manage to see objects from many different viewpoints at the same time (West 1997).

Gyarmathy (2000) refers to this as a marked feature of gifted dyslexics. 'Their more holistic ways of working can prove to be less effective in school activities, but in some instances they can even be more useful than a sequential approach' (p. 84). She suggests that we call such children 'different learners'. Morgan and Klein (2000) also refer to the dyslexic tendency to categorize, find patterns and learn from experience. 'Dyslexic people do not generalise and apply generalisations, but rather learn from experience and make connections through meaning' (p. 19).

Mackinnon (1962) studied creativity in architects, a profession in which over 50% of practitioners are considered to be dyslexic. He found in a test to identify patterns of embedded geometric figures that the most creative architects scored higher than any other groups he had studied.

Do dyslexic people have a creative gift?
Possibly – but there are two sides to this issue.

On the one hand, there clearly exists some evidence that dyslexics are particularly creative compared to non-dyslexics.

Everatt et al. (1999), for example, found that dyslexics consistently demonstrated greater creativity than non-dyslexics when performing tasks that required original insight, and that they had more innovative styles of thinking. There is also some evidence that dyslexics might congregate in certain creative professions. When Grant (2001) analysed the list of successful dyslexics on the BDA's website (see Appendix F), he found that 75% worked in a creative, rather than a practical, capacity, with an additional 13% working as innovators and 5% as inventors.

It is also true that many outstanding creators had problems with literacy. Einstein was a weak reader, as were Leonardo da Vinci, Nietzsche, Anatole France and Agatha Christie (these last two had terrible spelling), Pablo Picasso and WB Yeats. Benoi Mandelbrot, the creator of fractal geometry, could not count at all well. Their spatial and creative skills also make dyslexics first-class military strategists. Winston Churchill was severely dyslexic.

On the other hand, there is, however, a more circumspect view of dyslexic creativity. My own experience with dyslexic children and clients, for example, suggests that there is a distinctive creative and artistic bias to *some*, but by no means *all*, dyslexics. To assign a notion of innate exceptional creativity to all dyslexics is just too sweeping. Some are hopeless at art and design, just as some of them become literate quite easily – given the right help.

Miles (1993) also found that those of his subjects who were extremely gifted in arts and crafts, some of whom produced remarkable drawing and sculpture, pottery, painting and technical drawing, were in a minority.

Is there a link between creativity and the severity of the dyslexia?
Yes – I think there is.

My hunch is that, when there is a talent, it is considerable, but it is related to the most severe cases of dyslexia. The greater the dyslexia, the greater the creative talent and the more disorientated, distractible and 'spaced out' the dyslexic person can be.

Davis (1997), a dyslexic commentator writing on creativity, observed, for example, that he was at his most creative when he was at his most dyslexic.

Recent research on social cognition might be able to cast some light on this. Henderson (2003) reports on research in California that shows that there is an inverse relationship between language communication and social interaction, and the gifts of artistic expression and creativity. The indication is that the order and regulation in the brain needed for language and social behaviour can act as a brake on free expression. Subjects in this study, who had all lost their social skills through a rare form of dementia, all acquired new musical or artistic talents. One gifted linguist lost his command of language and confused the names of his children and pets but found a fluency in composing classical music instead. Others found original and wildly expressive artistic ability that was not there before they lost their social skills.

In this respect, it is interesting that dyslexics, particularly the most severe, can also have deeply faulty social skills and stunningly inept social cognition (see Chapter 4 and Section 4).

Whether there is a significant *pro rata* pay-off between a dyslexic's social deficits, the severity of their dyslexia and their creative talents is, however, unknown at present.

Why do dyslexics enter the creative professions?

I believe that this occurs not just because dyslexics have some particular creative talent but because it also suits them.

Dyslexics are not stupid – creative professions can enable them to be themselves and to use their talents. It is a choice that minimizes their difficulties, and it puts success and pleasure in their lives. It is a coping strategy and a rational case of 'goodness of fit'. Since dyslexics are not able to succeed in the more language-orientated subjects, so the creative, constructional, design and inventive fields are those principally left open to them: 'subjects at school which place emphasis on alternative means of thought, and require little in the way of written work, might well appeal to dyslexic pupils' (Grant 2001, p. 2).

In his case-study analysis of 100 dyslexic pupils, Grant found that, while art was the GCSE subject that occurred with the greatest best-grade frequency (30%), English (language and literature) and languages occurred with the greatest lowest-grade frequency (40%). He argued that dyslexic students choose subjects that are matched to their strengths and minimize their cognitive deficits.

This is a point also made by Miles (1993) who supposes that 'those talents which are least affected by the handicap will be the ones which tend to flourish. In particular, art is something at which a dyslexic subject can be successful without having too many dyslexic-type problems to overcome' (p. 146). In other words, creativity can be both a default option and one that does not perpetuate the pressure and anxiety of literacy.

I think that the following factors are also relevant:

Creative process

Grant (2001) believes that the multiple cognitive deficits of dyslexics enable them to arrive at creative solutions to problems. He found that a very weak working memory and slow speed of visual processing were particularly associated with high levels of abstract verbal and visual reasoning ability. These abilities, in turn, are linked to a capacity for problem-solving.

What Grant points out is that a weak working (short-term) memory will affect problem-solving ability because ideas will slip in and out of conscious thought in a random manner. 'It is as if there is far more information jostling outside consciousness than there is space for it in conscious memory. As a consequence, ideas can enter almost randomly, and, as they do so, other ideas disappear from consciousness. This results in a transient and chaotic experience – almost like an ongoing brainstorming session' (p. 6).

In addition, Grant observes, the dyslexic's visual and verbal abstract reasoning ability are functioning faster than incoming visual information. This will not only result in misperceptions of visually similar items but 'it could be hypothesised that, as a consequence of these two factors, dyslexics are likely to be more tolerant of ambiguity, which enables them to be more accepting of unusual juxtapositions of information and ideas' (p. 6). In addition, the 'brainstorming' experience can throw up unusual juxtapositions, 'with the consequence that serendipitous solutions are more likely' (p. 6).

Finally, Grant also posits that the dyslexic difficulty with semantic memory deficit may stem the use of analogies and encourage novel strategies and solutions.

Creativity is linked to hard work

As I have commented earlier, dyslexics, as a group, are unusually hard working, resourceful and persistent. They have to work harder than everyone else to reach the same standards, and they have to do so through tougher routes. Significantly, there is some evidence that this character trait is also linked to higher levels of creativity, and studies have frequently found a correlation between working harder, feeling different and creative genius (Grant 2001). Ochse (1990) referred to this as 'sweat as a style of life' (p. 134).

Creativity as a coping process and defence

The issue may not be that dyslexics are good at being creative, but rather that they are good at devising coping strategies. From this angle, creativity becomes a good answer to the literacy problems of being dyslexic, in that it deflects criticism while keeping self-esteem intact. 'The process of surviving schoolwork, avoiding embarrassment, failure and rejection ... may require the dyslexic to discover more creative/innovative ways in response to these challenges' (Everatt et al. 1999, p. 43). Dyslexics are brilliant strategists – including finding ways of getting themselves out of trouble.

The issue of 'gift' may also be a defence. The counsellor must be aware of looking at this without being patronizing or touching a nerve. Being creative might be a rich curtain to draw over the bare literacy cupboard.

My instinct is that, for every true dyslexic artist, there are many more dyslexics who would give up this 'creative and gifted' stereotype tomorrow in exchange for the chance to read and write competently. It is notable that the idea of the creative dyslexic is not one devised by dyslexics for themselves but by non-dyslexics on their behalf. It can have the slight whiff of a consolation prize, and I would include it in the infantilization of dyslexics that I shall discuss in Chapter 9.

Can dyslexics excel at written imagery?
Yes – enormously.

What is prevalent – and largely unacknowledged – among dyslexics is their striking abilities in writing poetry and creative writing. This seems so illogical that it is often overlooked in the rush to focus on the visual side of the dyslexic talent.

The poetry written by many – not a few – dyslexic children is often quite breathtaking. Miles (1993) also noted that many of his research subjects 'showed remarkable powers of literary appreciation and expression' (p. 147).

It is not conventional poetry that comes easily to dyslexics. For example, many dyslexics find rhyming almost impossible because a deficient language system forestalls sound linkages. What they can produce is the most moving and unusual imagery, and glorious language patterns. WB Yeats, for example, was dyslexic.

This paradox of dyslexia – among many – is that people who struggle so hard with written language should express themselves so originally in the written form.

Are there many famous dyslexics?
Many – and more are 'coming out' all the time, including some younger dyslexics in the music industry. Appendix F gives the BDA list of famous dyslexics.

Are difference and eccentricity linked to dyslexia?
This is certainly a thread of observation in the literature and, in working with dyslexic adults, I do find a definite off-the-wall quality to them much more than in non-dyslexic clients.

As a counsellor, I have often reflected on how and why I get this impression. Is it some type of transference or projective identification? It may be that I pick up some dyslexic internalized view of difference – which would certainly be socially and psychologically accurate. I also have a frequent counter-transferential response with this dyslexic strangeness that tempts me to treat dyslexics as rather precious and fragile, artistic and different.

There are a number of possible reasons for this. It may well be collusion with how dyslexics see themselves in a non-dyslexic world. After all, many dyslexics will have internalized the fact that their school peers saw them – and treated them – as different (see Chapter 11). It may also be a way in which dyslexics restore the balance of power – by wrong footing non-dyslexics and leaving us slightly dazed. Grant (2001) also suggests that appearing to be slightly weird may be a coping strategy by its power to deflect attention from potential failure.

There is also the real chance that being eccentric confers an identity, which can deflect criticism. It fits with the 'class joker' defence that kept a dyslexic from being bullied, and has become a way of life.

I have also noticed that a large number of my dyslexic clients dress in very odd, but charming ways. Some of this has to do with being disorganized and wearing what is on the top of the pile that morning. The fact that this weird mixture of clothing is usually charming and not repellently grubby does, however, hint at a more sophisticated strategy – capitalizing on a common dyslexic strategy to appear hapless to manipulate others.

Finally, it is important to note that the dyslexic's occasional weirdness may simply be an exaggeration of normal human traits during the effort of coping with dyslexic symptoms.

This is not an unusual observation in the literature on eccentricity. Deary et al. (1998), for example, found that the behaviour of eccentric people only differed 'quantitatively rather than qualitatively from others; and there is substantial overlap between normal and abnormal personality dimensions. There is much common ground between the two' (p. 647). Dyslexic eccentric traits are quite probably normal ones that are exaggerated to cope with the daily features of their handicap.

For example, someone who hears badly will often stare as they strain to hear and understand. Dyslexics can do the same as they struggle to process what you are saying, form a response and get it back to you before the psychological moment has passed. The concentration can appear manic at times.

Other dyslexics are excellent at obfuscation, or can purposefully under react in order to throw the listener off track while the dyslexic brain unpacks the situation. Such strategies temporarily allow the dyslexic to take control of an interaction. It is nothing to do with slowness – in fact the dyslexic brain is working far harder and faster than that of non-dyslexics most of the time. It is the logjam of information moving in and out that causes the strange physical presentation. This will be a life-long characteristic.

Is dyslexia linked to giftedness and high intelligence?
No. Dyslexia is not related to IQ.

Having said that, there is a sub-group of gifted dyslexic children and, for them, the discrepancy between their intelligence and their often-disabled cognitive abilities is particularly challenging. In fact, Congdon (1995) records his belief that dyslexic individuals scoring in the high ranges of the intelligence scale (IQ 150 or more) may have very special needs and 'the child who falls in both categories may be at a total loss' (p. 91).

He also notes that the gifted dyslexic faces a 'wintry climate of opinion' (p. 91), attracting prejudice from middle-class stereotypes of both dyslexia and giftedness. He considers the gifted and the dyslexic have been among the most neglected in our educational system. Being tagged 'lazy' or 'dull' is bad enough for any dyslexic but to be so when your IQ exceeds by 50% the person teaching you – and calling you these names – can incur particular resentment.

Self-doubt, public failure and humiliation collide in the early school years and, for the gifted dyslexic – who previously may have had high aspirations for himself – this period will be particularly traumatic. Congdon found that this group often acted out with temper tantrums, aggression or destructiveness and, since gifted children are often perfectionist and are satisfied with nothing less than their own high standards, sometimes destroyed what they had made or simply refused to participate. Some gifted dyslexics can also retreat into themselves or play dumb.

Brody and Mills (1997), in a research review of gifted dyslexics, noted that, in the last 25 years, it has become accepted that high ability and learning problems can both be present in the same individual. It is, however, the gifted component that is not always recognized. In fact, in one study, 33% of students with learning disability had unrecognized superior intellectual ability.

The worst-affected and largest group of gifted dyslexics are those in whom their abilities and disabilities mask each other. Such pupils appear to function reasonably well, and are only referred for help if they have behavioural problems. The gifted dyslexic can also suffer from the 'performance discrepancy' diagnosis criterion. In their case, their discrepancy should be compared with their absolute potential and not the population norm, which will often fall well below their potential ability.

What is very interesting is the suggestion that learning difficulty might be biologically related to such extra giftedness. 'The literature is replete with references to individuals with extremely high abilities and talents who also have a specific learning disability. Some researchers have even suggested that, at least for some individuals, the learning disability may be fundamentally associated with a gift' (Brody and Mills 1997, p. 3).

Gold (2002) is clear that dyslexia and high spatial intelligence are associated. High intelligence does not only exist in verbal forms. She gives examples of dyslexics, including world famous sculptors and architects, who score in the superior range in a test of spatial intelligence. This high spatial intelligence – seeing the big picture without having to go through all the steps, doing well on tasks involving abstract concepts and visualization, solving puzzles and problems, design, construction and mind-mapping (West 1997) – is also frequently linked to being poor at rote learning, phonics, spelling and computation.

This point is also picked up by Taylor (2001), whose definitions of high creative intelligence also describe dyslexic abilities, including 'flexibility and originality of thought', 'willingness to challenge the existing way of doing things', 'intensely curious and speculative', as well as 'setting high standards for one's work', 'self-confidence in ability to achieve' and 'perseverance, endurance, determination, hard work and dedicated practice' (p. 24).

Do dyslexics reverse left and right and east and west?
Yes – and this will have a direct bearing on the counselling process (see Chapter 11).

Directional confusion and sequencing difficulties are a central part of the dyslexic problem and intimately linked with their magnocellular deficit. The difficulties are so integrated with what, and who, dyslexics are that they are often unaware that there is a problem.

Miles (1993), for example, describes how one dyslexic research subject, when asked which hand he wrote with said scornfully 'my left hand' and held up his right. Another, when asked to point to the experimenter's left eye with his right hand, proceeded, after a long pause, to point to his own right eye. Directional errors were often consistent, and subjects regularly gave mirror images of the direction indicated; that is, always getting the tester's and his own hand or ear wrong. Miles quotes in full from one subject:

'Tester: "Show me your right hand." (Subject shows his left hand.) "Are you sure?" (Subject looks puzzled.) "Show me your left ear." (Subject shows his right ear.) "Touch your right ear with your left hand." (Subjects touches his left ear with his right hand.) "Point to my right ear with your left hand." (Subject <u>correctly</u> points to tester's right ear, though with his own right hand). In the notes taken at the time, [the tester] wrote: 'I think this is a <u>double</u> error. He's got his own side wrong; so by getting my side "wrong" he ends up by getting my side right' (p. 90).

Just as with mathematics, dyslexics can devise sophisticated compensatory strategies to cope with their sequencing problems. A large number of Miles' subjects, for example, made use of mnemonics, such as 'you write with your right hand', and recognized their right hand because they noticed that their pen was in it. Some recognized their left hand because their watch was on their left wrist.

Others had to carry out actual movements with their bodies, such as picking up a pen in order to ascertain 'right', or mimicking the action of using a knife and fork.

The use of such concrete stimuli was all the more marked when dyslexics attempted to discover the difference between east and west, including turning in their seats and drawing diagrams. Mnemonics such as 'WE' were used and 'Never Eat Shredded Wheat'.

Miles describes how one subject faced each wall in the testing room, using mnemonics as he went, pausing, gesticulating and turning until he found the correct direction asked for.

'His performance seems to me typical of the dyslexic subject in that it shows that the ability to make a step-by-step series of deduction and the ability to combine these deductions with use of the appropriate mnemonic' (op. cit., p. 99).

Do dyslexics confuse time and dates?
Yes.

I shall give some detail on this since it provides an important overlap with counselling, which rests heavily on the ability of clients to work in time sequences, arrive punctually at specific times and dates and to observe space and time boundaries.

It also illustrates how counsellors need to see dyslexic timekeeping problems as endemic to their physiology. Strange behaviour around time and dates cannot be simply categorized as acting out. It must be interpreted within the context of the dyslexic's individual differences.

First, dyslexics have a very poor conception of time because it is the ultimate abstract concept. 'It is difficult to estimate, and seemingly fixed periods appear variable' (McLoughlin et al. 2002, p. 112). Dyslexics are either late or early and have little idea of time passing. Appointment keeping is a nightmare. Sometimes, a dyslexic client will not allow anywhere near enough time to get to an appointment, while having imagined that they have. Some dyslexic student clients would ring me to say that they would be there in a few minutes while on the opposite side of the city from where the university was. Dyslexic conference speakers will often ask an audience member to keep time and warn them when units of time are up.

Second, technology helps dyslexics – but not that much. Those with poor timekeeping, for example, rarely wear watches. I know of hardly any dyslexics who wear a watch, simply because you have to have some idea of time to remember when to look at it. Dyslexics do not understand the sequential element of diaries, and a dyslexic diary would ideally have just one big space saying 'this week', 'next week', 'sometime in the future'. Diaries, because they require sequencing, writing and the entries need to be read, are, anyway, abandoned fairly quickly. Dyslexics prefer organizers that bleep and mobile-phone alarms, and will have no qualms about using other people, including the counsellor, as timekeepers. I have had to resist frequent requests to ring dyslexic clients to remind them when an appointment is due.

Technology, however, is only useful as long as short-term-memory problems do not lead you to forget to punch in the time needed and to check it regularly. Equally, these strategies are of no use if your sequencing problems with digits lead you to enter 3.40 p.m. instead of 4.30 p.m.

Third, time problems are linked to sequencing problems and confusion over days, months and years. Many dyslexics have difficulty remembering what day of the week it is and help themselves by anchoring the day to an activity and fanning the resultant days around this. It is also a feature of dyslexic subjects in psychometric testing that they cannot say the days of the week in order.

Dyslexics also experience confusion about years and months. Some of Miles' subjects did not know the date of Christmas, and another did not know what year it was. Some could not write year dates in sequence, while others did not know their birthday, although most knew the month. Being unable to recite the months of the year in order is one of the most consistent dyslexic characteristics. Some dyslexics omit months and jumble others. Some name some months but not all. Others can give only eight months, and sometimes one month can be repeated twice. Others can get to, say, August, then make up a random selection. There is considerable uncertainty over order. The most common mnemonic is simply to count to twelve months, even if some months are repeated. Saying the months forward is hard enough, so saying them backwards might seem harder. Yet, Miles recorded that some subjects were more successful at the reversed order. If sequencing is difficult, then it must be difficult in both directions and, by chance alone, the sequencing might be right whatever the direction. By similar logic, some dyslexics are as good at reading books upside down as the right side up.

To say the least, these problems with time can cause havoc with appointment keeping. One of the most memorable examples of this that I can recall concerned one of my very dyslexic clients who had an appointment to see me in mid-December 1999. He failed to turn up but appeared for his appointment in mid-January 2000. Uniquely, it was on the right day and at the right time, but in the wrong year, the wrong century and the wrong millennium.

One thing that does help dyslexics to manage time is the confidence to take control. Interestingly, work by Francis-Smythe and Robertson (1999) has shown that good time-management practices are linked to a sense of positive control and reasonable self-esteem. It works in reverse, too, so that those who learn to view themselves as good time managers become so. A sense of control is the significant feature.

This might explain my rather mystifying experience that, when a counsellor tenaciously holds the time boundaries in a deepening therapeutic relationship, a dyslexic's timekeeping can become spot on.

Are dyslexic people a political group?

No. Dyslexic people comprise the largest non-politicized minority group in the world, but they have little, or no, sense of group identity.

It is a strange characteristic of dyslexics that they operate largely as individuals, and non-dyslexic people take most of the action on their behalf. This occurs because the medium of political action – the spoken and written word – is something dyslexic people not only actively want to avoid but are also not skilled in manipulating. There are probably other reasons, but this subject is never discussed.

It could also be because of the infantilization associated with dyslexia. This occurs at a family level (through overprotection), at school (through inadequate socialization) and at a psychological level (through inadequate transition of the latency stage of development). This will be discussed in Chapter 9. What is clear is that dyslexics have the character of a subcultural minority without any of their associated political and economic rights.

If the dyslexic minority ever became organized, their effect would be significant. I would predict that most of the entrenched literacy problems – and the associated appalling waste of potential in dyslexics – would be solved within five years. After all, the number of dyslexics in any one constituency must be larger than the overall majority of most MPs.

SECTION TWO
SCHOOL

Introduction

Libby Purves (1996) wrote of five-year-old children:

> A child of four or five, starting school, is a profoundly important and beautiful creature ... Nowhere else do you find that combination of clear vision, considerable reasoning ability and utter inexperience. It is an age that learns fast, absorbs deeply and questions life with a serious awakening moral sense ... A child rising five stands on the threshold of the wider society: emerging from a dependent infancy to take his or her place as an individual in the world ... [they are] naughty and wilful, but nonetheless display a quixotic kindness which shames the adult world. Because of what they are and the simple and eternal values they embody, we owe them respect.

She goes on to make the point that if 'they trail clouds of glory, so do those who teach them'. Whenever I read this, I find myself adding 'unless they are dyslexic'.

It is a fact that many teachers do cherish the task of teaching, but others do not. More specifically, many teachers do not cherish teaching dyslexic children, and, by definition, these are the teachers that dyslexic children will endure rather than enjoy.

Generally speaking, the dyslexic child does not reach school and find someone who likes what they offer, or a system that values what they do.

This is tragic, since dyslexic children enter school with the same optimism as any five-year-old. As research reviews conclude: 'Global self worth is very high at school entry' (Sylva 1994, p. 163). The raw material is great. A lot of what happens next squanders every ounce of it.

It is absolutely essential for a counsellor to appreciate this range of experiences if they are ever going to empathize with a dyslexic client. Not to take account of a dyslexic client's school experiences is crass, because it is so important. Extending this point, it is essential to be especially vigilant about any dyslexic client who dismisses their school experience as 'fine',’OK' and 'I survived'. They themselves may have never been able to look at these experiences or be able to revisit them. They may be hidden under a blanket of shame or buried in a lead coffin. Either way, these school effects do exist and can emerge in the safety of a good therapeutic relationship.

CHAPTER 3

The effects of school

Summary

Good schools influence their pupils' attitudes to school and have good rates of attendance. Bad schools do the opposite. They are powerful places. Significantly, when children leave school at 16 years, they will have been there for two-thirds of their entire lives.

As Donaldson (1978) reminds us, 'When we make laws which compel our children to go to school, we assume collectively an awesome responsibility. For a period of some ten years, the children are conscripts' (p. 13).

School

How important is school?
Too important. When life goes wrong for a child at school, their life goes wrong for a long time after they leave school. The influence of school is profound.

Rutter (1985), in his seminal review of the influence of school, concluded that there were: 'powerful effects of the school environment on pupil behaviour and attainment [and] ... most important indirect effects as a result of the earlier school influences' (p. 362). Similarly, in her review of the massive literature on school influences on child development, Sylva (1994) observed that a principal influence of school was not on academic achievement but on the personality of the child. This intervening influence 'may be just as powerful in predicting later outcome as intelligence or school curriculum' (p. 135).

In short, the effect of school is less about what you learn and more about what you pick up along the way.

The nature of your schooling is like being forced to go for a ten-year, unpredictable route march through unknown and dangerous territory.

Whether it makes you fit or destroys you depends on a number of things. Were you well prepared? Was it energizing or exhausting? Did it make you fit or spark off an illness that debilitated you for the rest of your life? Did you make friends or stumble along alone and weary? Did you find your way or get lost? What did you find on the soles of your shoes when you got home?

Importantly, if it irreparably damaged you, how do you feel about those who forced you to do it or beguiled you into it by suggesting that it would be great; who then failed to help you, who took away your map, who tripped you up, who ignored you when you needed help? If you were an adult, you might have liked to have a few words with them. If you were a child, exhausted and disabled by the experience, you just wanted to survive. In both cases, you had to find strategies to cope.

School is not a safe place for some children, and bad experiences at school are very bad indeed. The types of abuse condoned at school would cause uproar if they occurred in the home or on the street. It is not surprising that a recent research review of school effects concluded that, 'adjustment problems at school are a risk factor for psychopathology' (Van den Oord and Rispens 1999, p. 417).

Donaldson, an educational psychologist who works with the effects of this psychopathology, is a little less smooth and disinterested in her conclusions. For many children, she observes, school is a place of 'bitter defeat'. When they leave school, they have not become people who rejoice in the exercise of creative intelligence. Instead, 'large numbers of them emerge ill equipped for life in our society and are inescapably aware of it' (Donaldson 1978, p. 14). She concludes: 'The present levels of human distress and wasted effort are still too high to bear' (op. cit., p. 15).

What are the general effects of school on dyslexics?
All dyslexic children – and this is not a loose phrase – experience some form of damage from school.

To be dyslexic means that school, in some way, has harmed you – sometimes in many ways. An unharmed, fulfilled dyslexic is one who did not go to school. It really is as simple and as awful as that.

I believe that the abuse of dyslexic children is accepted in the school system in a way comparable to that experienced by ethnic minorities before the earliest race-relations legislation. It is to the benefit of the school system that the huge dyslexic minority who could become politicized have not done so.

Obviously, dyslexics are not all the same. Some are better equipped than others for their long, long journey through school. Some just survive; others thrive in the half-hearted way of an etiolated plant that has too little light. Some fall by the wayside through nervous breakdown or suicide.

What is clear, however, is that most dyslexics spend their time at school veering between fear and outright terror. It is hardly surprising that they fail to thrive. As Maslow (1954) established, only a child who feels safe dares to grow forward healthily. His safety needs must be gratified.

Is this an overreaction?
No. Overall, for the vast majority of dyslexic children and adults, school has been a place of psychological, and often physical, torture.

School for them was destructive and humiliating. It was a nasty, degrading experience, sometimes of raw brutality, of which modern society should be deeply ashamed.

> 'The suffering that is endured by dyslexics in the current school system and the attendant psychological scarring is hard to quantify, but it impacts on the motivation, the emotional well-being and possibly the behavioural stability of the dyslexic. In many ways, it seems to me that dyslexics are working constantly at the limits of their endurance' (Fawcett 1995, p. 23).

Edwards (1994), after in-depth interviews with eight undiagnosed, severely dyslexic adolescents, found herself deeply shocked at the level of pain these boys were enduring. She concluded that they all bore emotional scars as a result of their school experience. Every one of them had been neglected and bullied by both peers and staff, and the barely adequate help they had from their teachers was laced with discrimination, humiliation and violence. They now had little confidence, were sensitive to criticism and experienced disabling behaviour problems including truancy, psychosomatic pains, isolation, alienation from peers and a breakdown in family communication.

Riddick (1996), in a review of the personal accounts by dyslexics of school, concluded that they provided 'compelling accounts of how dogmatism and ignorance can combine to provide poor and, in some cases, atrocious educational practice' (p. 34). She observes that these same themes of 'distress and humiliation' (p. 50) run though all other research in this area.

School also has a long-term effect on dyslexic children.

Parsonage (2002), a dyslexic, in a study of other dyslexics, writes: 'the troubles suffered by many dyslexics while in education have had a lifelong effect on both their confidence and their abilities' (p. 6). Although many dyslexics manage to survive and find their own way to literacy, they take with them problems from school which 'impinge on the performance of the dyslexic throughout life' (Fawcett 1995, p. 23).

George Bernard Shaw said that his schooling interrupted his education. This may well be true for many dyslexic children, but this is the lighter end of the spectrum. For others, school destroyed their education and, in the process, distorted their whole view of themselves and the opportunities life could offer them.

How do dyslexic children fail at school?
There are no surprises here. Basically, dyslexic children fail to do almost everything that school is designed for. They can fail in a rich variety of ways.

Failure to make friends

For a dyslexic, the failure to make friends or gain peer approval can have a lasting effect well into adult life. It is a major contributor to adolescent and adult depression (Fine et al. 1993). Much of this problem has to do with the aetiology of bullying, but it is also true that dyslexic children can be cut off from peer interaction through poor social skills. For example, dyslexic children have problems with information-processing delay, so, in conversation, they can still be furiously unpacking one lot of information while their peers have moved several sentences down the line. The blank look, which often accompanies this perusal of incoming data, is off-putting. It can make a dyslexic person seem uncommunicative – or even slightly simple – and discourages peer interaction. This point is significant, particularly for the counsellor, and it will be examined in more detail in Chapter 8.

Failure in literacy

Chapter 1 outlined how dyslexic children have fundamental problems in learning to read, write and spell. Dyslexic children fail in this area, and they fail spectacularly. They are up against children who are not dyslexic and who have the correct brain organization and neurology for learning to read, write and spell. You might just as well race an Alsatian against a greyhound. They both have useful qualities, and the Alsatian may well be more intelligent, but the defining element of the environment is speed, and the greyhound will always win because he is built for speed and the Alsatian is not. No matter how fit, hungry or well trained the Alsatian is, nothing can extinguish that essential difference.

Failing to read and write is a very public failure. It is experienced every time a dyslexic is asked to read, write or spell anything. He fails whenever he is required to act on written instructions, read from the board or read aloud – all of which happen dozens of times every day at school. Failure must also be anticipated at every examination and at every reading of test results. Many of my dyslexic clients find it traumatic to recall the anticipatory terror around these daily events, and recount the desperate strategies they devised for avoiding them. Some can still vividly taste their fear and remember their intense shame and embarrassment among the sniggers and jeers of the rest of the class.

Miles (1993) talks of the range of difficulties of dyslexic children at school including problems with organization, copying off the board, mathematics, losing their possessions, forgetting lessons and instructions, tripping, dropping things and, mostly, not understanding what is said or taught by teachers.

The dyslexic also fails to be liked or respected by a teacher since teachers do not generally care for dyslexic children. This is not only because they fail to read and write but also because the transference of failure, anger, guilt and hopelessness from the dyslexic child is acutely disturbing to teachers – as I shall note in more detail in the next chapter. Dyslexic children can also be irritating. Out of nervousness, or to help concentration, some dyslexic children use repetitive behaviours (foot tapping, squeaking, strumming), and the more hyperactive ones can fidget, wriggle and squirm for England. One teacher told me she was blue with bruises from one dyslexic child who could not stop kicking out involuntarily under the desk.

Most teachers do not really understand dyslexia, and the easiest and most comfortable response is just to vilify the child.

Failure to be attractive

Dyspraxia also adds its own type of failure. Eating, for example, can be a messy process for dyspraxic children who can end up with food over them, the table and their fellow eaters with eating utensils flying everywhere. Even the most tolerant of children can find this process disgusting to see and can express their revulsion dramatically and publicly. Additionally, although it is true that some do excel at sport, for many dyslexics their clumsiness, lack of co-ordination and poor sporting skills can add up to even more failure outside the classroom, and many dyslexic children are left out of play activity by their peers and politely passed over in sports teams by teachers.

Failure to get it together

There are also hundreds of other daily, small failures and opportunities for belittlement that can litter the lives of dyslexics. Problems with sequencing and perception of time can mean that dyslexic children fail to get to class, or they may go through the wrong sequence of doors to fetch up in some terrifying no-man's land. Illiteracy means that they cannot read signs, so, when they do get lost, they can't find their own way out. Timetables and instructions may as well be in Chinese, while clumsiness and fine-motor-coordination problems lead to frequent tripping over unfastened shoelaces and trails of dropped paper from files. Memory problems translate into lost work, forgotten deadlines, jobs half done, mislaid books, and even carefully prepared-for examinations missed. This social image is neither a successful nor an elegant one, and dyslexic children know it.

Transition

Does it help to go to a new school or a new class?
No. Dyslexics hate all types of change and transition.

It strains the child's weak points – particularly organizational skills – as well as opening up new avenues of failure. For dyslexic children and adults, transition is not a period of adjustment but a period of disruption.

At school, the dyslexic notion of self is never robust, but transition can only disintegrate what is there. 'Anyone who has ever found themselves in a strange culture will know how disconcerting and anxiety-producing it can be when the self-structure is challenged through contact with a different set of values or mores' (Tolan 2001, p. 21).

At a recent special-needs conference, I attended a talk on transition by a dyslexic educationalist. He regarded transition as the worst time for dyslexics because their cognitions are slow. Dyslexics resemble a combine harvester in that they need a long time and a lot of space to change direction and adjust to changes. All their old coping strategies have to be rebuilt.

What are the problems with school and class transition?
There are three issues. First, new material has to be absorbed. This affects the dyslexic's concentration, increases their anxiety levels and hampers their ability to focus.

Second, dyslexics also have to go through all the peer integration again and suffer new forms of exclusion and bullying when they had only just got used to the last lot. This is a realistic fear. The evidence is that bullying and aggression increase with the transition between and within schools. This is how children – particularly young adolescents – manage peer and dominance relationships in the transition to new social groups. The only way that victims are buffered by this is by friendship, but, since he is probably no better at forming friendships than in the last school, the new dyslexic pupil will have small hope of avoiding or being protected from this new set of bullies (Pellegrini and Long 2002).

Third, dyslexics soon start to feel vulnerable and uncontained, particularly if they have not learnt the new behaviour patterns or new building layout. They can feel bewildered and panicked with the primitive fear of being projected into a strange, alien land.

Is the transition to secondary school any easier?

No. In fact, the transition to secondary school is particularly bad.

Dyslexic children now have to move from room to room remembering books, direction and equipment. They must retain instructions, often given at speed. Written work increases, and they have to organize themselves and use a timetable. New school rules are terrifying to dyslexic children because they cannot read them and cannot interact with children who can help them.

The dyslexic child's spelling and poor reading will attract new attention, while his problems with numeracy will lead to overload not only in maths but also in other subjects such as chemistry and technical drawing. The pace of life also quickens: 'in the secondary context, where speed and productivity in written presentation are paramount, the dyslexic pupil is particularly disadvantaged' (Povey and Todd 1993, p. 194).

In extreme cases, 'the proceedings may become so meaningless that it is very difficult to pay much attention to the lessons. The impact of strange situations can even threaten to disintegrate the boundaries of the child's ego' (Dwivedi 1993, p. 54).

Do things improve when dyslexic children leave school?

Enormously. Leaving school always makes a big difference.

Riddick et al. (1999), reviewing two follow-up studies of dyslexic children, noted that 'there was a considerable drop in adjustment problems once individuals had left school' (p. 231). Although there was still higher anxiety than in controls, dyslexic students saw university as a more sympathetic environment. Hales (2001b), in his study on the personality of dyslexic adults and children, reached a similar conclusion. He found that the relationship between age and anxiety in dyslexics was curvilinear. Performance anxiety was higher at main school and lower in early school and after leaving school.

Reaction

Are dyslexics hypersensitive to criticism?

Excruciatingly so.

I would say that dyslexics become so flayed by their experiences at school that there is a period when they have no skin at all on their sense of self. Such a volume of negative feedback and criticism is hard to handle. Edwards (1994) identified oversensitivity to criticism as one of the common features of the eight dyslexic boys she interviewed. Oversensitivity can, however, be a rational and sensible response to a real problem. When you have been strafed several times a day, every week, for years and years, you are not 'being oversensitive' when you cringe at the sound of a plane's engines.

Riddick (1996) investigated whether dyslexic children received more criticism about their work than others, or if this was a perceptual bias. She found that dyslexic children received significantly more criticism of their work than other children. Some dyslexic children had over half their work criticized in some way, every time. Some always had work covered in red pen, with no praise ever. Rather understating their case, the dyslexic children found this overwhelmingly 'unfair' (op. cit., p. 137).

The criticism of dyslexic children starts early – from the first attempt at reading at five years of age. Although it had been thought until recently that children under the age of nine or ten were relatively immune to the effects of criticism and failure, recent work has established that children as young as four or five are affected. In one study, although some five-year-olds saw failure in 'mastery' terms – something to overcome – others already saw it as a reflection on them – a 'helpless' response. Nonetheless, all the children, even the most secure, demonstrated a drop in self-confidence. 'Five-years-olds ... were sensitive to criticism; they reacted significantly more negatively in response to criticised failure than in response to non-criticised failure' (Cutting and Dunn 2002, p. 856).

Does anxiety affect the work of dyslexics?
Most definitely – and it does this by amplifying the reactions that are normal in any testing experience.

Anxiety affects everyone's performance. An anxious person attends to fewer environmental cues, encodes information less well and his worrisome thoughts reduce his cognitive resources (Warr and Downing 2000). Stress also makes tasks more laboured and less automatic as anxiety makes us more self-aware and conscious of every action (Hardy et al. 1996). The dyslexic, however, has serious additional problems.

Anxiety jeopardizes the dyslexic's already thin organizational skills, increases his clumsiness and reduces further his facility for automaticity. The added stress also disables the dyslexic's fragile short-term memory so that he has effectively smaller working-memory storage or processing capacity to devote to a task.

In the face of this rapid loss of basic operating skills, the dyslexic's concentration, which is always holding on by its fingernails anyway, then disappears, and the dyslexic enters a panic/stress loop that can leave him, literally, immobilized.

The extent of this anxiety is emphasized by Davis (1997) who, writing about his own dyslexia, states that reading and writing will always be stressful to a dyslexic because 'the inability to read and write often seems life-threatening to a dyslexic person' (p. 31).

Consequently, as observed by Pumphrey and Reason (1991), dyslexic children perform badly at all school tasks performed under pressure, because their anxiety disables them. In this respect, it can also affect IQ test performance, leading to a significant underestimation of a dyslexic's intelligence.

Etkin (1993) also suggests that a child's performance anxiety is a problem that feeds on itself 'worsening as the years pass' (p. 21). It can even remain dormant and be revived swiftly by the smallest of cues. Dyslexic university students, for example, found that simply recollecting school had a negative effect on their performance when faced with literacy tasks (Riddick et al. 1999).

There will also be a carry-over effect for dyslexics from stressful to non-stressful tasks.

Everatt and Brannan (1996) gave adult dyslexics a spelling test – which would have terrified them – before a non-verbal memory task. Those who were given the spelling test first performed less well on the subsequent tasks. The anxiety caused by the spelling task carried over to the other tasks and impaired subsequent performance.

The problem of performance anxiety in dyslexics is difficult for teachers to negotiate. They have to manipulate the anxiety-risk ratio in children to arouse some, but not too much, anxiety to allow the child to take some risk so that he gains confidence. What is just the right amount of anxiety for a non-dyslexic child can, however, wipe out the test confidence and render almost catatonic a vulnerable dyslexic child.

Is dyslexic self-esteem linked to academic failure?
Yes – and not just in dyslexics.

It is a universal research result that self-esteem and self-image are compromised by academic failure (Burns 1979). Those with learning difficulties are most affected and, as a result, can consistently refer to themselves in a negative way: 'the experience of dyslexia at school has clear and demonstrable negative effects on the self-concept and self-esteem of children' (Humphrey and Mullins 2002, p. 199).

For dyslexics, the experience of failure also leads to further anticipation of failure and the distortion of self-perception – academically and personally. A specific study on this issue by Riddick et al. (1999) observed that the strongest relationship for dyslexics was between poor reading performance at school and low self-esteem. This was found to be independent of general ability and, thus, indicated 'the powerful mediating effects of literacy performance on how individuals perceive themselves and are perceived by others' (p. 241).

Literacy and low self-esteem in dyslexia are believed to be so closely linked that some practitioners suggest that literacy training and counselling should proceed side by side (Lawrence 1971).

This is, however, a complex area, and it is discussed in more detail in Chapter 9.

Do dyslexics idealize academic ability?

They not only idealize academic ability, dyslexic children also acquire the belief from school that being a good reader is significantly correlated with happiness (Thomson and Hartley 1980) and intelligence (Humphrey and Mullins 2002).

Thus, to a dyslexic, being good at reading means one is intelligent and happy. Conversely, not being good at reading (being dyslexic, in other words) means being stupid and miserable. Humphrey and Mullins (2002) also found that dyslexics believe being hardworking is associated with being intelligent. By a process of logic, this means that dyslexics have also internalized the notion that they are lazy if unable to read.

Do dyslexics feel out of control at school?

Yes – which is a pity since a large-scale national survey showed that believing oneself to be in control of one's destiny was more important to achievement than any other school factor measured, including facilities, teachers and curriculum (Burns 1979). Feeling out of control also goes against the fundamental, natural urge of children 'to be effective, competent and independent, to understand the world and to act with skill' (Donaldson 1978, p. 113).

What happens to dyslexics, however, is that repeated failure, despite huge effort, distorts their belief that they can control their world – at least regarding academic success. They learn to be helpless. 'The parallels between learned helplessness and children with reading difficulties are striking' (Butkowsky and Willows 1980, pp. 410–11).

Learned helplessness occurs when a person 'has learned expectations that external events are largely beyond his control and that unpleasant outcomes are probable' (Harrington 1995, p. 125). It is a learned, maladaptive passivity where the *expectation* of a loss of control starts to predominate. In its extreme form, it is typified by the rat who quivers in immobility after getting an electric shock, no matter what it does.

The main effect of learned helplessness in dyslexics is that they come to believe that others control what happens to them. Attributions become external rather than internal. Consequently, dyslexics eventually associate success with the inputs of others; that is external attributions. They do not equate success with their own internal factors, such as ability or effort (Humphrey and Mullins 2002). It is, thus, easy to give up when no one helps.

This externality is symptomatic of learned helplessness – and gives teachers a great deal of power in the dyslexic perception. Overall, the learned helplessness of dyslexic children means that, like all low-achieving children, they 'attribute their successes to factors beyond their control' (Hiebert et al. 1984, p. 1139).

What maladaptive behaviours do dyslexic children learn at school?
Dyslexic children learn avoidance techniques and defence mechanisms at school. Experienced teachers recognize these for the defences that they are; other teachers read them as negative or obstructive.

Dyslexic children get angry and frustrated. Humiliation causes resentment. Sometimes, they misbehave. Cooper et al. (1994) refer to how such children 'avoid the experience of repeated failure by acting out or challenging behaviour in the classroom' (p. 93). More usually, dyslexics simply despair and withdraw.

Gifted dyslexics have particular problems since boredom, and divergence from ability, can be hard to take when they may have been ahead in every area until they start school (Congdon 1995).

Do dyslexic children have the means to express their anger about school?
No – and this will be a life-long problem that can fetch up in the counselling room with the most virulent expressions of projective identification.

The dyslexic's language disabilities and peer problems mean that the verbal expression route is closed to them. Nor can dyslexics easily access the route of creative writing as a therapeutic form of expression. This is such a shame because dyslexics can write with great depth of feeling and, in my experience, often crave the private outlet of creative writing to describe their feelings about things that happen to them.

It is unfortunate, too, that writing about stressful events has significant benefits to psychological and physical health. Children who write about negative life events have a general reduction in symptoms of stress (Reynolds et al. 2000). Some good teachers let dyslexic children off the leash of literacy so that they can express their thoughts without worrying about spelling or presentation. This is, however, an uncomfortable experience for dyslexics, like running in ill-fitting shoes. You get where you're going, but the journey is too fraught with self-awareness to be relaxing.

Do dyslexic academic problems develop over time at school?
Difficulties with dyslexia vary with age.

Late primary-age dyslexic children see writing about things as their greatest difficulty. Secondary-age dyslexic children show increased concern with the speed and accuracy of their work (Hales 1994). All dyslexic children, at all ages, are particularly concerned with visible public indicators of their difficulties, such as finishing work last. In this respect, Riddick (1996) found that the worst stresses were dictation, having to read aloud and the general pressure to keep up. Most stress came from daily humiliations in the classroom.

Is isolation an enduring feature of school life for dyslexic children?

Isolation is an enduring feature of *all* life for dyslexic children. Sometimes they feel as if they are alone on the planet.

Feeling lost at school is the commonest cry from all school-failing children, although for dyslexics this is both a figurative and an actual problem. 'For many of the young people we interviewed school was a profoundly sad and depressing experience. Their images and depictions were powerful, suggesting that "I am very sad", "stressed out", "lonely", "depressed", "on my own". Many of the images are bleak, picturing isolated children and shouting teachers. A recurring image is of school as a prison from which children continually try to escape ... The children themselves appeared as lost, small voices crying for help, caught in a cycle of circumstances which they felt largely unable to influence' (Riley and Rustique-Forrester 2002, pp. 32–3).

The isolation of the dyslexic is one of their most significant problems, and is a recurring theme in their lives. This will be examined in detail in Chapter 9.

School organization

What about the education authorities?

Many dyslexics battle to be recognized as dyslexic by local education authorities (LEAs), but most are not only discouraged but also actively opposed by LEAs. This is because recognizing dyslexia means, under current legislation (see Appendix E), that LEAs will have to take action to help, and money will have to be spent.

Scott (2003), in a review of this problem, observed that 'local council officers are often complicit in denying disabled children therapies on the basis of cost, which directly contravenes the 1996 Education Act' (p. 47). Parents are often too exhausted to fight these decisions at special needs tribunals – which are often vicious proceedings – and LEAs rely on this. 'Local education authorities know that they will be challenged by only a tiny minority of parents – those with the knowledge, resources and confidence to stay the course. For the few who take on the stress involved in appealing, a hundred others will fall by the wayside, unable to cope with the time, potential expense and mind-numbing complexities of dealing with council lawyers' (op. cit., p. 48).

Hales (2001a), in his review of dyslexic experience with LEAs, concluded that there was, universally, an 'unwillingness to try and understand, and avoidance of responsibility, that are not the type of provision that most people would expect to happen in the twenty-first century' (p. 1). He gives, as examples, the refusal of one authority to act on the recommendations of another, the unwillingness of one authority to accept out-of-area findings, and general LEA indignation at parents' wanting to question anything ('we know best').

Concluding on how helpful the different professional educational bodies could be, Hales found that the least helpful were LEAs, schools, SENCOs and LEA psychologists. The quality of dyslexic experience with LEAs was 'bad' or 'very bad'. Most dyslexic children only obtained help after a 'struggle', 'battle' or 'discussion'. At college or university, help was more immediate and less likely to be after a struggle.

Notably, the most helpful professionals for dyslexics were non-LEA psychologists and college or university student-support departments. This is not unusual (see Chapter 10).

Are special classes in mainstream schools helpful for dyslexic children?
Generally, no.

Removing dyslexic children from class for special help in mainstream schools is not good for them, unless the school handles this very carefully indeed. Goldup and Ostler (2000), two very experienced dyslexia teachers, write: 'Dyslexic children – all children – hate to fail, hate to be different, hate to be singled out as having "special needs"' (p. 324).

Sylva (1994), in a short review of special education in mainstream schools, noted a researched relationship between special class assignment and subsequent police contact. She concludes that studies have found detrimental consequences of removing children from mainstream classes, including lower self-esteem, lower expectations, feelings of isolation, dropout and delinquency.

Other research shows that the type of teaching given in special classes is often inappropriate and in far too wide a range of abilities (Seeman 2002). There are, also, many personal observations by dyslexics of the humiliation of going to 'remedial' classes, where they learnt even less than in mainstream, or were given inappropriately low-level work in a 'dustbin' class. Some high-IQ dyslexics were left to colour-in all day.

Sinason (1993) observes that a school may claim to be integrated but this can often involve a child 'largely in a corner with an occasional support teacher and without gaining much attention, whereas the local special school would have provided much more' (p. 65).

As I shall return to in the next chapter, bullying of dyslexics is also far higher in mainstream than special schools.

Are special schools better for dyslexic children than mainstream schools?

Yes. The dyslexic child prospers in special schools, often for the first time.

Sinason (1993), a psychotherapist who specializes in the study of disability, favours the special school – and boarding school where necessary – since it provides a place of safety for a disabled child.

England has a large supply of special schools – 25% of all children with disabilities are educated in them compared to 7% in Italy and 5% in America. Where there is high morale, good leadership and good relations with parents, special-needs children do best of all in special schools.

I would suggest the following reasons:

Self-esteem

Some studies have demonstrated a dramatic increase in self-esteem among dyslexic children who go to a special school (Thomson 1990).

Crozier et al. (1999) also found that children with special needs in segregated units tended to have a more positive sense of self than those educated in mainstream schools. He concluded that teachers at special units were more likely to recognize the behavioural and self-esteem problems of dyslexics. The children with dyslexia in the special units revealed that they felt more valued and cared for than when they were in mainstream schooling. All his research led to the view that 'children with dyslexia in SpLD units develop more positive self-concepts and levels of self-esteem than those left in mainstream education' (p. 34).

Pumphrey and Reason (1991), in a similar comparison of the effectiveness of special units and mainstream schools for dyslexics, showed that self-rated ability for dyslexics in reading, writing, English ability and neatness were higher in a specialist unit than in a mainstream school. Dyslexics in mainstream schools were disadvantaged.

Less isolation

Special schools reduce the sense of isolation experienced by dyslexic children in mainstream schools. This reduces their anxiety and allows them to learn, free from distraction. In a special school, they are surrounded by like souls. They are fish in the same water. Riddick (1996) notes, 'particularly in schools where dyslexia was not acknowledged, children could feel very isolated' (p. 150). The majority of children in her study found it helpful to be taught with other dyslexics and celebrated 'the positive value of having close friends who were dyslexic' (p. 151).

Specialist provision

Sometimes, such as when a child has ADHD, special schools will use teachers who are trained in coping with disruptive behaviours. Such challenging children simply cannot be educated in ordinary classes without damage to the educational prospects of the other children. Thomson (1995b) writes of the 'failure of ADHD children to stay on task, their impulsive behaviour, disorganization and unpredictable reactions that exhaust adults, annoy other children and impede constructive learning. Almost inevitably they attract negative reactions and will often respond with attention-seeking behaviour which is unpopular in class' (p. 41). Such children suffer because they are not invited home by others, can be ostracized in school, and teased and bullied by exasperated peers. 'The social rejection of children with ADHD by their peers at age 10 to 11 is a damaging outcome [with] severe implications for the subsequent adolescent development of friendless children' (Lightfoot 2003, p. 46).

Special schools and specialist teachers not only know what they are doing with special-needs children but can give them far more social support. Children with ADHD are not popular in ordinary classes. The unexpressed and overt hostility from other children inflicts further damage on an often already battered, demoralized and helpless self-esteem. Special schools understand how to fulfil the social needs of such children.

School phobia

Do dyslexic children experience school phobia?

It is my experience that some dyslexic children have a history of refusing to go to school.

The actual number of dyslexic children who are so frightened of school that they refuse to go there is, however, unknown, although Riddick (1996) found that 70% of her sample of dyslexic school children said that they 'dreaded' (p. 124) having to go.

Intuitively, I believe that the number of school phobics among dyslexics is high – but not as high as common sense would dictate. Furthermore, the school phobia aetiology of separation and general anxiety, maternal enmeshment and terrible school experience are all related to the dyslexic condition. It would, not, therefore, be unrealistic to suggest that a sample of school-phobic children might well comprise a large number of dyslexics.

What is school phobia?

There is some debate.

The topic of school phobia has, for example, generated 25 times as many research articles as any other childhood phobia, and 'this is not surprising, given the tremendous distress that the condition causes not only to those children affected by it but also to their families and school teachers' (Blagg 1992, p. 121).

The condition has been recognized for over 70 years and, once upon a time, there were considered to be just two categories of school absence. These were 'truancy' and 'school phobia'.

Truancy refers to children who are not particularly worried about school, who have more attractive pastimes in mind and who engage in delinquent and disruptive acts in the company of like-minded peers. Although parents encourage some truants, a distinguishing feature is that truants attempt to conceal their school absence from their parents. This category is still defined in this way.

In contrast, the view on school phobia has changed dramatically. School phobics were once seen exclusively as children who had separation anxiety, that is, an overly strong mother-and-child attachment. More recently, a wider term of 'school refuser' has been used to describe all children who refuse to attend school for reasons other than truancy. A number of researchers in this field prefer, however, to use the term 'school phobia' with its more serious overtones of a learned fear response (see below).

The role of anxiety and depression in school phobia also differentiates it from truancy, and school phobia is seen, not as a single psychiatric diagnosis, but as an index of problems, including separation anxiety, social phobia, general or trait anxiety and depression, with many cases having multiple diagnoses. It should not be considered 'a unitary syndrome but rather one that is heterogeneous and multi-causal' (Elliott 1999, p. 1002).

In school phobia, psychological symptoms are often accompanied by physical ones, such as stomach ache, dizziness, headaches and nausea, that swiftly disappear if the child stays at home. Parents get very distressed by these symptoms and need reassurance that serious trouble is not present.

Who and how many are affected by school phobia?

Differing definitions do not help but, in 1975, estimates of 3.3%, 1.6% and 1.3% for truancy, lateness and general school refusal were each given (Elliott 1999).

In 2000, an estimate of 20,000 school refusers at any one time in England and Wales was considered a conservative figure. A figure of 1%-2% for all school-aged refusers is not considered uncommon. It is equal between the sexes and rare before adolescence, when it increases significantly. True separation anxiety is more a feature of young, female children, and fear of school more that of older, male children. Older children suffer from more severe disorders and have a poorer prognosis. There is no class bias, although the school refuser does not suffer from the same multiple adversities as the truant. Family size or being a single child is not related to the condition. It is often the quieter and more conscientious children who are affected by school phobia (Winkley 1996).

Is separation anxiety an important factor in school phobia among dyslexics?

My clinical experience suggests that separation anxiety is a feature, if not the cause, of school phobia amongst dyslexic children, since the aetiology of dyslexic families includes a high degree of maternal overprotection.

Psychoanalytic practitioners, however, consider the dependent-hostile child-parent dynamic to be a central feature of most school phobic cases. Bowlby (1991) was one of the first researchers in this field to observe this. 'Relations between child and parents are close, sometimes to the point of suffocation' (p. 300).

Winkley (1996) also argues that 'the main fear is often one of leaving home and being separated from the mother' (p. 170) and the children 'tend to be over-protected and over-dependent' (op. cit., p. 171).

Some of this makes sense for dyslexic children, but I find myself at odds with Winkley's (1996) assertion that 'fear of school is not the major underlying cause' (p. 170). Bowlby also overgeneralizes when he observes that 'what a child fears is *not* what will happen at school, but leaving home ... disagreeable features of school, for example a strict teacher, teasing or bullying from other children, are little more than rationalisations' (p. 301). For a dyslexic school phobic, strict teachers and bullying are not 'rationalisations' but are all too real.

Overall, it is fair to say that current theorists generally regard the separation anxiety cause in school phobia as overstated, and some studies have shown separation anxiety to be a distinct subgroup accounting for less than 20% to 25% of school phobics.

More attention is now given to school-related factors such as terror about the place and anxiety about what will happen there tomorrow.

How important to school phobia are fear and anxiety about school?

These are the central factors in school phobia.

There is now considerable emphasis on the school context as a source of fear and anxiety, since high levels of anxiety and associated depression have been found in most school phobics. In fact, anxiety and depression are now considered to be co-morbid with the condition. The organization

'Education Otherwise' has even campaigned for school phobia to be interpreted as 'acute school-induced anxiety', arguing that school phobics are reacting rationally to unreasonable and cruel pressures in school. School is, literally, unendurable.

Blagg (1992) explicitly prefers the term 'school phobia' to 'school refusal' because it conveys to teachers and parents the fear, anxiety and helplessness that often accompany the problem. 'School refusal ... sounds like a far less serious problem and, to the uninitiated, could even imply that the child has simply decided that school is not for him or her' (p. 121). He sees school phobia and the concomitant school refusal as a rational response; that the child who is continuously subject to ridicule and criticism from peers or teachers has legitimate problems. Elliott (1999) also quotes research showing that many school-phobic children were afraid of a strict, sarcastic teacher or of academic failure. Such children find it difficult to cope with school, and have real worries about class work and social interaction.

Social-skills deficits are seen as particularly important. School phobics include many children who lack the social skills and self-confidence in order to mix with other children (Spence et al. 2000). This is an important point that I shall return to in the next chapter.

Is school refusal a rational learning response?

Yes. This is the leading view in modern research.

This approach de-emphasizes the symptoms of school phobia and, instead, focuses upon the effects it has on the child's life, particularly the advantages it bestows. School phobia is seen as a useful, learned response – a form of coping strategy – that can be replaced with other, less maladaptive coping strategies.

The reasoning is that a child becomes school phobic because parents are seen as safe and school as unsafe. Children return to parents when they feel frightened or uncertain. Parents reinforce this reaction by their concern and by offering safety. There is a push and pull: push from a toxic school environment and pull from a safe, rewarding home.

With dyslexic children, the parental relationship – usually with the mother – can be especially close and overprotective (see Chapter 6), so the pull is already strong.

This is a useful model that also forms the basis of the behavioural treatments that have a high rate of success.

What is the best treatment for school phobia?

Behavioural approaches, focused on how the child has learned to be school phobic, are considered to be the most effective treatment.

During this treatment, enforced return to school is usually effective, although 25% of school-refusal situations remit spontaneously. Blagg (1992), in a review of treatment, found that 93. 3% of the group who received behavioural treatment returned to school and were attending regularly without any further problems at a two year follow up. This compared to 37% of the group who were hospitalized and 10% of those who received psychotherapy and home tutoring.

Treatment of younger children is good irrespective of the treatment type, with success rates of 95% or more. Older children's reactions are more unpredictable and dependent on the type of treatment. Outcomes for hospitalized school phobics is poor and is also the most intensive and costly. In fact, it was 'so appallingly poor that this kind of intervention may inhibit spontaneous remission or, even worse, reinforce the school phobia' (p. 134). Although prognosis for the older children is poor, some studies have produced highly impressive treatment results, maintained at follow-up. These include:

- a problem-solving approach, unique to each case, involving child, family and school in a systematic approach (see Chapter 12)
- examining rational and realistic concerns and medical problems before labelling them 'irrational concerns'
- attending to practical issues at home and school, removing blocks so immediate return is effective
- a vigorous and energetic approach to treatment in which there is never any question of *if* the child will return to school but only *when* and *how* it will be accomplished, even using an escort system and legal intervention
- a watertight system of attendance checks and follow-ups with particular care after holidays, weekends and illnesses

After a two-year absence from school, if the school refusal is chronic or linked to depression, treatment of the condition is limited. Without a remediation of the problems at school, however, no treatment will have much chance of success, and may be seen as abusive.

CHAPTER 4

The effects of teachers and peers

Summary

If school is the malign incubator of the dyslexic child's problems, it is his relationships with teachers and peers that provide the nourishment and oxygen for those problems. If a dyslexic child had a productive, warm and supportive relationship with a teacher and was valued, played with, had fun and giggled in the bosom of a good group of friends, he would cope really quite well with his literacy problems. He would also avoid most of the worst long-term effects of his dyslexia.

Unfortunately, it is the norm that a dyslexic child has significant problems with both teachers and peers at school. These problems, more so than his dyslexia, make him unhappy and store up relationship problems for the future. In fact, it is my position that it is the relationship problems associated with dyslexia – rather than the literacy problems – that cause most of the damage to his psychological functioning. Counsellors will work with these old relationships in the transference of therapy. It is, therefore, useful to look at how they are formed and acted out in the life of the dyslexic child at school.

Teachers

How important is an individual teacher to a dyslexic child?

Very important – because no dyslexic child has a relationship with a system. Any problems that dyslexic children take from the learning environment are not located in the school curriculum, the education authority or in any expectations of society. Their learning problems are specifically located in a relationship with a teacher. Furthermore, it is not an exaggeration to state that an individual teacher can make the difference between psychological life or death to the dyslexic child at school.

Every dyslexic has a relationship with some teacher and, usually, that teacher has a name. In fact, one of the most singular characteristics of counselling dyslexic adults is how they can remember and name – sometimes decades later – the teacher who damaged them. That name has the same power to terrify them as it did decades ago.

One woman – an iconoclastic, fiery businesswoman – still refers anxiously to 'Mrs Lyon'. In the manner of child clients, she assumes that I know Mrs Lyon, that this person has a universal, huge identity known to every person on this planet. 'Who taught you English?' 'Mrs Lyon.' It is not 'this elderly lady, I think her name was Mrs Lyon' or 'dunno – some woman in a blue cardigan' but – bam! – 'Mrs Lyon', as if I should know this woman, as if her presence and influence is still so enormous that I could not possibly not know her. It is individuals such as Mrs Lyon who harm dyslexic children. It is the relationship between such teachers and dyslexic children that carries the means of harm, and this relationship is never forgotten.

Having said this, I do not think that it is of the slightest use to subscribe to some two-dimensional view of such teachers as 'good' or 'bad'. This is how our dyslexic clients see their teachers because they were children when the relationship was formed. Counsellors work with relationships. They know enough about them to perceive that, at some level, the teacher's behaviour must have made sense to him or her. Counsellors also know enough about the importance of relationships, particularly early relationships, not to realize that there had to be two sides, two transactions, two histories, two transferences operating between teacher and child. A counsellor also knows that such a powerful teacher-child relationship might well be acted out with her in the rather similar counsellor-client relationship.

How do teachers have such power to influence a dyslexic child?

The obvious answer is that they are seen in the same category as parents – as figures of authority. My work with dyslexic children also suggests four other significant reasons.

The class

Teachers control the primary system of dyslexic contact: the class. It is the Petri dish of the class rather than the laboratory of the school that carries the teacher bacterium and its effects – whether benevolent or toxic. Van den Oord and Rispens (1999), for example, found that the psychosocial adjustment of children was more affected by the structure of a class – which is under the direct influence of an individual teacher – than the school as a whole.

The class regulates immediate peer reaction and the daily dose of criticism or praise. The class atmosphere is also equivalent to the atmosphere of the child's home, and in this school 'home' the teacher is 'parent'. No matter how amiable the head teacher, it is this powerful human being, this teacher/parent, who either welcomes and values the dyslexic child or jails and destroys him. Unfortunately, the dyslexic child is closeted in these teacher relationships for all of his most important primary-school years of personality development and literacy training.

The expectation of hope

The teacher holds the eternal power of redemption for the unhappy, school-failing pupil. Just as a child never quite gives up the fantasy that a critical parent will, one day, offer those words of praise, so do all rejected and criticized school children eternally hope that the teacher will, one day, approve of them, notice them, praise them and admire them. Thus, no matter how truly terrible his relationship with a teacher has become, the dyslexic child continues to hope for acceptance and admiration from her.

I believe that this unreleased hope informs the return of dyslexics to higher education and much of the subsequent acting out of appeasement and skilled adaptation to other authority figures in a dyslexic's life – such as employers and counsellors. Whether the disapproving teacher transaction is a re-enactment of a disapproving parental transference or has impetus of its own is less relevant than its continuing power in the life of a dyslexic.

This hope for redemption from a teacher can survive the most terrible discouragement. In a study on excluded pupils who had all felt that their teachers had singled them out for blame, de Pear (1997) found that most of them expressed a strong need to be accepted and to gain positive attention from their teacher. This was despite the fact that 'few had experienced any real feeling of being seen as competent and responsible by their teachers' (p. 19). All were keen to learn how they could 'improve' sufficiently to return to those teachers in mainstream school.

Riley and Rustique-Forrester (2002), in asking EBD children what would make a difference to them, found that an overwhelming majority of pupils wanted more help and support with schoolwork. Other students said they would like to try and 'deal with the problems with their teachers better' (p. 37).

Teaching as power

The power and authority attached to teaching can be part of the job's attraction to an individual. If this is the case, it will be the enforcing of power and authority rather than the teaching that will be the primary, unconscious motivation to teach. Jacobs (1986) explicitly observes the direct harm that can be done by teachers who are not just insecure but who have profound authority problems of this nature.

The sadistic, overcritical teacher can even overwhelm the influence of a child's benign home environment. By being a parent substitute, such teachers 'plant a strong negativism in the child, and reinforce the super-ego, often prejudicing a child's view of any activity that is called education' (p. 127). Where both parents and teachers are cold and critical 'the task of achieving confidence and self-esteem becomes doubly difficult' (p. 127).

The bestowed and unearned authority of teaching will also be seductive if a teacher felt powerless at school as a child. By reinventing themselves in the role of teacher, such adults are revising the context of their powerlessness to create a different outcome. This last point is relevant in the light of research that demonstrates that up to 75% of teachers were bullied when they were children (Tattum 1993). This unexamined motive will be acted out in the transference with different children, and is discussed in more detail below.

Significantly for the counsellor, Jacobs (op. cit.) warns that the dyslexic client who has experienced a variation of this authority influence from teachers will be afraid that the counsellor, too, will be critical. Such a client will not mention the things that arouse feelings of shame or guilt. He may fear to suggest ideas or take the initiative. Any counsellor who is drawn to certainty, who tends to see things in black and white or who has authority problems of her own will set up a harmful collusive spiral that will act out the client's teacher experiences in the abuse of power.

The power of expectation

An enormous body of research shows that a child's behaviour and academic performance at school largely mirror what their teacher expects: 'children modify their behaviour for better or worse in response to the way they *feel* themselves to be perceived by their teachers' (Greenhalgh 1994, p. 84). Burns (1979) in a similar review showed that high teacher expectations 'lead to high pupil self-esteem and performance' (p. 303), but the opposite will also apply.

The effect of low teacher expectation, observed historically in racial and gender research, is similarly observed in the dyslexic field.

Dyslexic children do not, however, reach school already handicapped with cultural stereotypes. Their problems start when their emerging difficulties in academic performance start to ease a wedge between them and the good performers. This leads to a parallel widening of expectations between teacher and child from which neither party escapes. Each little increment of failure tarnishes the teacher's expectations of the dyslexic child, and this poor view then creeps into other perceptions of the child's behaviour. Adams et al. (1999) found, for example, that teachers take a negative view of children who underperform academically when their behaviour does not conform to the perceived norm, whereas such behaviour in high achievers may be overlooked.

It is not long before these negative opinions are internalized by the dyslexic child, who helpfully gives back the teachers the disruptive, 'difficult' child that they think is expected of him.

Can the personality of the teacher have a negative effect on a dyslexic child?

Yes. The character and problems of a dyslexic child can trigger conflict with a teacher by resonating with any pre-existing personality problems and low self-esteem that the teacher may have.

These problems remain dormant when teaching 'normal' children but are activated both by failing and uncooperative children or the creative, eccentric, non-conforming, non-learning behaviour of a child who is dyslexic or gifted.

Schlichte-Hiersemenzel (2000), a psychotherapist working with gifted and disturbed children, writes: 'I have the impression that it is not the child who should be the patient ... At times, perhaps, the teachers concerned should instead be the patients' (p. 51). Any difficult behaviour by the child is only one side of the coin. 'I have learned that teachers are often psychosocially unbalanced. They often seem to be controlled by difficult, unreflected feelings that they are unaware of, or cannot deal with, or suffer from long-term problems. Intrapersonal conflicts seem to be acted out in the relationship with [an unusual] child' (p. 51).

Children who do not respond to a teacher's authoritarian style will also challenge a teacher who has low self-esteem. In this respect, there is ample research to demonstrate that there is a relationship between low self-esteem in a teacher and academic performance in a child. Teachers who respect and like themselves are able to do the same for pupils – no matter how difficult they may be (Lawrence 1996). These high-self-esteem teachers encourage pupils to develop more divergent and evaluative approaches to schoolwork.

By contrast, those teachers who have a low, or insecure, sense of self will need the external validation of a child's success to validate themselves. Thus, a child's failure – and apparently vexatious failure to learn – will provide a good reason for rejecting him.

Teachers with low self-esteem also talk more and listen less. This prevents interaction with the child and, therefore, understanding. Such teachers are also more rigid, want 'right' answers and use convergent thinking. A child who needs a different style – such as more informality and a more intuitive teacher response – will be a threat. He exposes inadequacy and inferiority in those who do not have a strong sense of self.

Burns (1979) reviews the research on this: 'The facilitator of learning must be above all else a secure person. The person with low self-evaluation sees those with whom he interacts through the distortions of his own needs, fears and anxieties' (p. 306).

Why can the relationship between the teacher and dyslexic child be so intense and difficult?

I think that the answer lies in transference.

I do not think that it is just the dyslexic child's problems with learning which lead to such strong teacher antipathy towards them. Helping a child with learning and overcoming their problems underpin the whole point of being a teacher, and this must have been a central point in their wanting to teach. What occurs in a teacher–difficult-child interaction is a powerful and unexamined transference between them. I think that this transference is central to understanding not only the malign effects that teachers have had on dyslexic children but why they can choose to behave towards dyslexic children in such strikingly negative ways.

How does this transference occur?

The child transfers onto the teacher all his difficult feelings of guilt, failure, anger and frustration, and the teacher not only picks them up but is also highly likely to act them out.

When this happens, the sensitive teacher will find themselves bewildered at their own irrational behaviour: 'shouting when one did not intend to, or saying something unintended which just seemed to "pop out"' (Greenhalgh 1994, p. 47).

The teacher's reaction is complicated by their own counter-transferential feelings from when they were at school. This counter-transference can become quite viciously straightforward if the teacher was either a bully or a victim, or failed in some way when he was a child. The amplified transference and counter-transference between a teacher and dyslexic child can gain resonance and velocity, as well as explicit persecutory aspects if the child is also mired in victim.

Does it compare to counsellor transference?

It is probably identical, but with one major difference in process.

A counsellor who experienced strong feelings of anger, frustration, hopelessness and defeat with a particular client would incubate these feelings, examine them – perhaps in supervision – and then decide how to use this transference for the beneficial growth of her client.

A teacher does not usually have the training and essential personal therapy antecedents to recognize this transference and interpret his or her own counter-transference in response. They do not examine the strong feelings that this dyslexic child inexplicably sets up in them, and can often simply react. This can set up a spiral from which neither child nor teacher might escape. The feelings must be overwhelming.

It is worth the counsellor reflecting on this, since this pattern of transference and acting out may have become both a collusion and a habit for the dyslexic client who will expect to act it out again in the similar counsellor-client relationship.

Do teachers acknowledge this transferential aspect of the dyslexic child's education?

No. The lines between teaching and therapy are clearly drawn and rarely crossed.

Some would regard them as battle lines, and it is true that the role of the school counsellor is not only little understood but almost never extends to those who most need it – the teachers (see Chapter 10). Teachers are not in the habit of identifying a child's feelings in themselves. No inferences are drawn from the obvious fact that different children arouse different feelings in them. Whereas a counsellor makes the assumption that every client will elicit different feelings in them, and looks to the relationship between the client and herself to understand this, a bewildered teacher too easily looks to the child alone as the source of the problem. The child then becomes the repository not only of their own problems but also of those of the teacher. The child is doubly loaded with responsibility, and the teacher is comfortably lightened of hers.

Cooper et al. (1994) succinctly address this notion of failed-child-teacher transference in their discussion of the notion of 'maladjustment', of which many dyslexic children, even today, are accused. They argue that a distinction must be made between a disturbed and a disturbing child. Most children attract teacher attention not because they are disturbed but because they are disturbing to the teacher.

What types of transference and counter-transference can occur in the teacher–dyslexic child relationship?

I would suggest that the following feelings are common:

Failure and hopelessness

Teachers working with dyslexic children are pulled into a halo effect of failure and hopelessness. They will be a container, and will receive the split-off projection of the child's unwanted feelings of failure and all the associated feelings of guilt, anxiety, helplessness and hopelessness. The child will also convey the feeling that he is useless and invisible and the teacher will pick this up as feeling unskilled and irrelevant.

Dwivedi (1993), who is one of the few writers who gives serious consideration to the role of transference between failing dyslexic children and their teachers, suggests that the helping professionals can become objects of infantile hopes of relief from distress. 'They are frequently used as containers for excessive mental pain and have to be receptive to this level of emotional communication' (p. 55). The child's demands may seem unreasonable, but they need to be acknowledged and contained or they will become more out of control the more the child's pain is uncontained. Such a child can lead to teachers becoming over-involved, idealized and denigrated by turn.

'When such an intolerable intensity of pain or confusion is dumped into a receptive teacher by a pupil, the teacher is then possessed by the feelings of being inadequate, helpless, stupid, frightened and confused' (op. cit., p. 55).

Counter-transference of teacher failure and guilt

A dyslexic child not only transfers his own horror at his own level of failure, but he can also tap into a teacher's fears about her own professional ability, if that ability is insecure, or she has her own feelings of failure. 'The teacher may blame her or himself for failure to achieve any worthwhile improvement in the skills of the child' (Fawcett 1995, p. 15).

This counter-transferential anxiety about the teacher's own failure to help the child, which may be conscious and professional or unconscious and personal, can then lead to a rejecting and self-protecting anger towards the dyslexic child, or the acting-out of the same overprotective guilt that the child finds in his mother. I have no doubt that, in this instance, the child may also be engendering a parallel process of what he finds in his family: mother guilt and teacher guilt resonate in harmony.

Transference onto the home

Teachers can also avoid the guilt of their pupils' underachievement by splitting off these feelings and projecting them onto the dyslexic child's parents. In this case, the teacher will blame the child's home for his failure at school. This distances the teacher from the responsibilities of the situation. They can comfortably send the difficult split-off feelings from the child back to his home in a symbolic parcel of unwanted goods.

Difference – the dyslexic as 'outsider'

Dyslexic people report, almost universally, that they have always felt different from their peers. In the most extreme forms, this becomes social phobia and neurotic isolation. I have no doubt that teachers can pick up this notion from a dyslexic child and collude with it, even to the extent of isolating the dyslexic child in the class. This is sufficiently common for Goldup and Ostler (2000) to insist: 'the dyslexic child must be at the heart of the classroom action. Too often he feels he is an outsider in his own classroom and his peer group; alienated and marginalized' (p. 310).

This sense of difference will also be encouraged if a teacher is bewildered at the dyslexic pupil's erratic motivation patterns, the clear discrepancy between their verbal and literary skills and their ease in using visual, creative or obscure views of the world which differ from the teacher's own.

What does not help, is that dyslexic children, in terms of personality and skills, are also *in reality*, very different from teachers themselves. Dyslexics do not have the teachers' facility for linear, verbal thinking. Teachers are also comfortable in the school environment and dyslexic children are not.

Since 'teachers may find it relatively easy to empathise with children who appear similar to the way they were themselves as children' (Greenhalgh 1994, p. 88) and, by contrast, will find it hard to empathize with those children who were not similar to themselves as children, it is likely that the clash of the teacher and dyslexic child cultures goes very deep. Other children will pick up this disharmony so that the whole class – teacher and pupils – can collude in treating the dyslexic child as different.

Linked to this point, we are also attracted more to those who evaluate us positively and dislike those who provide negative feedback. Thus, a dyslexic child who reads a teacher as disliking him will not respond warmly. This further pushes the relationship between them into the cold.

Stress

Dyslexic children are mildly or severely stressed most of the time.

Unfortunately, so are teachers – and for very similar reasons. For example, Morris (2001), a counsellor who works largely with helping professionals, reports that teachers not only comprise 63% of her practice, but are bringing the types of problems that I find also afflict dyslexics; that is, burnout, stress-related physical conditions, disintegrating relationships, low self-esteem and excessive tiredness.

Thus, both teacher and child lug the same wearisome stresses into school, where the teacher feels the same stress in teaching a dyslexic child as the dyslexic child feels from being taught. Both parties bat stress between each other, colluding in parallel processes of feeling out of control and overwhelmed.

Ironically, it may be that it is only in dyslexic children that stressed teachers find some resonance with their own problems.

How do teachers act out these feelings towards dyslexic children?
Some teachers can use these transferred feelings from the dyslexic child for an empathic, creative and helpful response.

Unfortunately, others – perhaps the majority of teachers, 'discharge them in a manner that can be very damaging' (Dwivedi 1993, p. 55). A measure of a teacher's own self-esteem is how well they can hold onto these feelings and act reasonably on them, or split them off and project them onto the children who are failing. Wearmouth (1999) describes how this teacher splitting and projection happens in the face of behaviour they find worrying, disturbing or uncontrollable in the child. The child's failure is seen as a rejection. 'They are likely to attribute this rejection to some kind of personality defect within the pupils and may then go on to interpret the pupils and their behaviour as deviant' (p. 20).

Any negative behaviour of the teacher towards the child is then justified and acceptable. Deviant behaviour must, after all, incur a penalty. This provides a comfortable rationale of any subsequent abusive behaviour from a teacher to a child.

A dyslexic client will have received a rich variety of penalties from teachers for his 'deviant' behaviour at school. These responses by teachers will have informed his sense of self and distorted his already fragile confidence and personality. They will include the following:

Shame

Dyslexic children are daily embarrassed, both deliberately and incidentally, by their deficiency in literacy. They are embarrassed because teachers publicly draw attention to their inadequacies.

Teachers can be sadistic to dyslexics. Seeman (2002) recalls how she was made to recite in every assembly so that 'the laughter that resounded at my inevitable mistakes would "encourage me" to study harder' (p. 4). This is a very common observation in the literature on dyslexic experiences at school. Riddick (1996) found that both children and their mothers mentioned how often they were shown up or humiliated by teachers.

Labelling

Teachers have verbally and/or physically abused most dyslexic children. Pollock and Walker (1994), in a review of case studies of dyslexic adolescents, found that the vast majority had had extremely negative experiences at school before they had been properly identified. Most worryingly, many of these experiences involved their class teachers calling them stupid, lazy or slow.

Although name-calling is the most common form of abuse of dyslexic children by other children and by teachers, and teachers commonly address dyslexic children as 'lazy' and 'stupid', it is this last label that makes dyslexics the most angry.

What hits deepest is the sheer unfairness of these names when dyslexic children 'input considerably greater resources in all skills not just literacy skills to achieve the same level of performance as other children' (Fawcett 1995, p. 14). The problem is that these labels are not only internalized by the dyslexic child but are spread over his persona like ants over jam. Soon, no one sees anything but what these labels indicate.

The literature on EBD children has a term for this labelling: 'signification' (Cooper 1996). Signification occurs when pupils come to be labelled by the key elements of their behaviour so that the individual child or adolescent comes to be identified with a factor of deviance. He is objectified as an 'EBD', 'yob' or 'bully'. The deviant acts come to be seen as that person's most significant acts. The label has the effect of a self-fulfilling prophecy, whereby the individual internalizes then acts out the label that is projected by others. Also, pupil reputations are notorious for being passed on from one teacher to another, increasingly determining the child's performance for good or bad.

Riley and Rustique-Forrester (2002), in a study of EBD pupils, found that 'many pupils stated that they would like to change their own behaviour, but they found this difficult because they had been labelled as "the awkward squad"' (p. 36). Wearmouth (1999), in his article on labels such as 'maladjusted', calls this 'an unstructured, careless, authoritarian approach' by teachers (p. 20). He also observes that teachers never consider that such behaviour 'might be a rational reaction to stressful circumstances' with pupils acting in a self-defined 'perfectly reasonable manner' (p. 17).

Ignorance

Apart from specialist training courses, teachers are not taught enough about the known aspects of dyslexia. Seeman (2002) found that remedial courses were still teaching that dyslexics have low intelligence, and most did not deal with behavioural problems. Dyslexic herself, she observed how she was bracketed together with a brain-damaged child as the 'dummies' of the class. Pumphrey and Reason (1991) found that teachers still failed to accept the existence of dyslexia, preferring to label their dyslexic adolescent pupils as 'disruptive' or 'dim'.

Riddick (1996), in a study of dyslexic children, reports on teachers who, before they knew about dyslexia, remembered that there were children in their class who mystified them. It was only in retrospect that they realized that these children were dyslexic, and many of them felt guilty that they had done so little for these children. In my opinion, it is outrageous that any teacher, anywhere in the current education system, should be 'mystified' by the presenting symptoms of dyslexia when Russia was identifying and treating the symptoms for dyslexia nearly a century ago.

Critical, cold and bullying behaviour

Teachers can be competent and subtle bullies. Bad teachers can bully dyslexic children to destruction. Riddick (1996), for example, reports how one teacher routinely gave a dyslexic child 20 hard spellings a week. The child's mother said: 'He was worrying himself sick before the spelling tests. In fact, he started bed-wetting because of the pressure of the spelling tests. She destroyed his confidence' (p. 136).

Edwards (1994), in her study on dyslexic adolescents, found that they had all received responses from teachers that were violent, unfair or discriminatory. Most had experienced deliberate abuse and humiliation.

What is more, it is not just being screamed at or hit that is harmful.

The more subtle type of degradation can be worse because it is more pernicious. Like a virus compared to a bacterium, it is harder to spot and harder to eradicate so that, very slowly, the 'strong grip of constant demeaning squeezes out the last drops of self-confidence and worth' (Burns 1979, p. 292).

Insensitivity and criticism

Common complaints from dyslexic college students about teacher contributions to their work include: 'correcting spelling and grammar with a coloured pen', 'putting me at the back of the class', 'putting me down in public', 'emphasizing my bad points, never my good ones', 'placing me in a learning-difficulties group full of disruptive children who did not want to learn as much as I did', 'not helping me with bullying', 'blaming me for my phonetic spelling and saying I wasn't trying', 'marking down my work because it was difficult to read and full of errors', 'marking down other subjects because I wasn't any good at spelling' and 'blaming my parents for not caring about my spelling' (Dyslexia Institute 2002).

Incidental, insensitive comments by a teacher are also powerful; for example, 'John, you never get it right, do you?' or 'Frank, you're a strong boy. Help me move this desk'. The normal run-of-the-mill verbalizations of the teacher are fraught with evaluations and expectations of the pupil. 'But few teachers have realised how potent it all is' (Burns 1979, p. 288).

Unfortunately, it is the children with the lowest self-concept who tend to get more behavioural criticism from their teachers and are also less favourably evaluated than their high-self-concept counterparts. Criticism can also be non-verbal. It can occur through omission as well as downright rudeness.

Perception and not *reality* will inform behaviour. Children modify their behaviour for better or worse in response to the way they feel themselves to be perceived by their teachers. A grade can be read as a comment on the person rather than the work. Similarly, ignoring or having low expectations of a dyslexic child – which is the tendency in secondary school – implies that the teachers have given up on the child. The message is that this dyslexic child is worthless.

A similar message is sent by insincere praise: that the teacher cannot be bothered to be congruent. Not only does this add to the incongruence that dogs all the life of a dyslexic but it is also patronizing and disrespectful. These children are dyslexic, not thick: 'not even a young child depends entirely for his judgement on the views of others. For he can often see quite well for himself how he is doing' (Donaldson 1978, p. 114).

Lack of sensitivity also allows the teacher to forget that those with least approval need it most. Burns (1979) found that those who are the most dejected by, and hostile towards, criticism and failure are far more likely to glow when praised. They are also much more dependent on the evaluator's judgment. When criticism – even the mildest – comes, then 'the influence will be greatest on those who are least able to bear the cross' (p. 247).

How have teachers been helpful to dyslexic children?
A good relationship with a teacher really makes its mark on the life of a dyslexic child. A counsellor can usefully be informed by those teacher characteristics that help to empower and encourage a dyslexic child.

Practical help

If a teacher is motivated, they can give important advice and practical help to a dyslexic child. For example, they can set up extra time in examinations, which undoubtedly benefits slow writers (Bishop 2001), and plenty of help with SATS tests and public examinations such as GCSEs (Turner 2000b).

Flexibility

The best teachers for dyslexics are agile and flexible in their teaching methods. The gifted ones will turn on a sixpence to catch a teaching opportunity, like a bird wheeling onto a dragonfly. Rawson (1996), who is unquestionably the guru on the subject of teaching dyslexics, always valued flexibility and devised some useful aphorisms on the subject. Her most famous ones were: 'teach the language as it is to the child as he is' and 'go as fast as you can, but as slowly as you must'.

Warmth and acceptance

Research suggests that how teachers interact with children has more influence on their progress than organizational differences such as whether they are in a mixed-ability class or not (Riddick et al. 1999). Warm support is the main therapeutic teaching dimension, just as it is the most enabling and positive maternal response (see Chapter 6). Well-organized, focused, psychologically secure, creative, enthusiastic, encouraging and prepared teachers cope best with dyslexics. Sylva (1994) also reviewed evidence that good management and an engaged, empathic, clear and business-like manner in teachers were significant characteristics in the progress of all pupils.

A good relationship to challenge the bad view of self

Hay (2000), in a recent review of students suspended from school, showed that the quality of the teacher-child relationship and its connectedness was as crucial as that of the parent-child relationship. Bonding was more important than any school-based factor. What was important was 'students' perceptions that teachers cared and were fair-minded' (p. 348).

This particularly applies to children with emotional and behavioural difficulties. Cooper (1996), for example, in a review of such children and what makes their teachers effective, concluded that a good relationship with staff was the single most important factor: 'It was through these relationships that pupils were often first exposed to an image of themselves which challenged their low opinion of themselves as bad and worthless individuals. It was the reflection of themselves that they saw in others' response to them that enabled them to develop a positive self-image. This, in turn, gave them the confidence to take on new challenges in the knowledge that they would be accepted and valued by others, even if they failed in mastering those challenges' (p. 104).

High expectations

Teachers contribute to children's self-esteem. Sylva (1994) reviewing the 'enormous literature' on how teacher expectations can influence pupil achievement, concluded that expectations and attainment were strongly correlated. By contrast, 'if a child is defined as a failure, he will almost certainly fail and perhaps later he will hit out very hard against those who so defined him' (Donaldson 1978, p. 114).

Acceptance

Coopersmith (1967) showed that a teacher, by accepting the child with all their strengths and limitations, allowed the child to internalize all the good and bad bits of himself. This was particularly so because the acceptance came from a powerful person about whose opinions and judgement the child cared a lot.

There are, not surprisingly, significant positive correlations between the teachers' perceptions of their pupils and the pupil's own estimates of their class positions. This does not have to be openly stated. It can be conveyed by something as small as a gaze held or not held, a smile given or not given, a hand touched briefly or shaken in congratulation. Children notice these things. They get the message.

The acceptance by other people of the skills that a child has to offer is also important to a young child and has a powerful effect on his self-esteem. Unfortunately, what dyslexic children have to offer is not what teachers want, or know how to accept. As Donaldson (1978) observes: 'within the educational system ... there is certainly strong social approval of competence in the more disembedded skills of the mind' (p. 113). The child who succeeds in these is accepted and valued by teachers, and the one who fails is not.

Peers

Are peer relationships important to children?
Very much so. Good peer relationships empower children.

Woodward and Ferguson (2000) reviewed a body of literature, which showed 'a growing acceptance of the importance of good childhood peer relationships for children's optimal social, behavioural, and cognitive development' (p. 191). On the other hand, bad peer relationships destroy children. Hawker and Boulton (2000) reviewed 20 years of research on peer victimization and recorded its destructive effect: 'victims of peer aggression suffer a variety of feelings of psychosocial distress. They feel more anxious, socially anxious, depressed, lonely and worse about themselves than do non-victims' (p. 453). This effect occurs with both sexes, in all age groups and with all subtypes of aggression.

Do dyslexics have good relationships with their peers?
Generally, no.

This will be a constant theme throughout this book since it impinges directly on the counselling relationship with a dyslexic client.

It is easy to jump to the conclusion that dyslexics have peer problems simply because they are failing at school but this, alone, is not the reason. Many children fail at school and can be quite popular, particularly if they are good at sports. In certain school cultures, failure can even be the reason for popularity where there is an anti-academic ethos. I believe that the dyslexic academic failure becomes a catalyst for further peer rejection because of other, pre-existing characteristics. These are:

Poor relationship and social skills

This is the most serious reason for peer rejection. Dyslexics are not sought out as peers because they are not very good at making friends, nor are they very skilled at the things that encourage friendship.

For one thing, the dyslexic's skills at peer interaction are often eccentric, their reading of, and reaction to, non-verbal cues can be truly terrible, and some dyslexics present to others in a way that varies from the unusual to the downright weird. Dyslexics can also have significant language problems so that normal communication with other children is seriously handicapped. Poor social skills are also considered to be the main reason for peer-group rejection of all disabled children (Eaude 1999, Gurney 1988).

Clumsiness, sport and exclusion

Dyslexic children who are dyspraxic or just clumsy do not get selected for school sports teams, and they are often excluded from playground games. This is a particularly poignant form of peer rejection which has been recently examined by a number of researchers who found that movement difficulties are related to patterns of play and social interaction in young children (Smyth and Anderson 2001).

Children with movement impairments have been shown to be more isolated than others in their school playground. Compared to more agile controls, they were not selected to take part in games, had poor social competence, fewer friends and low self-esteem. They were found to be alone in the school playground more often, were onlookers more often and were moving around aimlessly more often. Both boys and girls took part less often in team games (e.g. football and rounders) and informal games (e.g. playfighting or skipping).

Another problem for dyspraxic and clumsy dyslexic children is that doing several things at once can be overwhelming. The attention given over to simply staying upright and dignified means that attention to smiling or other social interaction goes by the wayside: 'Poor coordination makes physical activities more attention demanding ... increasing the likelihood of perceived incompetence within that world' (op. cit., p. 411).

Working with peers in class

In a mainstream school, dyslexic children are deprived of the cosy experience of working with peers in a class setting. Not only can dyslexic children be socially unpopular but also a non-dyslexic can find their work and thinking style hard to understand. This is a social and academic loss since working together with peers enhances the cognitive capacity of children and really helps those children with learning difficulties (Watson 1999, Firman et al. 2001).

Dyslexic children can also miss out on the social interaction involved in working with peers. According to Piaget (1932), this joint activity between children decentres their thought processes, breaks down their cognitive egocentrism and encourages the development of operational thought. Piaget believed that, without this interaction with other children – and the disagreements and wrangling that go with it – then the thinking of young children would be trapped within the relativity of their own perspective. Young children need other children to disagree and argue with them rather than someone who just demonstrates a correct solution. Disagreement is essential.

Finally, dyslexics cannot even have the option of cheating effectively by glancing at others' work – since they cannot process or read fast enough. Also, they cannot experience the flattery of being copied from since their work is very hard to read. Unfortunately, the work of other children can be a useful aid to learning. Butler (1996) found that attending to peer's work was helpful both to 'reduce uncertainty about one's capacities' and 'acquire information relevant to clarifying task demands or to promote mastery and self-improvement' (p. 1). This resource is denied to dyslexic children who are locked in a lonely, desk-bound cocoon.

What is the effect of peer-relationship problems for dyslexic children?
The single, overwhelming effect of the poor peer relationships that dyslexic children have at school is that they are bullied – regularly, viciously and far more often than non-dyslexic children.

Twenty years ago, Tattum (1993) called bullying 'the most malicious and malevolent form of deviant behaviour widely practised in our schools'. He noted then that it was 'widespread and persistent' (p. 7). It is even more so today. Things have not changed. Childline listens to 1.5 million children a year. In 2002, among the under 11s, the largest category for calls – as it has been for many years – was for bullying (30% or 450,000 calls). Last year, the number of children who rang Childline about bullying was far higher than the number ringing about family abuse (23% or 345,000 calls).

What also does not change is that dyslexics tend to be disproportionately on the receiving end of bullying. In fact, no counsellor can work with a dyslexic client and not take this experience of bullying into account since the probability approaches certainty that, if a client is dyslexic, then he was bullied.

This also means that the counsellor will find in the bullying aspect of dyslexia not only a powerful victim transference but also some of the strongest feelings – real and transferred – of helplessness.

Bullying

Background

Are dyslexic children more likely to be bullied than non-dyslexics?
Yes. Dyslexics are bullied far more, and more severely, than other children.

McDougall (2001) found that 48% of a sample of dyslexics had been bullied at school, but only 10% in the non-dyslexic group. My own survey of dyslexic children found that 80% had been bullied prior to arrival at East Court School, a proportion that is between two and three times the norm reported for non-dyslexics (Rigby 2002).

In this respect, dyslexic children receive no different treatment from all children with learning difficulties and disability. Such children are at a universally increased risk of bullying of which the most 'common and hurtful' bullying is deliberate 'exclusion from activities in which they could take part' (op. cit., p. 186). Other studies have found that children with special educational needs are more susceptible to bullying than their peers and are more likely to have few friends and to be rejected (O'Moore and Hillery 1992, Martlew and Hodson 1991). Clumsiness is a particular problem (Smyth and Anderson 2000).

A disabled child's chance of being bullied is greater if his disability is more visible. While dyslexia is not itself visible, its associated elements – hyperactivity, clumsiness, slowness, introversion, anxiety, low social competence, difficulties in speech, reading and comprehension – definitely are. These are as visible – and as inviting – to a bully as a wheelchair.

Do dyslexic children bully others?

Yes. It is a serious and complicating factor when counselling dyslexic children that they come to the bullying problem from both directions.

It is not just a feature of dyslexia, but of all disability. Rigby (2002) observes that disabled children can be as likely to bully as be a victim of bullying. They may be bully/victims. Whitney et al. (1994) found that dyslexic children who had been bullied previously in mainstream schools tended to retaliate at first by bullying other children. Children with special needs 'may be at greater risk of being bullied if not of bullying others' (p. 216).

A number of studies have also shown that bully/victims are often the most disturbed of all bully categories. They are also more likely to have attachment problems and punitive parenting. Wolke et al. (2000) found that not only are bully/victims a sizeable group but they also had the highest rate of behavioural and psychological problems.

Does bullying occur more in mainstream schools than special schools for dyslexic children?

Yes.

Children with special needs are bullied in mainstream schools far more frequently than other children, and dyslexic children may be more damaged psychologically by being in mainstream units than in special schools.

Whitney et al. (1994), for example, reviewed research showing that children in remedial classes in mainstream schools were more likely to be victims of bullying, particularly of frequent bullying, were teased significantly more than mainstream children and formed fewer friendships. Nabuzoka and Smith (1993) also found that children with learning difficulties were more likely to be selected as victims (33%) than those without (8%). Mainstream children were also more likely to choose friends among other mainstream children rather than children with special needs.

Visibility is an important factor in bullying, and the child with learning problems is more visible in a mainstream school: 'just being different in a noticeable way can be a risk factor for being a victim' (Whitney et al. 1994, p. 213). Being visible also comes from being alone at playtime or not having many friends. This is, in itself, a self-selecting risk for being bullied. The lack of peers is both a cause and a result of being bullied: 'children who are alone at playtime, or do not have many friends (often the case with learning-disabled children), run an increased risk of being victims of bullying' (Nabuzoka and Smith 1993, p. 1437).

Learning disability also tends to amplify any problems that are already there. Ordinary children who have few close friends are merely neglected and left alone. Those with learning disabilities are actively rejected. In addition, the reaction to the dyslexic child's behaviour is different. For example, Nabuzoka and Smith (op. cit.) found that dyslexic children were no different from other children in terms of being disruptive or starting fights. It was just that when they did these things they were seen as even more unpopular than non-learning disabled children.

How are dyslexics bullied?

In the same way as everyone else. They can be hit, pinched, burnt, kicked, have their work destroyed and their possessions stolen.

In my own survey of dyslexic children, I found that they had been, variously, kicked downstairs, left on the floor with a bleeding mouth and nose, been sprayed with lighter fluid and set alight, kicked, grabbed by the legs and swung around, had their fingers bent back, picked up by the neck, thrown over a wall, poked and thumped in the genitals, tripped up over a top step, had their head pushed down a lavatory and their hands stamped on, shoved and shut into a cupboard so strenuously that a shoulder was dislocated, punched to the ground and urinated on by a group of boys. A quarter had been bullied every day, a third up to three times every week.

Does their dyslexia feature in the bullying?

Yes – and those who bully consider it to be sufficient justification for anything they do to a dyslexic child.

Half of the dyslexic children interviewed by Riddick (1996) said they had been teased specifically about their dyslexia: 'many of the children lived with the constant fear of being teased about their difficulties and put a lot of their energies into covering up their difficulties or trying to divert attention away from them' (p. 149).

In my own study, most of the dyslexic children had grown up with being called names associated with their learning disability such as 'dyslexic dick', 'spastic cunt', 'you dyslexic little prat', 'just a spastic idiot – no one will talk to you', 'he's stupid – he can't spell', 'you're so dumb, your mother should have put you down', 'you big fool, you're at the bottom', 'you're so slow' – and so on. This was a sample of 40 dyslexic children on one occasion. Up to 6 million dyslexics have regularly received such bullying – both physical and verbal – through most of their school years. Dyslexic children are still experiencing this torment, right now, right here, in a school near you.

What effect does bullying have on dyslexic children?
It causes suffering.

All the studies on the subject conclude, variously, that victimization makes people ill, anxious, depressed, angry, terrified, vengeful and withdrawn. It annihilates self-esteem and destroys any assumptions that the world is benevolent or meaningful. Reviews of the research conclude that victims have low self-worth, are non-assertive and have poor social skills. They are psychologically introverted, relatively uncooperative, uncompetitive and are not group orientated (Rigby 2002).

Being bullied makes children feel bad about themselves, find bullying reassuring, get upset if told they are good, destroy their own work, say no one likes them, become oversensitive, lack humour and startle easily (Elliott 1999).

Severe bullying also induces post-traumatic stress disorder (PTSD) (see Chapter 7). In line with the effects of PTSD, victims can clearly recall details of their bullying five years or more later, including the type of bullying and its location (Rivers 2001).

In the long term, bullying spoils adult relationships, including sexual ones. Smith (1991) found that 80% of 'love shy' heterosexual men, who had difficulties in their relationships with women, had experiences of bullying or harassment at school.

Help against bullying

Who do dyslexic children go to for help?
Not teachers or counsellors.

In fact, dyslexic children who are bullied rarely go to adults for help.

Studies on bullying report that only one-third of children would tell an adult, one-third friends. Parsonage (2002) reviews a study in which only 20% of children reported to teachers when they were being bullied, and Whitney et al. (1994) found that a lunchtime supervisor was as likely as anyone to be told about bullying. Less than 50% of bullied children asked for help. This still means that most children, most of the time, suffer in silence.

Children do not tell counsellors and clinicians about bullying, even when this is the main reason for their referral. The clinicians also do not ask. In one study, examination of clinicians' case notes showed that only one-third of the 64% of children who had been bullied could be identified from the notes. Furthermore, only a tiny number of the bullied adolescents felt that the clinic had seen the bullying as relevant. Even fewer had been able to discuss their experience of bullying with the doctor, social workers or psychologist who first assessed them (Quinn 1996).

Do teachers help?
Generally, no. There are four reasons for this.

First, teachers greatly underestimate the amount of bullying that goes on in schools. O'Moore and Hillery (1994), for example, noted that only 24% of the total number of bullies in one school were identified by the victims' teachers.

Second, pupils are reluctant to inform teachers when they are being bullied. Over one-third of children do not tell their teacher and, generally, most victims endure their plight or try to ignore it (Rigby 2002).

Third, worrying research by Pepler and Craig (1998) found that teachers are in the frame 11% of the time when a bullying incident occurs and intervene only 4% of the time. Lane (1992) also found that 25% of teachers feel that it is sometimes helpful to ignore the victims. This attitude apparently hardens with the teacher's length of service, so that those with the longest service have the least sympathy for victims (Boulton and Smith 1994).

Finally, a significant number of adults despise victims and have pro-bully attitudes. They 'see bullying as socially undesirable, but this is not the same as considering it [socially] incompetent' (Sutton 2001, p. 532). In a school with a male ethos, bullies and aggressive children are often secretly admired.

Do friends help?
Peer support systems encourage telling.

Dyslexics have no peer support, so there is no one to encourage them to tell. Their own helplessness and language problems also make asking for help physically and psychologically difficult. Dyslexics are, thus, unlikely to seek help from teachers or peers. This reluctance to ask for help occurs even in schools with well-established support systems and whole-school bullying policies.

There is another less acknowledged issue. Literacy and bullying problems start to affect dyslexics when they are between eight and ten years old. Unfortunately, this is also the peak age for unhelpful behaviour among children, particularly boys. Terwogt (2002), in a study of helping behaviour among school-age boys, found that a friend's sad behaviour was given as a specific reason for *withholding* help. A boy's sadness made his peers feel inadequate and guilty.

At ten years of age, children are also not that interested in altruism: 'none of our happy ten-year-olds referred to [helping another child] as a way of prolonging happiness. In their eyes, happiness clearly does not need improvement. Helping someone in need might only threaten its maintenance' (p. 143).

Terwogt also reported that younger males were less likely than younger females to respond to a peer in need of assistance, while Berndt (1981) found that boys were less helpful towards close male friends than others. Jackson and Tisak (2001) found that age of participants was important. The nine- to ten-year-old group was highly unlikely to comfort a friend, or feel bad about not doing so. They cared little about negative judgements for not comforting.

The problem is that close male friendships among eight- to 11-year-old boys involve a strong element of competition. The *Just William* philosophy prevails: 'Open display of fear ... is often unacceptable in boys' (Terwogt (op. cit.), p. 134). Demonstration of fear is regarded with scorn. Even explicit awareness of a friend's fear is not sufficient reason for helping them.

Children are also concerned with what is useful and visible. Roberts and Smith (1999) found that non-disabled children were most likely to be friends with disabled peers who had the most control over their actions. Interaction and friendship needed to be easy. By comparison, when children thought such behaviours would be difficult, even when they expressed positive attitudes to a child's disability, they reported fewer intentions to interact. Children at this age do not want interaction that involves extra effort. This is also a useful explanation for why dyslexic children in the 7–12-year age group might struggle to retain friends, even among those children who are positively disposed towards them.

In short, the age at which a dyslexic child is in most need of friendly support from peers is also the exact age when he is least likely to receive it. This significantly increases the effects of social isolation (see Chapter 11). It is also clear that an important inference to be drawn from this research is that unhappiness is, in itself, an unattractive social handicap at this age. Unhappy dyslexics will be shunned simply because of their mood.

There is, therefore, some merit to the argument that teaching social skills to a dyslexic child so that he knows how to respond in a happy way – or present a fearless exterior to other children – might have positive benefits in social acceptance (see Chapter 12).

Does anyone help a bullied, dyslexic child?

On the whole, no.

The dyslexic child who is physically and emotionally abused first by other children is abused again by adults who fail to help him. As La Fontaine (1991) observes, 'doing nothing is the worst reaction to being told about bullying that an adult can have. It causes the victims more pain without solving their problems' (p. 29).

For a dyslexic, it also confirms his belief that he is helpless, unimportant and worthless.

It is, furthermore, an abuse of trust that can carry over into the counselling relationship. With some justification, a dyslexic client might wonder whether a counsellor will be as unhelpful and abandoning as everyone else has been.

There is clearly rich ground here for testing of the counselling relationship and for the counsellor to feel deskilled in the transference.

The context of bullying

What is the main personality difference between bullies and victims?

My hunch is to go with the newest line of research evidence and suggest that social cognition is the main difference – a variable that underpins many other differences between the two groups.

Bullies positively brim with social cognition while victims almost universally are deficient in it. It may even be that the experience of bullying is educational and may even aid in the bully's development of social cognition. Bullying is social-cognitive-skills training in itself.

For example, a recent study by and Sutton et al. (1999) has shown that, contrary to the widespread view that bullies are ignorant oafs who lack social skills, they are superior to any other subgroup in their ability to read the minds of others, thus enabling them to be manipulative and domineering. A well-developed theory of mind, with a good grasp of mental state and the emotions of others is a very useful skill in bullying; for example, in spreading gossip, social exclusion, organizing gangs and avoiding detection. Overall, the evidence is that bullies should not be seen as isolates or incompetent.

Victims of bullying, on the other hand, often demonstrate poor social skills and deficient social cognition. There is a negative correlation between victim score and social cognition, and it is possible that the deficient social cognition skills of victims contributes to their experience. In this respect, it is important to note that dyslexics can also have very poor theory of mind, social cognition and social skills (see Chapter 8).

Is bullying a social activity?
Yes. It provides the framework for social cognition.

Bullying is a 'complex social labelling process' (Lane 1992, p. 146), a group rather than an individual activity. Sutton (2001) describes bullying as violence in a group context in which pupils reinforce each other's behaviour. It is a collective action in which relationships are important. Sutton asserts that bullying has too much been based in the aggression literature and fails to take account of the social context and methods of bullying.

Are there different types of bullying?
There are two broad types.

First, there is 'social' bullying. This is the more common and involves physical and verbal abuse. It takes place in a social setting where peers are present 85% of the time (Pepler and Craig 1998). These peers take several roles. They may instigate attacks on other children (bully), help the bully (assistant) or reinforce him through laughing, watching or shouting encouragement (reinforcer). Alternatively, other peers may stick up for the victim (defender), or remain resolutely uninvolved (outsider). It is possible to assign one of these roles to 87% of children (Sutton et al. 1999).

Second, there is 'relational' bullying where there is a deliberate attempt by a bully to destroy friendships or isolate an individual from close friends. This can be achieved by spreading rumours, inventing lies about the victim or threatening their friends.

Half of female-to-female, and one-third of male-to-male bullying takes place within a friendship or 'relational' network (Sutton 2001).

Bullying of boys is more likely to be linked to power-based social relationships, and girls to affiliation activities or relationship aggression. Having said that, there is increasing evidence that boys are also affected by relational bullying too but report it less, and Rigby (2002) believes that we are in danger of underestimating the effect of relational aggression on boys.

Overall, relational aggression causes more distress than any other types of bullying. Schafer et al. (2002) say it causes 'substantial distress' (p. 282), particularly to female targets. Rigby (2002) calls relational aggression – being excluded, breaking up friendship, ganging up on others – 'the most hurtful [of] aggressive acts' (p. 64). Being hit or kicked was way down the list.

Action against bullying

What can be done about bullying and dyslexia?
I wish I knew for sure.

Unfortunately, the whole topic of bullying generates more research, but fewer solutions, than any other issue in the social sciences. As Mencken famously observed: 'For every complex problem there is an answer that is clear, simple and wrong' (quoted in Rigby 2002, p. 233). No solution to bullying has ever been produced that is clear, simple and right.

What does the literature on bullying suggest?
The bullying literature is huge, unhelpful and mired in a vast, depressing, 'ain't it awful' ethos.

I have been following this literature for 15 years, and it has not moved forward in any practical or useful sense. I believe that there is a parallel process in the research which reflects the helpless, angry, frustrated and impotent view of victims. In other words, the research on bullying reflects the perception of victims that nothing helps, nothing gets done and no one understands.

A similar exasperation permeates the conclusion of the latest enormous review of peer-victimization research. While observing that all these research studies 'reveal patterns of distress that can no longer be ignored', Hawker and Boulton (2000) go on to say 'enough is enough'. They conclude: 'It is clear enough already that victims are distressed ... it is time for victimisation research to move on' (p. 453). What was needed now were interventions to reduce victims' distress. If more researchers devoted themselves to addressing this, then the practitioners 'may begin to make a serious impact on the distress that children feel when they are bullied' (p. 453).

I have considerable sympathy with this point of view. There are, for example, several thousand studies that agree on how distressing it is to be bullied and how bullying can have appalling long-term consequences. There are another few thousand studies which agree and disagree – about equally – on the characteristics of victims and bullies, their family aetiology, psychopathology and degrees of conduct and personality disorder. There are also a few dozen inconclusive reviews on this vast literature. Rigby (2002), for example, has written the latest of these tracts. His last chapter on who should be blamed for bullying is a furious rant around the victim, the bully, the parents, the school, the system and the whole of society before coming to an exhausted, angry conclusion that, basically, he hasn't got a clue.

Is there any evidence on what actually works to stop bullying?
Unfortunately, no.

There are perhaps only a dozen studies that look objectively at why bullying occurs. There are no studies whatsoever on exactly what works to stop bullying. There are, certainly, suggestions of strategies of what might work: such as, Circle Time, Whole-School Policy, Shared Concern and No-blame approaches, but none of them has been tested in any rigorous way. There is a conspicuous lack of useful empirical evidence. As Lane (1992) observes, there is 'a considerable amount of descriptive material in the literature to suggest that effective action is possible ... [but] there is a substantial shortage of experimental evidence' (p. 150). Furthermore, I have tried most of these anti-bullying strategies and, like the Curate's Egg, they are good only in parts.

Take Circle Time. The principle of this strategy is that the group meets to discuss the bullying of a child. Both bully and victim talk, empathize, agree, weep, shake hands and leave with an eagerly expressed determination to form a new relationship. Within a short time, the bullying starts up again, sometimes with worse violence than before. I thought I was the only one to find this. Then, while running seminars on bullying, I heard a number of teachers and counsellors also observe – tentatively – that they found it didn't work. Like the emperor's new clothes, we were pretending the solutions were there – but they were not.

Torrance (2000) makes a similar observation. 'More recently, research has focused on addressing bullying rather than simply studying its existence, although many intervention strategies have been disappointing in the extent to which they reduced bullying' (p. 16).

Can a counsellor do anything at all to help a client who is being bullied?
Yes – but I believe the counsellor must be clear about her objectives.

I think that there are two problems here, and they get tangled up with each other. First, there is the wider school and social problem of bullying – the macro problem. Second, there is the individual's problem of victimization – the micro problem.

First, the macro problem involves understanding the social role of bullying. This is the school-wide problem, and may well respond to tactics based on manipulating the social roles surrounding bullying (Sutton 2001). To be blunt, however, my own experience is that the only macro-response that always works is to exclude the bully after the proper sequence of warning, parent involvement, constant vigilance and decent communication. After such exclusion, not only does the whole atmosphere of the school change but also the act of exclusion significantly discourages other potential bullies. My own research into bullying found that over 80% of all bullying is done by just one or two individuals. These children manage to terrify the vast majority of the other pupils either by actual harm or by fostering an atmosphere of anxious, head-down behaviour among the rest. After the removal of these children, their acolytes fade away, and it is possible to see a huge difference in morale.

This, of course, is hardly within the remit of the counsellor, although she can do her best to try to effect change by pursuing the matter directly with the school. I have had anecdotal evidence of counsellors working with parents of bullied children to take civil and criminal action against schools to have the bully excluded. In these respects, the counsellor was able to short circuit the usual helplessness that seems to drown any effective action against bullying.

Second, there is the micro problem of an individual's victimization – which is the one that faces the counsellor in one-to-one therapy. Here, the question is how to help the client during the normal counselling process. In this respect, I believe that we can also look at the social model of bullying but from the perspective of how the client is acting out a victim role in the group.

There will be a tacit assumption in this micro-counselling perspective that, when the client stops being a victim of bullying, the bully will just move onto another target, if the macro problem of school-wide bullying is not solved.

How can a counsellor use the counselling process to help a victim?
What I find can work in the traditional counselling setting is to use a two-pronged counselling policy.

First, it is important to establish a therapeutic relationship in which the child feels safe and supported. This, itself, is empowering. Second, the counsellor can use what is known of the social context of counselling to help her client to present as a person who is not bullied: to extinguish her client's victim-like manner, self-talk, and physical demeanour. In this way the child becomes less 'bulliable'.

My view is that both bully and victim are operating in a social dance. I think that they have a transaction, an implied contract and a learned relationship that the counsellor can unpick. As Lane (1992) observes, the therapist cannot act on bullying without addressing its social context. Therapy for the victim 'cannot take place or be effective without impacting on the context in which the problem occurs' (p. 153).

Ignoring the social context, anchoring the problem in the personality of the individual alone, is to ignore the oxygen that gives bullying its vigour and the victim his identity: 'the form and perceived effects of bullying are socially constructed and there is a danger that when bullying is divorced from its social context, investigations become limited to dry questions and answers' (Torrance 2000, p. 16).

Focusing on the bully, alone, is also a waste of time because the bully is really oblivious to the feelings of the victim. What is important is to understand that, to a bully, the victim really does not exist as a person. What is useful to a bully is that a child should present as a victim, look like a victim, act like a victim and, therefore, act as a tool to maintain the bully's social role. The victim can be child A or child B. If child A stops looking and acting like a victim, the bully will use child B. In an important way, the bully can honestly say to the victim – 'nothing personal'.

Bullying for the bully is satisfying and pleasurable. It establishes dominance, and it is an easy and effective social strategy. 'So it makes sense to them – it might not to us, but it does to them. Bullying is just one of a range of strategies available to create a reputation' (Sutton 2001, p. 532).

The micro-approach to helping the dyslexic victim through counselling can build on these insights. Details on the counselling strategies mentioned below are given in Chapter 12.

Options for action by the counsellor can be summarised through three scenarios.

Scenario 1: The social fantasy of the bully needs someone to act like a victim

The bully constructs a social fantasy based on a relationship with a number of children. This fantasy is maintained by threat of harm or exclusion. Bullying is the means by which he maintains the fantasy, but it can only live through strong group cohesion. There has to be a sense of 'us' and 'them'. The notion of 'us' can only be defined strongly if there is a 'them'. Victims are 'them'. Victims are valuable because they represent difference from the group – by their psychology, behaviour or self-selection. They mark the line between 'in the group' and 'out of the group'.

In these respects, dyslexics, all learning-disabled children and even children with chronic illness (Meijer et al. 2000) self-select as victims because they are not only different in actuality but their disability makes them behave differently. They are, in effect, ready-wrapped as victims.

Hodges and Parry (1996), for example, found that learning-disabled children were rejected simply because they were needy, submissive, vulnerable or inadequate. Being shy, uncooperative, seeking help and being in need of help were, in themselves, violations of the social rules of the group. Even simply being a 'victim of bullying' and needing help from adults was itself a reason for the role of victim, since this was a sign that the child was socially inept and incompetent at interacting with others.

In short, dyslexic children are bullied simply 'because they have not managed to understand how to avoid being victimised' (Nabuzoka and Smith 1993, p. 1446).

Action: Improve the social cognition, confidence and social demeanour of the victim by social skills and social cognition training (see Chapter 12).

Scenario 2: Children need peer-group support

Bullying can only succeed because children need friends. To be a good victim you have to be excluded and you have to care about it. What, therefore, is useful is to consider those children who are never bullied, who opt out of the bully's fantasy and who do not care about group approval. These children – variously described in research as onlookers, rescuers, outsiders and loners (see Chapter 11) – are merely neglected by, rather than excluded from, the group. They often have a strong internal locus of control and good self-esteem.

Action: Improve the victim's self-esteem through the counselling relationship. Encourage improvements in literacy, since dyslexic self-esteem improves when reading and writing improve (see Chapter 12).

Scenario 3: Victims, bullies and bully/victims are learned relationships with others

Victims are essential to define and maintain the bully's control and the cohesion of the group. In their own way they are powerful in that, without a victim, the bully could not operate. Victims, too, can use bullies to maintain their own identity.

Victims and bullies – in a bizarre, toxic and fascinating way – need each other. Sometimes this need is complicated when the victim accepts the role of victim as a valuable social role, when no other is on offer. Victims also watch the success of bullies – whether at home or school – and, when they get the chance, try to emulate it. Those who are most likely to see bullying as valuable, who have envied the role and power of the bully will, given the chance, try it out for themselves. This, I believe, explains the high rate of bullying among former dyslexic victims.

Action: Challenge and reframe the victim role through classic counselling particularly the use of challenge, and techniques of Cognitive Behavioural Therapy.

SECTION THREE
FAMILY

Introduction

Everybody's family is exactly like our own.

That is the assumption made by every dyslexic child as they grow up. There is no other point of comparison. This is the *normal and correct* family, and the way it has of doing things is the *normal and correct* way of doing things.

What a family says or does to a dyslexic child has, therefore, the power of oracle. The older child may challenge this view later – and it is healthy that he should – but for the young and growing child, their family's way is the *correct* way in which they should be treated and spoken to. It is how any *normal* person would act.

This child thinks: 'They must be right. This is how I am and how I should be. Therefore, this is how I shall live my life.' If his family treats the dyslexic child as a fragile, helpless puppy – or as a disabled, incompetent idiot – the child will come to believe that this is all he is or all he can become.

If, however, his family treats him as a normal, happy, healthy child who just happens to have the inconvenience of dyslexia, or as someone who has a problem but who also has the strength and resources to deal with that problem, the dyslexic child will also come to believe this information about himself and live his life accordingly.

All children are sensitive to the 'particularities of the emotional climate of their own family and they encode those particularities from an early age' (Harris 1994, p. 23). In the same way, the dyslexic child internalizes his family's message and carries it, in unconscious form, through to adulthood. Locating the family pressures on a dyslexic child, whether from parents, siblings or the whole family dynamic, is, therefore, central to understanding a dyslexic client.

This section identifies those aspects of a dyslexic client's family life that can be usefully explored during counselling and that may also – in the nature of transference and the therapeutic relationship – be acted out in the counselling process.

CHAPTER 5

In the home of the dyslexic child

Summary

In his seminal review on how a child's behaviour develops, Rutter (1985) described the influence of family as 'important' and 'sizeable'. This is hardly surprising news to a counsellor. What is reassuring, however, is that the family influences on a client may be important but they are not set in stone. These influences are transactional, and will vary by the individual's personality, so that 'recurrent opportunities to break the chain continue right into adult life' (p. 365).

Without this last flicker of optimism – and given what most counsellors learn about what passes for normal family life – the counsellor's job would be impossible. The extent to which a counsellor can help to break the chain of any toxic family influence on a dyslexic client depends, however, on some understanding of two factors: first, how the intrusion of dyslexia can permanently change the family dynamic and, second, how the relationships within a family are altered when a child is diagnosed as dyslexic.

The arrival of dyslexia: changes in the home

Will family relationships change when a child is diagnosed as dyslexic?
Yes. Things are never the same again.

The diagnosis of dyslexia leads to the formation of new dyadic relationships within the family, and other family relationships reform to accommodate this. Since the different dyads within the family are interdependent, the dyslexic child's behaviour cannot be understood by studying any one dyadic family relationship in isolation.

Generally speaking, problems in the family usually arise 'when the balance of give and take between parents and children or between fathers and mothers is disturbed' (Mathijssen et al. 1998, p. 477), or – importantly –

when the balance of what is fair and just is distorted. The risk of emotional harm and the development of problem behaviour in a dyslexic child are then multiplied with each hot spot of hostility in the family.

In the most extreme cases, for example, the dyslexic child can take on the role of family scapegoat, accepting in the family politic the scorn of both siblings and parents and, eventually, internalizing all the 'bad' things in the family.

Are the family influences on dyslexic clients unusual?
Yes. In fact, what is central to understanding the dyslexic client is that the family influences to which he is now subjected are not only complex but involve large amounts of unexpressed negative material from both siblings and parents.

This results in a significant degree of acting out by all family members that contaminates the dyslexic's view of himself in quite specific ways. Most family effects on our clients have at least been overt – extending the courtesy of open and measurable abuse. The key to understanding the dyslexic client's family influence lies in the fact that much of the abuse can be denied, covert and, worst of all, well meaning.

In order to understand these influences, it is important to go back to the beginning, to the time when the family gradually realizes that it has an illiterate and troubled dyslexic cuckoo in its midst.

How does the family first realize a child is dyslexic?
Three very experienced observers of dyslexic children and their families have given insightful overviews of what it is like for parents to discover their child is dyslexic.

> A few months after beginning school, the once happy and contented young child may not be quite so settled. Often, parents develop vague feelings of unease about their child's development, but they will probably not be able to put their finger on what is wrong. They will be baffled by their child, who seems so able and bright in some contexts but so poorly skilled in others. He may have trouble remembering how to write his name, or he may be the only one who has not been given a reading book because he hasn't learned how to recognize the key word flash cards. Behaviour problems may appear as he rebels over having to conform to the class rules. He may start wetting the bed, having been dry for two years or more, or he may become reluctant about attending school. As he falls farther and farther behind his peer group in literacy skills, his self-esteem may suffer and poor behaviour, mood swings, introversion or depression may become manifest (Goldup and Ostler 2000, p. 326).

> Apparent failure at school does not pass unnoticed by the parents, who start to become anxious. In their turn they too are confused. Often there was

little concrete evidence before their child started at primary school that anything was amiss. Some clumsiness, a quaint way with words or failure to
remember instructions could easily be ascribed to general immaturity. The
parents' increasing worries reflect on the child. If there are other siblings
without learning difficulties, the parents may be tactful enough not to make
direct comparison, but the child will usually be aware of the discrepancies. A
deep sense of unease begins to grow and the child becomes conscious that
he is disappointing his family. Stress for the dyslexic is not confined to school
but permeates home life as well. As it grows it can lead to such manifestations
of emotional disturbance as temper tantrums, aggression and bed-wetting.
An element of guilt may be set up in either child or parents, whose management of the child becomes increasingly uncertain. Pressure creates further
stress, but acceptance of failure can appear to be demoralising patronage,
and a middle way is hard to find (Thomson 1995b, p. 41).

Does a home have to be organized for dyslexia?

Yes – and parents have to put a lot of effort into coping with a dyslexic child
at home. There is always a degree, however, to which this is resented – especially as the problems do not diminish as a child becomes older. Parents
must, for example, learn to deal with the associated problems of dyslexia,
such as timekeeping, organization and the encouragement of coping
mechanisms. They must also help their dyslexic child take control of himself and his routines as well as involve themselves in the educational
management of their dyslexic child. 'When these objectives are met, parents can see they are making a difference in the life of their child' (Goldup
and Ostler 2000, p. 330).

This may, indeed, be great for those who relish such challenges, but
many parents do not enjoy doing this at all, and, if there are other children
or an enjoyable job, all the extra family help for a dyslexic can seem an
unending chore. Many parents are surprised to find that they are not alone
in resenting, rather than revelling in, such extra routines.

Some of the work is irritating in the extreme.

Dyslexic children need help with the peripheral handicaps of dyslexia,
including losing books and sports clothes, forgetting messages and
appointments, confusing the days of the week, the incomplete following of
instructions, the inability to read what the homework requires – let alone
do it – and general wild disorganization.

One mother confided that it had been easier to look after her dement-
ed, 70-year-old mother with Alzheimer's disease than her highly intelligent
ten-year-old son with moderate dyslexia. If the dyslexic child also has dyspraxia or ADHD, the organization problems can increase exponentially.

In order to survive, the parents must learn strategies, such as providing
checklists tabulated with two boxes to check if something has been found

and a second to indicate it has been named, daily lists detailing lunch money, reading book, pencil case, art materials or musical instrument. Schedules must be worked out and glued in appropriate places, such as in the dyslexic child's diary or locker. Bulletin boards and organizers must be bought and problems endlessly anticipated. There must also be back-up strategies for every eventuality, such as having the telephone number of a school friend who can be relied upon to help with homework details, and having copies to hand of all school timetables detailing clothing and equipment needs.

These extra planning demands are hard for non-dyslexic parents – but for parents who are dyslexic themselves, particularly a mother, this can be a nightmare. Her own anxiety will rebound back onto her child who will then feel unhelped and panicked. He will then make even more demands on her already stretched organizational resources leading to even greater anxiety for both of them. They exist in an endless, amplifying corridor of stress-reflecting mirrors.

It is sometimes the unremitting demands of looking after their own dyslexic children that finally sends a dyslexic parent into the breakdown that has been waiting in the wings all their lives.

The cycle of damage is thereby dramatically perpetuated.

Does a rigid or relaxed family structure help the dyslexic child?
Rigid helps every time.

In fact, it is not hyperbole to say that an army routine must be put in place. The family must adopt a new type of controlled and organized home environment run on very strict lines. This should not, however, be regarded by the counsellor as maladaptive or pathological family functioning but the opposite: effective, adaptive family response to the demands of dyslexia. It is axiomatic in working with dyslexics that the adults caring for them must be 150% organized because dyslexic children are only 50% organized themselves.

Margalit and Heiman (1986), for example, in a study of the homes of learning-disabled children found that the more rigid, controlled and ordered families of learning-disabled children 'can be viewed as an adaptive reaction to ongoing stress related to excessive demands for care of the exceptional child' (p. 844).

This was also found by Kappers and Veerman (1995). Parents of dyslexic adolescents discovered that their children coped better with control, discipline, fixed-role relationships and clear rules. This type of organization meant that there was a near absence of emotional and behavioural disorders among their children. The more rigid the organization of family life (as opposed to a more liberal regime), the more beneficial it is to dyslexic children.

Strong systems also make dyslexic children feel safe. This emphasizes a point discussed in more detail in Section 5 – the importance of quite rigid therapeutic boundaries for dyslexic clients.

To say the least, this process of home adaptation can be stressful for those parents who, prior to having a dyslexic child, might have had a more relaxed and laid back family lifestyle. While some struggle on with an increasingly desperate and tense attempt to be laid-back, it is my experience that parents usually face up to the inevitable choice of living with dyslexia: organize or disintegrate.

Do the family and school unite to help the dyslexic child?

In everyone's dreams. The reality is that almost primitive warfare can break out, with the parents and teachers acting more like children than the dyslexic child.

A dyslexic child's school problems rebound on home life and vice versa in an increasingly uncontrolled ping-pong of influence and blame. Teachers, for example, can attribute many children's difficulties to adverse home circumstances and assume that the parents do not care about their child's education, when the parents can be as bewildered about the child's problems as is the teacher. Riddick (1996) found that half of the parents in her study felt they had been stereotyped and blamed in some way by the school for their child's difficulties. Both parents and teachers can form inaccurate stereotypes of each other based on partial information.

Inconsistent teacher response and failure to respond to them can also lead to frustrated anxiety for parents of a dyslexic child who resent the fact that teachers seem not to understand the reality of what home life is like for them. This leads to rebarbative communications flying back and forth between home and school, with the wretched dyslexic child in the middle feeling that he is annoying everyone, which, in fact, he is.

This is sad because there is much evidence to show that the partnership between home and school can make a positive and significant difference to dyslexic children, and teachers can provide the very best support for a dyslexic child.

Unfortunately, children will always tend to give greater weight to what they find at home: 'children will always be able to distort what they find at school, because they will be expected to find their home environment either reproduced there or else represented by its opposite' (Winnicott 1965, p. 203).

Is it a good idea to teach a dyslexic child to read at home?

No. In fact, this is a very, very bad idea.

Almost any other type of help would be better. Living with a dyslexic child can be extremely stressful. Trying to help a dyslexic child at home with any sort of teaching is unimaginably so. It is like the worst type of driving lesson with a close relative. It also does not help one little bit if parents are using inappropriate teaching methods.

This situation has great potential for volcanic rows and spectacular disagreement with both parties ending up, literally, in tears. Neither does it help if a teacher gives a dyslexic child homework and is insensitive to the fact that the parents themselves may be insecure readers.

Parents who have tried to teach their dyslexic child at home can fall back before the onslaught of short-term memory problems, rage, frustration or their child's skilful use of sabotage, avoidance strategies and sly charm.

On balance it is better to leave well alone: 'Learning support might be given by a parent, but it can give rise to much tension and disagreement between parent and child. An older sibling, relation, neighbour or babysitter could be a viable option. Parents must be reassured that it is not unusual for support to be sometimes better when given by someone other than themselves' (Goldup and Ostler 2000, p. 332).

Acceptance, love, a sense of humour and reading lots of books to a dyslexic child are far more useful offerings from a parent.

Are there particular problems with hyperactivity (ADHD)?
Yes. Living with a hyperactive, dyslexic child can be a particular nightmare.

Such a child must have medication and specialist support if the parents can ever cope with the experience. Hyperactivity makes the parental reaction to straightforward dyslexia much more aggressive. Woodward et al. (1998) describe, in the cool tones of the academic, what it can be like to live with an ADHD child. Such children are less compliant, more off-task, more negative, more attention-seeking, more talkative and more demanding of their parents.

From what parents tell me, a nearer description might be 'living hell', both for the parents and siblings who have to endure the torment of the hyperactive behaviour and for the child who has to live with his own uncontrollable impulsiveness, manic energy and the awful reactions it produces in those around him.

It is perhaps not surprising that, in response, mothers of boys with hyperactivity 'tend to be more commanding and negative, and provide their children with greater structure and supervision than do mothers of control boys. They are also less responsive to positive or neutral child communications, and more frequently reprimand and punish their sons compared to mothers of control boys' (op. cit., p. 161).

This research study also found that parents of ADHD children did not cope at all well, and they obtained little satisfaction from the parenting role. They also felt considerable hostility and anger towards their children and were more depressed, anxious and socially disordered than controls. These reactions, unfortunately, also exacerbated their child's hyperactivity. In addition, parents of an ADHD child are conspicuously unsupported. They are socially isolated because no one wanted a hyperactive child in their home and, since their family are none too pleased with the idea either, they have little contact with extended family.

Such parents also feel out of control. This may be a transferential response to similar feelings in their child but, in reality, the parents are not in control of their children, just as their child is not in control of himself.

There is some evidence that parent training can improve child behaviour and, thus, parental response to the child. Such training encourages more proactive and authoritative child-management techniques to replace the use of raw power.

Most of all, what such parents need is empathic counselling that includes not only respect for their love and loyalty but also acceptance of the fact that they can also hate their child and sometimes wish that he had never been born. When all these mixed feelings are expressed and integrated, the parent's tension, which arose partially because of these unexpressed incongruent feelings, can reduce significantly, to their benefit and to that of their bewildered, beleaguered child.

Siblings

How are siblings important in understanding a dyslexic child?
Siblings are important in all child development and in the development of subsequent behaviours – some pathological.

Siblings are important because most children grow up with siblings (80% in USA and UK) and, in their early years, spend more time interacting with each other than they do with their parents. In many cultures, children are raised by their siblings. Most psychologists argue that what siblings learn from each other can affect child development in unique and dramatic ways (Piaget 1932). Siblings also share more reciprocal and symmetrical relationships and, therefore, have the ability to understand and support each other better.

Siblings are also particularly expert at tormenting each other, and they are responsible for a great deal of the bullying of dyslexic children. Siblings can also collude with the parents in whatever dynamic the family builds around a dyslexic child.

The most challenging relationships are between dyslexic and non-dyslexic siblings. Where both siblings are dyslexic – and because of the genetic component this is quite common – the siblings' dyslexia seems to neutralize the effect, and they operate pretty-much like any normal siblings would. It is the mismatched dyslexic and non-dyslexic sibling dyads that create most problems.

Overall, the effect of siblings on a dyslexic client is enormous. When counselling families of dyslexic children, the sibling dynamic cannot be ignored.

How do siblings cope with the dyslexic child's disability?

They cope with reluctance and with great ambivalence – something that the dyslexic child has no trouble in picking up.

There have been many studies to investigate how a disabled sibling affects family life (Tunali and Power 1993, Coleby 1995, Newman et al. 1997). Such studies have shown that the siblings of a disabled child have more emotional and behavioural problems than children with non-disabled siblings (Newman et al. 1997).

Important points in this research are:

Information

Siblings know little about the condition that disables their brother or sister and are keen to receive information. Their communication needs are substantial, but they often feel unable to discuss things with their parents, who tend to talk to each other rather than to their children. Various studies put at up to 48% the number of siblings who talk to no one. This lack of information allows them to project all types of fantasy onto the disabled child.

Communication

Parents repeatedly overestimate the coping abilities of siblings. This is often because they are preoccupied with the problems of the disabled child. They also consistently miss the needs of siblings to be reassured, or miss that they feel concerned or worried. Boys are particularly vulnerable. Substantially more boy siblings than girls screen positive for psychological disturbance in the families of a disabled child. Counsellors might find it helpful to encourage parents to communicate honestly with all their siblings, since studies show that siblings want their parents to be the source of all information.

Phases of family adjustment

Using the model of family adjustment to chronic disorder proposed by Rolland (1987), a 'crisis' phase occurs when the parents and siblings of a dyslexic child realise that he has walked back into the home with a new identity. Whether the family then treats him as if he were carrying dyslexic fleas or dyslexic flowers is obviously going to determine the nature of this 'crisis'.

After a while, however, the disruption diminishes – this is the 'adjust-ment' phase – and the child is transformed into a 'dyslexic person'. The family then moves into the 'chronic' phase. It is this family phase that, in my experience, introduces the time of greatest revenge attempts by non-dyslexic siblings. This is when the non-dyslexic child feels most ignored, and the needs of siblings within the family most overlooked.

It is no fun competing with a dyslexic sibling

Rivalry between siblings becomes distorted when one child is disabled in any way. Competing with a disabled sibling is deeply unsatisfying. While every child wants to be the cleverest, strongest and most attractive in their parents' eyes, 'children want to win in a fair race' (Sinason 1993, p. 40). It is mistakenly assumed that children with a problematic sibling would feel successful by comparison. This is not the case. When your sibling has prob-lems, it means that competitive ideas and wishes are very difficult to acknowledge openly, and success has no real value at all.

The pressure to be 'normal' is tough

The non-dyslexic siblings can feel some pressure 'not to be dyslexic' and 'not fail at school' and 'not be a pain to my parents'. Such children can become as emotionally disturbed and needy as their disabled siblings.

Non-disabled siblings can also be overwhelmed by the pressure to be 'good' and 'successful' to make up for parental disappointment. They may present as extra mature, sensible and adjusted for their age but, under-neath, they desperately want to be cared for themselves (Carpenter 2000).

Such non-disabled siblings can act out their projected need for care by joining the caring professions.

What is the normal reaction of siblings to each other?

Violence is normal.

The sibling relationship is always ambivalent, and it is usual and healthy for it to involve conflict. In some studies, siblings and their mothers spent around a quarter of their time together in conflict (Stallard et al. 1999). It is also important to remember that siblings are fighting on one of human-ity's oldest battlegrounds. It is a no-holds-barred relationship that can be both vicious and merciless.

A recent study on sibling violence in a varied group of 11- to 19-year-olds found that four-fifths of children physically attack their brothers and sis-ters: 'sibling rivalry has turned to violence in many more families than previously thought' (Keane 2002, p. 11). More than half the children inter-viewed said that they had punched, or tried to strangle, their siblings in the

previous year, with girls behaving as badly as boys. Most minor forms of violence, such as slapping and shoving, had been used by 80% of the sample.
Just over a fifth said that they had hit siblings with heavy objects, and guns,
knives, burning and hanging had been attempted by one sibling on another. A sixth said they had seriously beaten up a brother or sister. The study's
originator said: 'We had no idea the levels of sibling violence would be so
high' (Keane 2002).

Do dyslexic children attract violent and aggressive sibling behaviour?
Yes. Violence between siblings may be normal, but what is not normal is
the degree to which a dyslexic sibling will be on the receiving end of it.

Sometimes, a dyslexic child is being bullied as much at home by siblings as at school by peers. I have no doubt that this is because the
dyslexic child takes up far more parental attention than what the non-
dyslexic sibling deems to be fair. Where siblings pick up parental
ambivalence towards the dyslexic child, this makes matters worse because
the siblings read this as implicit parental approval for the torment of
their dyslexic brother or sister.

The most severe sibling violence occurs when the dyslexic is the younger
one, and the older sibling feels an even more intense variety of the jealousy
that he has probably felt since this child was born. There are other more specific reasons for the dyslexic child's disliked status among brothers and sisters:

Non-disabled sibling neglect

Mothers, particularly, can ignore non-dyslexic siblings to a greater or lesser
degree. The needs of these others then tend to be unexpressed and sublimat-
ed. This parental reaction 'may be helpful, or may distort family functioning,
arousing jealousy in their siblings, and there may be frank parental neglect
of the non-traumatised siblings' (Newman et al. 1997, p. 141).

Triadic relationships

Sibling conflict varies in the context of particular relationships. For a while,
a dyslexic child can form a triadic relationship with a parent – usually the
mother – against the other parent or the other siblings. I shall refer later to
the effect this can have on the father, but, for other siblings, this can be a
nightmare of favouritism and abandonment.

In this situation, Engfer (1988) suggests that there might be compensatory influences between two relationships. A positive relationship with her
child may compensate a mother for a troubled marriage. This, then,
becomes a cause for increased conflict between the enmeshed, dyslexic
child and his siblings.

There is also evidence that mothers are more likely to take the side of the victim in sibling relationships (Hay et al. 1998). In this case, the more the other siblings attack the enmeshed, favoured dyslexic child, the more the mother will also defend him and take his side in any conflict. It is not hard to see why the victim relationship in dyslexic children both starts and is maintained. In family-relationship terms, it is highly profitable and can be very powerful.

Unhappy mothers favour dyslexic and disabled sons

Favouritism towards a dyslexic child can also be heightened in the context of maternal illness. When women are depressed, the evidence is that they favour, and are most likely to protect, their sons (Hay et al. 1998). This is another reason why unhappily married women with dyslexic sons tend to become enmeshed with them.

An astute additional explanation of this feature of dyslexia is offered by Abramson et al. (1978). They point out that depression is sometimes accompanied by an acute awareness of an unjust world, and perhaps a depressed person identifies with the targets of others' criticism. Hay et al. (1998) also observed this phenomenon: 'it is perhaps not surprising that the depressed mothers were likely to adhere to a principle of alliance that supported the rights of protesters, rather than provokers, of a dispute' (p. 536).

Is there a pattern to sibling conflicts with dyslexic children?
Sibling conflicts are usually asymmetric, with older individuals objecting to younger ones rather than the other way around, particularly when children are left to their own devices (Hay et al. 1998).

It is normal for first-born siblings to feel some hostility and ambivalence towards their younger siblings. When, however, the younger sibling is also more successful, reads better, has a lovely smooth interplay of basic literacy skills and – worst of all – gets more parental praise, the jealousy of the older dyslexic child can be incandescent, and the humiliation of performing worse than a younger sibling, crippling.

The reverse – the favouring of the older child – usually happens when the mother feels that the older dyslexic child has greater specific needs of survival in the education system than a younger child. Somehow, this does not produce the same violent sibling reaction – perhaps because it taps into the 'natural justice' of family life where younger children normally defer to older ones.

Do the effects of sibling relationships outlive childhood?
Yes. Sibling relationships last a lifetime.

It is a longer relationship than between husband and wife, and parent and child. Sibling relationships show continuity over time and can be fraught with conflict throughout life. Anna Freud (1981) believed that the birth of a sibling can become the turning point of development to which all later pathology can be connected. For this reason, it is important that counsellors examine sibling relationships not just with children but also with dyslexic adults of all ages.

Vanzetti and Duck (1996), in their review of research on sibling relationships, show that those children with poor sibling relationships in early childhood are particularly likely to be disturbed later on. Also, children's self-esteem in middle childhood and early adolescence is related to how friendly or hostile their siblings had been some years before.

Furthermore, unfriendly behaviour from a sibling in the early years is linked to internalizing behaviour (worry, anxiety, depression) several years later, especially for second-born children whose older siblings were distant or unfriendly when they were pre-schoolers. Sibling aggression also fosters other aggression.

What happens if a dyslexic child is not favoured over siblings?
When parents do not show favouritism to a dyslexic child, he has a much better chance of favourable relationships with other siblings and some worthwhile lifetime support from them.

This sibling support to dyslexics can include reassurance over problems at school, refuge during parental conflict and kindness over general worries. Interestingly, there is also some evidence that it is the overprotective, enmeshed favouritism of the mother that contributes – in itself and through damaged sibling relationships – to the poor social cognition of dyslexic children and, thence, their bullying from peers (Foote and Holmes-Lonergan 2003). Fairer mothers, by contrast, did not have this effect.

Dunn et al. (1991) also showed that a child who had a more friendly, responsive relationship with his siblings performed better in tests of understanding other minds – social cognition – and of understanding emotion. This, in turn, enabled him to *improve* his social cognition and *reduce* his chance of being bullied.

An overprotective mother causes far more direct and indirect damage to her dyslexic child than she could possibly imagine.

Disability

How do parents react when they realize that dyslexia is a disability?
Many parents of dyslexic children are greatly relieved when their child is

diagnosed, and they don't care whether it is a disability or not. They are just pleased to know. For others, this semantic grenade, this totally unexpected slant on the problem, is a profound shock.

This usually occurs when parents – often with no dyslexia in the family – have had no reason to think that there is anything amiss with their child at all. Discovering that he is having difficulties because of a physical problem, a disability that can actually be categorized – not just 'laziness' or 'bad teaching' – hits them hard. Then, close on the heels of this information, comes the realization that they have lost the normal child they thought they had. Still reeling from shock, they are faced with the wrench of bereavement. At this point, these parents need as much help as their dyslexic child.

In some ways, it is worse for parents of dyslexic children to come to terms with the notion of 'disability'. They have had seven or eight years of 'normality', whereas parents of children with other disabilities have often been forced to come to terms with their child's limitations since birth.

This is not a particularly original observation in the literature on disability, but it is a point often overlooked in the literature on dyslexia.

For a while, all that these parents can think of is 'disability'. This concept is like a stop sign suddenly erected in front of both them and their child. Their lives come to a halt until they can get some traction on what it really means to be dyslexic.

For this reason, I think it is useful to look at what is helpful for those parents who must suddenly see their 'normal child with a few problems at school' transform into a child – not just with dyslexia – but with the *disability* of dyslexia.

Does parental reaction determine how a dyslexic child copes with their disability?
Yes – and I would estimate that it the most important factor of all.

Obviously reactions do vary. 'Some children with disabilities will bring pleasure and inspiration to their parents. Others will bring burdens. Most, like ordinary children, will bring a mixture of both' (Sinason 1993, p. 74).

Unquestionably, the most useful reactions by the parents are a sense of control – a belief in their own problem-solving ability – and optimism. Positive emotions predict favourable outcomes

Outside support – practical and loving – is also important, but, as Wallander and Varni (1998) note, this is most beneficial when it gives the parents the feeling that they can pick themselves up and access some adaptive, coping strategies in and for themselves. When parents simply believed that they could cope, and knew that others believed that they could cope, this 'was associated with better adjustment' (op. cit., p. 40).

Wallander and Varni also found that parental 'adaptive solution focused' methods ('Who do I know who has a dyslexic child?') were more successful than 'palliative-emotion-focused' methods (booze, chocolate and 'poor me') that were more likely to lead to maladjustment in the disabled child.

Putting it another way, a positive, optimistic parental attitude will determine whether the dyslexic child sees himself as a 'disabled person' or as someone who just 'has a disability'.

Do parents determine a dyslexic's self-image?

Not entirely.

School plays a significant, and often unhelpful, role in how a dyslexic child reacts to his disability. The child's personality also has to play a part.

Where parents can help is by being aware of the mirror that they hold up to their child. If the mirror reflects a proud and positive image, this can, at the very least, act as a counterbalance to all the other tarnished images that the child is forced to face at school. In particular, a child gets a very strong sense of self through the mirror of his mother's eyes, her facial expression and manner towards him.

What is so hard for dyslexic children is that their new mirror image – their change to the status of 'disabled' – happens suddenly. It is a shock. In addition, they not only have to deal with their own shock at this new image but also its catastrophic effect on their parents. This can be far harder.

As Sinason (1993) points out, we all need that parental mirror to say that we are the fairest of them all but, where parents are depressed or feel guilty, then the child can look into depressed eyes 'and take in an image of himself as someone depressing. Where the parent takes a long time to recover, [the child] takes a long time to trust there could be anything worthwhile in them' (p. 28).

To a child, his parents' mirror can also, of course, reflect the fact that his parents no longer really want him or particularly like the child they now find they have. I wish I could say that this is a false belief – a faulty perception by an anxious child. Unfortunately, it is often an accurate belief and an accurate perception. The child may not have got it wrong at all.

Can helping the mother to cope help the dyslexic child to cope?

Yes – very much so.

As I shall note in more detail in the next chapter, it is the mother who matters most. She is critical. If she is coping, then everyone else does. What helps the mother are a good marriage, social support and practical resources, such as dyslexia support groups. For this reason, I often recommend to mothers of dyslexic children that they might like to have counselling themselves. Like the last domino in the row, she has to be backed up to a brick wall to stop everyone else from falling, and counsellors can make a good brick wall.

Where there is a strong, resilient, humorous, well-adjusted mother, the dyslexic child has the best possible chance of dealing with whatever his disability brings to him. The difference between maternal support and maternal overprotection is, however, crucial – as will be discussed in the next chapter.

Does it help if parents are informed?

Yes. Precise understanding of the nature of dyslexia as a disability is important.

Reading about what is normal behaviour for a dyslexic child prevents angry misattribution of the child as being 'difficult'.

Chavira et al. (2000) showed, furthermore, that this is a particular problem for parents of children with developmental disabilities. Working out whether their child's behavioural problems were directly linked to the disability or to the child's deliberate wilfulness, was crucial, and 'played a significant role in determining family members' emotional reaction' to the child (p. 246).

Those parents who believed their child to be 'doing this deliberately to be difficult' were more likely to report feeling angry, and interacted negatively with their child. Correctly attributing the behaviour to the disability, rather than seeing it as an act of deliberate naughtiness, led to a more measured parental response.

When a parent understands about their dyslexic child, they no longer attribute every problem to the child's conscious will. If, for example, they know about a dyslexic's short-term memory problems, they can change their attitude to their child's constant losing of things as something relatively out of his control. They no longer see it as their child being deliberately vexatious or 'lazy'.

Are disability feelings transferred from the child to the parent?

Often, yes. This is usually where the parents find it hard to acknowledge their child's disability; for example, if they feel ashamed.

This disabled transference can make parents feel helpless and useless. They rarely see that these feelings might be coming from their child – that they have picked up the disability message themselves: 'parents' lack of confidence in their child may have been related to the child's own lack of confidence' (Barrett et al. 2002, p. 605).

Parents also need to recognize that they can feel disabled in the literal sense of being unable to function properly.

Coping with a difficult child is not easy, and a child's disability can cause parental distress, including increased depression and anxiety (Barrett et al. 2002). In their extensive review of research on chronic paediatric disorder, Wallander and Varni (1998) concluded that mothers of children with chronic disorder report more negative symptoms than mothers with well children, and mental-health treatment was two to three times more common. Mothers were more likely to have depressive and internalizing/ affective disorders.

Do parents give up play?

Yes. Having a disabled child usually means that parents have to give up that anticipated pleasure of children – playing with them.

Many parents have a secret desire to live through their own children by doing things they enjoyed as children. This is far less of a problem for parents of dyslexic children than, say, parents of an autistic child, but it does exist.

For example, dyspraxic dyslexics who have profound coordination problems will find some childhood toys impossible to use. Sporty parents of dyspraxic children can find sports departments particularly painful. Sinason (1993) quotes a father who explained how he could not bear to go past shops selling children's football boots and tennis rackets. Sports were his life, and it hurt every time he saw the sporting gear that his son could never make use of.

Similarly, buying books for a dyslexic 12-year-old with a reading age of seven can be a difficult, if not humiliating, experience for both parent and child. These problems can go on for years, and each has attached to it a little pocket of hurt. 'These experiences can highlight again the initial feeling of shame and failure. They remind the parent again of the difference between normal development and ... handicap' (Sinason 1993, p. 43).

Do dyslexic children cause problems in public?

Not often, but strange mannerisms and clumsiness can make it difficult to feel at ease in public with a dyslexic/dyspraxic child.

Dyspraxic dyslexics can, for example, have dramatically messy mealtimes, and many dyslexic children are clumsy, look sartorially odd and have problems in language and speech development. Dyslexic social skills can be abnormal, while some dyslexics can also have quite fixed facial expressions and body postures, along with some strange compensatory behaviours. Some dyslexic children, when confused or embarrassed, can regress to childish mannerisms, including repetitive, squeaky sounds and excessive fiddling. Where ADHD is involved, parents often have to scoop their child from various fixtures and fittings, bring them down from climbable objects or simply distract them long enough to eat a meal. It is not really surprising that parents of some dyslexic children find it easier to give up social activities completely. Even as adults, a dyslexic's public behaviour can present as eccentric.

Are parents of dyslexic children isolated?

Yes. Sometimes, disability can lead to isolation.

I have observed how this is the case for dyslexic children in school, and it can also be the case for their parents. It is not so much a case of being the tall poppy, as being the short one. There is in many people a need to be average, to be invisible, to be the same as everyone else. Disability in your child changes all this, and, for every parent who becomes defiant and empowered by this, there are other parents who resent the loss of privacy and predictability of their former lives.

Disability has the unusual effect of being both common and isolating. Sinason (1993), for example, points out that, within the United Kingdom alone, nearly six and a half million children and adults have some kind of disability. Wallander and Varni (1998) quote epidemiological surveys that show that 10%-20% of children in the West have a chronic disorder. In the world, over 1% of all new babies born will be disabled. When we add to that figure the families and friends involved in the lives of disabled people, a large, if powerless, group emerges.

These figures notwithstanding, the parents of a newly diagnosed disabled child can feel as alone as if they were the last people on the planet.

The shock of this solitude – this abandonment by normality – approaches the existential isolation known well to therapists but rarely discussed by anyone else. Sinason (1993) frequently acknowledges the isolation of disability, and the importance of human support: 'Most parents manage to weather the storms of bringing up a human being without being too ground down. Where the compass isn't clear or the bad weather continues too long, parents should recognize that help is needed. It may not provide dry land but it will provide support for the journey' (p. 74).

Does the disability of dyslexia harm the home?

Disability can break a marriage.

This can happen because of the economic pressure of caring for, and educating, a disabled child. It can also happen when fathers – many of whom care loyally for their family and disabled child – leave because they find the situation unbearable. This may be because their wife is now totally involved in caring for their child – this is not at all uncommon in the families of dyslexic children – or if he is 'unable to bear the signs of what his potency has created' (Sinason 1993, p. 30). Additionally, the father can just retreat psychologically, burying himself in his work or hobbies and leaving his wife to deal with the day-to-day management of their child.

Does the dyslexic child's disability affect the sex life of his parents?
Yes – far too often. This also, of course, introduces another loss and another potential source of resentment.

Sexual problems in the dyslexic child's parents arise not simply because of the pressure of the child's disability but also because of unexpressed anger and resentment between the partners, particularly when any unacknowledged blame is floating around (see Chapter 6). Sinason (1993) believes that it can go even deeper than this. Since it was 'an act of lovemaking that created the baby, there can be a primitive fear that lovemaking is in itself damaging' (p. 31).

Also, when a woman is pregnant, she can have many fears and negative ideas that she never shares with anyone. According to Sinason (1993), these kinds of thoughts are all forgotten in the presence of normality but, in the presence of disability, come back with a vengeance for both the mother and the father.

Does family life ever return to normal?
When the disability is just dyslexia, it does.

When hyperactivity or dyspraxia complicate a child's dyslexia, life in the long term is more problematic. Being a parent is normally regarded as a time-limited activity. Whether this is viewed with relief or sadness depends on one's disposition to parenting. It can, however, be easy for parents of a disabled child to feel that being a parent will never end. If this is so, they must also give up any idea of being parented by their children in old age.

Parents of dyslexic children sometimes appreciate being reminded that they can give up parenting in a way that parents of other disabled children perhaps cannot. The fact that some parents of dyslexic children can, but choose not to, give up their caretaking role for their children is something that features quite regularly when counselling dyslexic clients. In fact, some of these dyslexic clients – particularly those in their late twenties – can be driven to distraction by protective behaviour from parents who believe that they must remain on duty as an active parent for longer than most.

Do parents of a dyslexic child rediscover normality?
Yes – but blinded by the child's disability, parents temporarily forget their child's normality. They will later come to see, for example, that their child is *only* dyslexic but, initially, every action, every cell, every last gene, bacterium and microbe in their child is dyslexic, as if he were entirely contaminated by this disability. Later on, they will notice that their child's capacity for emotional intelligence and wonderful, lively individuality is still there, and always has been. As Sinason (1993) observes, no matter what the nature of a child's disability, the parents cannot forget a child's natural

ability to 'make sense of the environment and develop a capacity for love, hope and emotional development' (p. 11).

Do family members want to make the dyslexic child 'better'?
At first they do – but this can fade.

At the beginning, when the disability is new, it is natural to wish to make the dyslexic child 'better'. It takes time to remember that dyslexia is not an illness, and they can accept their dyslexic child just as he is. During this early time, it is common to try to take control of the condition by controlling the dyslexia. If this continues for too long, however, it can introduce a large disability where there was only a small one originally.

What also needs to be emphasized is that the dyslexic child, too, can have a strong wish to his make parents better, to make them more happy and less sad. He may cover up his own distress to make his parents happy.

What are the parents' most difficult feelings about dyslexia as a disability?
Shame and embarrassment – although there may be a number of other unspoken and unacknowledged feelings about a dyslexic child, including anger, hatred and resentment.

Family shame about disability is common in certain cultures, but shame can also be a strong factor in academically successful homes. There may also be difficult feelings of shame in one parent if they think that they carried the 'bad gene' – and this is not more so than with dyslexia. 'A baby is a joint product and each partner hopes that the best of them will go into the recipe' (Sinason 1993, p. 28). When one partner introduces a bad ingredient and spoils the whole dish, it is easy for both partners to collude in the 'bad' partner's deserved shame; that he or she is totally responsible for the 'problem'.

Needless to say, dyslexic children are quite capable of picking up this underlying message about shame and contamination. Sinason quotes Professor Sheila Hollis of St George's Hospital in London, who suggests: 'The key issue is to know your child for who he really is, not as who you would have liked him to be' (op. cit., p. 44).

This, however, is not as easy as it sounds, and an awful lot of unspoken negative feelings have to be waded through and discarded – with an honest and accepting listener – first.

Are there feelings that a counsellor might find hard to acknowledge?
Yes – and, as always, these are the most unacceptable feelings of all: the wish that the child were dead and the full extent of the parents' distress at their child's disability.

Disability and the death wish

Disability has always got a death wish attached. Mannoni (1973) argues that any disability will always have an aftertaste of death about it, of death denied, of death disguised. He argues that 'the idea of murder is there even if the mother is not always conscious of it' (p. 4).

The unconscious, parental wish that the disabled child had never existed can leave the disabled person with a very strong sense of being an outsider, of not belonging – something which is remarked upon in many different contexts of dyslexia, including their tendency to be isolates (see Chapter 11). At worst, a disabled person might feel that they *should* not exist, and act on it.

Disability is distressing

This seems to be an obvious point, but the counsellor, in rushing to make things better, and to look at all those complicated issues of ambivalence and guilt, may forget to acknowledge that dyslexia as a disability can seem unbearably sad for both parent and child. They will not always feel like this, but, while it is there, that feeling needs to be heard and understood.

Parental distress is not proportional to the extent of the disability. It is the perception that is important. For example, it is the high-flying, sporty father who can be devastated by a case of quite mild dyslexia, and another father, perhaps dyslexic himself, who takes it all in his stride.

Does counselling help with the notion of disability?

The evidence is that it does (see Chapter 12).

Parents of a child with dyslexia will cope far better if they are allowed the necessary emotional space to understand the impact of their child's disability on themselves. I have often noticed that one immediate effect of counselling the parents of dyslexic children is that the children themselves start to relax.

In fact, I would suggest that counselling the parents is one of the most efficient routes to helping the dyslexic child. Many of his problems are due to the mixed messages he receives at home so, when these bewildering parental transmissions disappear, he is much more able to cope.

I am reminded of a research study during the last war, where children felt far safer during an air raid in the arms of a parent in the open air, than alone in an air-raid shelter. When the parents are strong and safe, so can the child cope better. When the parents stop acting out their own problems, they have space for those of their child. Where counselling helps in particular is in normalizing and accepting the dyslexic disability, which helps the parents to accept it.

In fact, Segal (1996) believes that the way forward for parents of any disabled child lies in accepting the disability. This is crucial, and bound up with recognizing the new reality and grieving for what has been given up. It takes about two years to accept these changes.

For this reason, the notion of disability is always associated with that of bereavement.

Bereavement

What is lost when one gains a dyslexic child?
A number of things – some tangible, some abstract.

Most of all, the advent of dyslexia is seen as the loss of a possibility, the loss of the ideal of fitness and normality: 'not many parents lie awake hoping their child will be born with a disability. However loving, inspiring or gifted the child turns out to be, and however strong the bonding and the pleasure, it needs to be acknowledged that very few parents anticipate the possibility with pleasure' (Sinason 1993, p. 15).

This bereavement is what dyslexic children also pick up: the accurate suspicion that Mum and Dad have lost the perfect, successful and untroubled child that they thought they had – at least until that perfect child went to school. Normality, dreams, choice and a sense of control are also lost for both parent and child. Staudacher (1987) saw this as the loss of 'your own connection to the future [and] some of your own treasured qualities and talents' (p. 101). It is the loss of your own power. It can also mean the end of parental independence – and not everyone likes the idea of bringing up children for the whole of their life.

The dyslexic child is also bereaved. The parents may have lost their fantasy of a perfect child, but the child loses, sometimes permanently, the normality of his parents and the family life he had before his diagnosis. In effect, parents and child lose each other and the relationship they once knew.

Some of this may eventually be seen by the parents of a newly diagnosed dyslexic child as an overreaction. After all, unlike other disabled children, the dyslexic child will eventually be quite capable of living his own life. At first, however, these worries are real for his parents, and need to be acknowledged before any attempt to challenge or change them.

Does the grief for a 'normal' child ever end?
No. The grief at loss of a normal child is unending; it is a grief without closure.

As Carpenter (2000) observes, 'although many of the similarities between grief and parenting a child with disabilities may be endorsed, the reality at the sadness of having a child with disabilities is constantly renewed regardless of the pleasures gained' (p. 138). For this reason, the bereavement associated with disability can be termed 'non-finite loss'.

Bruce and Schultz (2002) specifically equate non-finite loss with intellectual or developmental disabilities, such as dyslexia. This is the life-span grief. It is a loss that retains a physical and psychological presence. It also includes a crisis of self-identity: 'Ultimately these experiences of non-finite loss generate a sense of disconnection from the mainstream ... [It is a] unique form of grieving' (op. cit., p. 9).

The grieving is ongoing, and there are incessant triggers that activate it. It can also separate parents, with the mother becoming isolated and the father withdrawn. The mother can be overdosed on loss and the father can be underdosed, experiencing, instead, delayed or sporadic grief. The father can sometimes become desensitized, while one-fifth of mothers can experience PTSD.

Following the shock surrounding normal finite loss, there are normally periods of yearning and searching for what has been lost. In non-finite loss, however, yearning and searching cannot be extinguished. Parents instinctively continue to seek what is lost. In mourning a loss through death, searching behaviour that continued for some years would be considered pathological. In non-finite loss, this would be considered as normal and cannot be 'simplistically labelled as denial' (Bruce and Shultz 2002, p. 10).

This yearning continues partly because there is no ritual for non-finite loss. There is no physical death to mourn and 'the grief is disenfranchised' (op cit., p. 12).

After diagnosis, some parents cope by relying on avoidance. Others are overwhelmed. This is why assessment of dyslexia needs follow-up counselling. A diagnosis introduces its own type of shock, and professionals can 'underestimate the emotional impact of the information that they deliver to parents' (op. cit., p. 11). The professional's compassion or indifference can even be retained as a life-long memory for the parents of any disabled child.

Which family member needs bereavement counselling?

The family member who will most need bereavement counselling is the one who has taken on the coping role, relieving others of responsibility. This may be a parent, but it may also be the dyslexic child himself. He will grieve, too, for old fantasies and an old future lost for ever. He will also have lost the security of the notion that life is predictable, and his belief in certainty will be shattered. Many such children can become anxious, vigilant, clingy and angry.

What are the signs and stages of bereavement?
The classic signs of normal bereavement may be present in different family members.

For example, there is the denial of loss and the reluctance to accept the reality of the loss (the father who won't accept diagnosis), and there may also be the normal reactions of shock, numbness, yearning, searching, anxiety, anger and guilt (the overprotective, or 'tiger', mother) for some months after diagnosis. There may be, in later stages, apathy and loss of identity for both parents and child.

Healing and full acceptance can take up to two years. Then, the dyslexia of the child will be integrated into the family. It is usually at this stage, however, that a second child's dyslexia is becoming apparent but, this time, everything goes much more smoothly, and all the stages of action are taken at the run. At this point, the loss no longer feels like an appalling tragedy. The family can settle into new circumstances and regain interest in things other than dyslexia.

Does pathological mourning occur?
Yes – and, sometimes, the grief can move into more serious forms.

These can include a persistent and unconscious yearning to recover the lost child, and intense, persistent anger or reproach towards various people (a partner, the school or a 'contaminating' dyslexic relative).

This loss of the 'normal' child of their own can also reawaken in a dyslexic parent the loss of their own normality in their own parent's eyes, and bring many old memories to light.

Pathological mourning can also express itself in obsessive care of the dyslexic child, or care of vicarious figures. There can even be complete denial of the dyslexia followed by serious defensive processes. For example, the parent can undertake continual reassessments of the dyslexic child, investigating allergies, brain damage and dietary factors. Some parents buy endless vitamins, herbal and homeopathic remedies, and obsess over 'alternative' therapies, and can be prey to all sorts of quack solutions.

When a parent is narcissistic, the loss of the 'normal' child to dyslexia can even be seen as loss of an extension of the self. To admit the loss would then necessitate confronting a loss of part of oneself, so the loss is denied.

The symptoms of abnormal grief in the parent of a dyslexic child can be an enduring preoccupation including crying a lot, not crying at all, disassociation and depression. There may be phobic symptoms, persistent and intense guilt and hypochondriacal conditions, including symptoms similar to those of the 'lost' person; that is a parent starts to 'discover' that they are dyslexic too.

Needless to say, a counsellor will consider what else the diagnosis of their child's dyslexia must mean to such parents.

CHAPTER 6

The parents of dyslexic children

Summary

Fawcett (1995), writing on stress and dyslexia, reviews the problems of school then comments darkly, 'This brings us to the second potential source of stress – the parents' (p. 14).

I know exactly what she means. My experience with dyslexics – adults and children – is that their parents can be unhelpful in a variety of imaginatively awful ways.

There is some complaint in the literature on dyslexia that there is a tendency to pathologize the parents and families of dyslexic children. As a counsellor, I would say that that tendency is entirely justified.

I see many dyslexic children whose problems have come principally from their parents. School and peers may exacerbate these problems, but it is the dyslexic child's parents who often start, maintain and stoke them. By contrast, when dyslexic children are blessed with good parenting and supportive families, they do not need counselling. Such dyslexic children can cope very well indeed.

What I give here, therefore, is a review of the common types of familial behaviour that cause problems to dyslexic clients, and examples of some of the ways in which a child's dyslexia can get mixed up in the parental relationship to negative effect on both sides.

In truth, this whole area is such a tangle that it is hard for a counsellor to tease out neat threads, and the problems outlined below will not be mutually exclusive. What is certain is that some of these problems will be present in the family of an unhappy dyslexic client some of the time. For the most ill-starred and damaged clients they will have experienced most of the problems, most of the time.

Parental reaction to their child's diagnosis of dyslexia

Do parents feel guilty?
Yes – and dyslexic and non-dyslexic parents feel guilty for different reasons.

Dyslexic parents feel guilt in two ways: first, that they have passed their difficulties onto their child and, second, that they might not have the necessary literary skills to help him. When non-dyslexic parents discover their child is dyslexic, their guilt comes out of the horrified realization of how unfair they have often been to their hapless child.

Before their child's diagnosis, many parents, dyslexic and non-dyslexic, may have been abusive and exasperated by what they interpreted as the laziness or unwillingness of their child to apply himself to schoolwork. The later guilt after diagnosis is also made worse when the parents have colluded with the negative views of others. One mother was devastated after her son's diagnosis because she had 'accepted the view of his teachers that he was lazy, in spite of the fact that she knew he struggled for two hours in his room to produce one page of writing and then crumpled the paper up because it was not good enough' (op. cit., p. 93).

Over the years, I have heard many parents express mortification and guilt about their earlier, uninformed reaction to their dyslexic children, and how they would have responded differently to their child had they been more knowledgeable about dyslexia. I really feel for them and, as a counsellor, am happy to reassure them that it is never too late to help.

What is the main response of dyslexic parents?
'Never again.' Then these parents go into battle. The warrior reactions of dyslexic parents are extremely formidable, but their motives are complex.

Watching their own children deal with dyslexia can help dyslexic parents make sense of their own earlier experiences, especially when they did not have the benefit of a diagnostic label. This is a poignant experience for such parents who recognize their own lost opportunities and can feel sad to see their own problems coming around again.

Most counsellors can work out for themselves that such parents might well feel guilt.

What is not always appreciated is how their child's diagnosis can also hand these dyslexic parents the means to expiate their guilt through the cathartic pleasures of revenge. Action diverted from decades of pain and loss can be very focused indeed, and dyslexic parents can be formidable warriors as they settle virulent old scores under the guise of defending their children.

These parents seem to siphon anger out of their memories, then spray it over those who would seek to harm their own children in the way that they were harmed themselves. It can be impressive and alarming: 'Parents who are themselves dyslexic often become powerful advocates for their children because they are determined that the education of their dyslexic children does not mirror their own negative school experiences. Acting as a role model and fighting for their children's rights to have their difficulties identified and addressed affords such parents the opportunity to redress the balance of their own unhappy past' (Morgan and Klein 2000, p. 88–89).

What has happened? The bewildered response of non-dyslexic parents

Non-dyslexic parents of dyslexic children have a particular challenge, in that they are forced to find out exactly what the problem is. They must not only grasp the psychological and scientific aspects of dyslexia but also understand their child's struggles in order to get hold of the most effective help for him. They must also send a benign virus back through their memories of their child's behaviour and reformulate those thousands of times when they might not have responded with kindness and understanding.

Do dyslexic parents have to 'come out' about their dyslexia?

'Have to' are the operative words. This is a phrase that can cause problems in its own right.

Dyslexia runs in families, but I have often encountered the situation where a dyslexic father or mother has been too ashamed to reveal their own problem. They little understand how helpful it would be for their child to know that they are dyslexic too. What is also a problem is that some people do not tell their partners that they are dyslexic, and when a dyslexic child appears, it not only stirs mud for the dyslexic partner but also introduces an element into the marriage that was not there before. It is like a forced coming-out.

Any negative effects on the partnership can also be transferred unconsciously onto the unwitting dyslexic child whose arrival opens up a vein of problems. If the dyslexic child is troublesome, and the non-dyslexic partner's life is badly affected by this, then he or she may also project their resentment back onto the dyslexic partner who so 'deceived' them. Eventually, both partners can see the child as the source of all their problems.

It must be appreciated that dyslexic people may not always reveal their disability. When they do, however, Morgan and Klein (2000) warn that: 'When an adult has been successful in hiding his or her problems, the partner's response when weaknesses are revealed can be a major test of love and loyalty' (p. 77).

Parenthood can also lead to a crisis of 'coming out' or of being 'found out'.

This often constellates around the literacy demands of a new child: 'parenthood frequently becomes a catalyst for unveiling difficulties, when the embarrassment of not being able to respond to children, either through reading aloud to them, or helping them with school work forces the adult to acknowledge his or her own problems' (op. cit., p. 77).

This inability to read to their own child is one of the commonest causes of regret among dyslexic parents. Often it is the motivation to get literacy help for themselves.

Parental reaction to their dyslexic child

What is the initial reaction?
Having a diagnosis of a child's dyslexia can be like poking a hornets' nest.

The reactions of all the family members fly out in a sudden burst of unpredictable energy that swirls around in confused and angry chaos until a new stability is found. This puts pressure on dyslexic children because they not only have to cope with their own problems but must also negotiate bewildering new behaviour in their parents. Both parents and child upset each other. Both sides are caused anxiety by the other's distress and frustration. Tension in the home is rife. Dyslexia has hit the fan.

Do parents defend their dyslexic child against school?
Not always.

Although some enlightened parents would defend their offspring at all costs, there are other parents who, far from countering the negative stressors of school for the dyslexic child, 'take on board the negative perceptions of the school, and endorse them. The situation for a child who is misunderstood at school and at home is particularly stressful' (Fawcett 1995, p. 14). This dyslexic child has no escape. In my experience, he can be the most emotionally disabled by his dyslexia, with an external locus of control, poor sense of self, high dependence, relationship problems and excessive anxiety.

Does dyslexia cause marital difficulty?
Yes. This is not at all uncommon. The dyslexic child easily gets caught up in the parental relationship.

I have often encountered the situation, for example, where a mother anxiously and guiltily overprotects her dyslexic child, to the envy and resentment of her husband, something that becomes much worse if the father is dyslexic himself and did not have his own mother's support. This fight over the mother/wife's attention, this acting-out of very complex relationships, can lead to marital break-up for which the dyslexic child can feel responsible, adding to his burden of guilt. There are many other similar scenarios that I shall return to during this chapter. (Also, see Chapter 5.)

What about the genetic inheritance of the dyslexic gene?
Partners can indulge in genetic guilt.

They can collude in the attitude that one partner should take the chromosomal blame for the dyslexic child's disability. A parent who believes himself to be responsible for the problem, or who accepts this blame, can really clog up his child's ability to deal with their disability by forming an exclusive, enmeshed alliance with him or, by contrast, displacing onto him his own anger and guilt. This is a significant problem in dyslexia because of its high heritability. The dyslexic child is very likely to have one parent who is dyslexic too.

In this respect, an unspoken thread in the counselling process with dyslexic children's families can be the blame that the non-dyslexic parent can attach to their partner for their child's disability. The non-dyslexic's anger is split off onto the dyslexic 'other side of the family'. Their dyslexic partner then becomes representative-in-chief of this other side. This resentment is often unacknowledged and can lie humming between the partners, fuelling anger and guilt like a low-level electrical charge.

What is the role of parental anxiety?
Parents of dyslexic children can get very anxious.

Riddick (1996) believes that this anxiety is linked to uncertainty and apprehension about the dyslexic child's future. It is touching that many of the mothers in her survey were fearful that the degree of worry that they expressed would be seen as 'inappropriate'. In other words, they were worrying about worrying about their children.

Unfortunately, there is considerable evidence that parental factors play an important role in the development and maintenance of child-anxiety disorders. Children of parents with anxiety disorders are at higher risk than controls of developing anxiety problems. The pathway of anxiety transmission between parent and child involves a 'complex interaction between genetic and environmental factors' (Spence et al. 2000, p. 715).

This is particularly the case when there are dyslexic children and dyslexic parents, both of whom are affected by the anxiety of being dyslexic (see Chapter 7).

Then, there will be a self-perpetuating family dynamic whereby each generation of dyslexics is predisposed to promote anxiety in the next. If, as recent evidence also indicates, the parents of anxious children are also more likely to engage in overcontrolling, overprotective and overcritical behaviour – that is independently associated with increased anxiety in children (Spence et al. 2000) – it is easy to see how anxiety can take residence in dyslexic homes, becoming more firmly entrenched generation after generation.

What is very important is that each dyslexic generation also transmits its own inadequate *coping strategies* for anxiety. Such parental behaviours undermine the child's natural ability to solve his own life problems. The fearful, anxious parent also encourages the dyslexic child to focus upon the threatening aspects of the world, rather than the helpful ones.

The fall-out of this is that: 'parental behaviours that model, prompt, or reinforce anxious, rather than coping, behaviour play a significant part in the development and maintenance of childhood anxiety' (Spence et al. op. cit., p. 715). Consequently, work with anxious, dyslexic children can usefully be linked to parental training in child-management skills as well as parental anxiety management, communication, problem-solving and social skills. Parents and children need treatment together, and parents need to revise their own behaviours towards their child: 'By implication, treatment involving the child is unlikely to be effective unless these parental behaviors are changed' (op. cit., p. 715).

Are parents emotionally abusive to their dyslexic child?

Yes. It is a sad fact that many parents with dyslexic children have little more understanding of their children's needs than, say, their school or peers.

Misunderstanding their children's problems as laziness and stupidity is a surprisingly common parental reaction. It can also be based on a misguided desire to help. 'Qualitatively, emotional abuse may well have at its core the targeting of the child's emotional and psychological well-being ... [the parents' intent] may not be actively malevolent and the harm often occurs by the failure to attend to the child's needs and rights' (Glaser 1995, p. 74).

Central to this problem are mistaken parental beliefs about dyslexia, in particular the interesting idea that persistent denigration of a dyslexic child will encourage him to succeed.

A more complex motivation for emotional abuse can occur when a child is perceived as similar to a scapegoated, dyslexic sibling of a parent, or some other family member who caused harm to the parent as a child. Such misattributions are given as an explanation for the child's behaviour, and are then internalized by the dyslexic child himself, who acts out his parent's family history in a cross-generational parallel process. An example of this would be the dyslexic son who resembles his father's overprotected and maternally enmeshed, dyslexic younger brother. The father's old jealousies towards his brother can be revisited on his son.

What about ambitious parents?

Dyslexic children can be keenly aware that they are failing their parents, and they have no problems in picking up when they are a disappointment to them.

Like most children, dyslexic children want to please their parents, but many have to face the fact that, for some utterly inexplicable reason and despite some strenuous effort, their parents are not at all pleased with what they do and who they are. Thus, a significant factor in dyslexic problems can be the expectations of the parents themselves.

It is, however, a matter of degree, and parental distress is not necessarily proportional to the extent of the disability. 'I have known parents dismiss serious cases of dyslexia whereas others will overreact to mild or moderate cases. When their child fails to live up to expectations, the disappointment can be marked' (Congdon 1995, p. 93).

A highly successful, non-dyslexic father can, for example, be quite clear to his non-achieving dyslexic son how lazy, stupid and useless he appears to be, while some dyslexic fathers, who had good parental support themselves, can be really very easygoing and accepting about their dyslexic child's difficulties. As we shall see later in the section on 'Fathers and the dyslexic child', this difference in attitudes can be crucial to whether or not the dyslexic child successfully negotiates his experiences.

Conditional parenting, based on parental ambition, is, in my opinion, cruel. It makes the dyslexic child's secure place within the family contingent on them learning to read, write and spell competently. It is, unfortunately, a tragic and common belief among dyslexic children that continued academic failure will lead them to lose their parents' love. Dyslexic adults also recall this belief, but often as a painful certainty.

Parental pressure is particularly difficult for gifted, dyslexic children. The parents of such children, not unreasonably, have high aspirations for their children. They see the potential in their offspring and may have already had a fantasy of high standards of attainment when the child enters and leaves school. 'When this is not forthcoming, the disappointment and disillusionment can be traumatic for both parent and child [with] ... parents becoming vexed, angry and unkind towards the child whom they see as careless and poorly motivated. Some children are the victims of bullying by disappointed fathers' (Congdon op. cit., p. 93).

What about unambitious parents?
In this situation, the family might have little experience of dyslexia or just lack interest in education. The parents may even choose to use the child's dyslexia as a reason to avoid developing his potential. Surprisingly, dyslexic children can often achieve quite well in these circumstances since they are not handicapped by anxious, overambitious parents. They seem to make their own decisions and, even if they do not achieve at school, many find their way to university or other skills. 'Such children may find that, although they cannot become literate, there are other socially acceptable school or out-of-school activities and they can concentrate on becoming competent in these' (Congdon op. cit., p. 94).

As a university counsellor, I found that a significant number of my dyslexic student clients had made their own decision about their abilities when their parents just let them be. Trusting a dyslexic is far less harmful than the effects of conditional or invasive parenting.

Are there problems with damaged dyslexic parents?
It depends.

Dyslexic parents revisit their past in their dyslexic child. Sometimes this awakening of old memories can be converted into positive action on behalf of their child. Where the parents are depressed and dyslexic, however, the evidence of their child's dyslexia can be extremely upsetting to them and, subsequently, damaging to their child.

Undiagnosed and unhelped dyslexic mothers or fathers who have experienced the trauma of poor school experience, bullying and peer rejection, as well as rejection by their own parents, have a high probability of depressive tendencies. Although the experiences of dyslexic children today are not always good, such children in the past had a perfectly terrible time. As a counsellor, I have encountered many instances of dyslexic parents, many still undiagnosed, who have been, or are, clinically depressed.

There is an extensive literature on the role of depressed parents in the upbringing of children. Significantly, parental depression – particularly maternal depression – can leave a child feeling isolated since the parent is unable to recognize and respond to their child's attachment and emotional needs. When this happens, a dyslexic child can display all the characteristics of a 'parent-child', something that is not uncommon among children with alcoholic parents (see below).

For many dyslexic parents, their dyslexic child can also bring back some well-buried memories about their own hated dyslexia. These feelings can be split off and projected onto their son or daughter, to the extent of disliking and rejecting their child, who now embodies their own childhood dyslexic traumas. Such parents, particularly those who are depressed and disturbed by this revisiting of their own dyslexia, may also withdraw psychologically from their dyslexic child.

'For many parents, the difficulties their child suffers are an unpleasant reminder of their own experiences in school. The feelings of ineptitude and frustration that they suffered at that time, when the education system was less sympathetic to dyslexia, may render them impotent to deal with their current situation' (Congdon 1995, p. 14).

Do dyslexic children have to parent a dyslexic mother or father?
Yes. The problem of the dyslexic child-parent with a parent-child is

particularly common when the parents are dyslexic, depressed, alcoholic or, as often happens, all three.

In this family, a dyslexic child fulfils the psychological needs of his parents. The parent's poor sense of self, their related self-centredness and their preoccupation with their own emotional needs are to the detriment of the child's personal development. In this case, the counsellor will find a profound problem with boundaries and will encounter a child who is coping both with his own dyslexia and the parenting needs of his parents.

In this situation, Glaser (1995) identified five characteristics of problematic parenting. It is my experience that these five characteristics present frequently among the dyslexic parents of dyslexic children.

> '• premature imposition of physical and psychological responsibility on the child
> • inappropriate or inconsistent expectations of a young child in terms of understanding, behaviour and internal controls
> • failure to protect from inappropriate experiences
> • confusing communication and distortions of "objective truth"
> • overprotection and failure to provide age-appropriate opportunities for cognitive and emotional learning experiences' (p. 77).

Commonly, the alcoholic dyslexic parent is also found in this family dynamic.

Again, we must look to the genetic inheritance of dyslexia and not be surprised that the parents of dyslexic children have chosen alcohol in their flight from the anxiety associated with their condition. Unfortunately, the child inherits the responsibility from which his parents are fleeing.

When, as the counsellor, I encounter this situation, it usually involves some major collusion between the family members. Not at all uncommon is the enmeshment of the mother with the son and the father with the daughter. In one recent case of a ten-year-old dyslexic boy, his alcoholic, dyslexic father was physically abusive to the boy's mother and the dyslexic son regularly slept with his mother as 'protection'. He often wished that his father were dead, and, when the father did die, his mother, free of this family dynamic, rejected her son. The horrifying and complex mess that dyslexia had brought to this family was a therapeutic nightmare from any theoretical position.

Generally speaking, when the co-dependence of alcoholism tangles with the collusion of dyslexia, the destruction inherent in the dyslexic child's family is extremely hard to treat. It is the therapeutic equivalent of getting chewing gum out of hair, and, sometimes, the therapist may only be able to minimize, rather than remediate, any damage to the dyslexic child.

Mothers and the dyslexic child

Who is the main carer of the dyslexic child?
The mother.

In his extensive review of the resources and strategies of parents caring for a disabled child, Beresford (1994) established that, in the majority of cases, mothers are responsible for their child's care. Carpenter (2000), in a Nordic study of 1,000 mothers of disabled children, found that they had increased their care-taking responsibility, had often amended their life goals, leisure activities and work patterns and, when they did work, they had high levels of sick leave. In her international study, Mittler (1995) found that mothers typically remained the major carers throughout all regions of the world.

Who picks up the child's dyslexia first?
Mothers.

There is no doubt that it is the mothers of dyslexic children who spot the problems of dyslexia early on, and who endure their child's distress, night-mares and bed-wetting before the diagnosis of dyslexia gives a label to the problem.

From then on: 'At a day-to-day level all the mothers in the sample thought that they had the major responsibility for dealing with their child's dyslexia' (Riddick 1996, p. 163).

Mothers also reported that 75% of their children had gone through a time when they had displayed considerable distress of one sort or another, and saw making improvements in this as their main parental task.

Who acts to solve the dyslexia?
Mothers.

It is also mothers who have to push to have their child diagnosed and to get help. 'Mothers often find it easy to accept that their child is struggling and is in need of learning support. They are less likely to feel their child is being lazy and not trying hard enough' (Goldup and Ostler 2000, p. 328).

It is mothers who, variously: begin the detective work by painstakingly eliminating all options until it is only dyslexia that remains; challenge teachers – who clearly see them as fussy, demanding, overanxious and con-frontational; demand action from headmasters, local authorities and educational psychologists – despite their own fear of the educational sys-tem; are patronizingly reminded that 'the professionals know best' or 'children develop at different rates' or 'your child is not ready to read yet'. Fathers, particularly dyslexic fathers, can find any contact with their child's school unbearable, particularly the humiliation from teachers.

How does the child's dyslexia affect his mother?
It worries her sick.

She is bewildered, frustrated, helpless and angry. Then, she usually rallies. She develops a thick skin, and goes into battle on behalf of her child with a wide range of burgeoning skills, including diplomacy, education, politics, psychology, duplicity, targeted flirting, blackmail, manipulation, intuition and straightforward threat. Humiliation, however, often goes with this territory, and Riddick found that many mothers had to deal with the hostility of others.

Edwards (1994) notes how the parents of a dyslexic child face the continual strain of having to watch helplessly while their child suffers at school and the authorities blame them for the literacy problem; something, she observes, that would be unthinkably brutal with any other form of handicap.

Does she give practical support to her child?
Very much so.

Mothers, in Riddick's study, 'were keen for guidance and advice on the sort of support they should give. They first looked to the school for advice. When this was not available they used trial and error to try and find out what would work ... Once their child was identified as dyslexic, some mothers turned to the specialist literature for advice and also to specialist organizations' (Riddick 1996, p. 116). By default, they used commonsense.

The types of practical support offered by the mother, in order of frequency, were reading, games, homework, books, phonetics, story tapes, computers, flashcards and writing. This was despite the fact that many of these mothers worked full time, had other younger children, were single parents or had husbands working away from home. Many became very expert. What was striking was the level of responsibility that these mothers had, and the total absence of any explanation from within the mainstream school. 'What clearly emerged was that nearly all of the children were left to fend for themselves with mothers offering what support they could in the background (op. cit., p. 148).

What about emotional support?
Riddick (1996) found that mothers gave two main types of emotional support: one was countering negative feelings in the children, and the other was boosting their children's self-esteem or confidence by offering encouragement and dwelling on the positives. 'It can be argued that mothers were responding to negative images that children had received largely from outside the home' (op. cit., p. 111). These mothers worked hard to improve their child's confidence, although it was quite difficult to do this for

children who had physical problems, specific cognitive impairments or poor verbal fluency.

What positive effects does all this have on her child?
First, these mothers are superb role models of how to be hardworking and persistent.

I cannot help but wonder whether it is these resourceful, formidable mothers who provide the template for the persistent, bloody-minded and brave characteristics of many dyslexics. Also, such mothers model for their children that adversity can make you tough. I have often observed in mothers with two or more dyslexic children that they operate much more ruthlessly when the next child starts to have problems.

Second, dyslexic mothers can demonstrate coping strategies for their dyslexic children.

Mothers who have successfully dealt with their own dyslexia, whose own parents encouraged them to cope or who meet with professionals who believe they can cope are more likely to deal successfully with a dyslexic child in their own life. He will then internalize these attitudes and use them himself (Beresford 1994).

Poor coping by mothers has, however, the opposite effect. Bifulco et al. (2002) found that poor maternal, psychosocial functioning led to a four-fold higher rate of disorder in their children. Maternal vulnerability 'provided the best model for offspring disorder' (p. 1075).

What is the most helpful maternal quality?
Maternal warmth.

This is the one factor that many studies identify as the most beneficial for a dyslexic child. Dyslexic children thrive with a happy, reassuring, affectionate maternal style. This seems to serve as a protective factor in preventing the development of behaviour problems, in contrast to children whose mothers are cold and rejecting.

Warm, responsive mothering is also associated with children's positive beliefs about their own competence, and the development of a warm, outgoing style that modifies problems in peer relationships at school.

High maternal criticism is, however, linked to depression and conduct disorder (Vostanis et al. 1994).

What are the problems faced by dyslexic mothers of dyslexic children?
Dyslexic mothers can have their own problems of disorganization and depression stemming from trying to cope with their own negative experiences.

This will lead to problems with all their children but especially with a dyslexic child. This child becomes a mirror to his mother's problems, and the two of them can spiral downwards, out of control, like two drowning swimmers. Rejection of the dyslexic child by a dyslexic mother occurs when she – who has all the usual problems of dyslexia – finds it hard to cope with just about everything.

The dyslexic tendency to short-term-memory problems and disorganization are real hindrances to bringing up children. If the dyslexic mother is also depressed, as many can be, she may be unavailable emotionally for her child, and he will be unable to gain the reassurance, support and encouragement that are essential to him. His basic needs will be met in a functional way without reference to his feelings, and he will not engage or attach securely with his mother. All the energy in such a child may be directed towards trying to attract his mother's attention, though if this fails he may develop his own rejecting responses.

If he adopts attention-seeking strategies to ensure that he is noticed, his mother's rejecting behaviour will increase as she becomes more pressured. Alternatively, the child may withdraw, making fewer and fewer demands. The mother's emotional unavailability also makes the dyslexic child anxious. To reduce this, he has the option of taking control by adopting the parental role.

Any experienced counsellor can visualize the opportunities for testing behaviour, boundary violation and over-enmeshment in a counselling relationship with this type of dyslexic.

Fathers and the dyslexic child

Is the father as relevant and present as the mother?
No. As a recent review of disability research concluded, fathers are seen as 'hard-to-reach' parents simply because they are so often excluded from the mother-child relationship (Carpenter 2000, p. 137).

The father is excluded for two reasons. First, overprotective mothering (see below) marginalizes the father. Second, with disability, there is no normal separation and individuation between mother and child. Both these situations 'can result in a cutting-off, or excluding, of the father' (Bungener and McCormack 1994, p. 368).

Thus, as the researchers' terminology has just unconsciously conveyed, the father is, in effect, castrated by the arrival of dyslexia: the potent, relevant, needed part of him is cut away by the mother. He is surgically removed from the relationship with his wife, his child and his sense of himself as a man. With a dyslexic son, the father can see himself replaced as the preferred male partner, the provider or the protector.

This can only heighten the conscious and unconscious resentment that the father feels towards his own child. I think that this is also one more reason why the mother tries to keep her dyslexic child constantly young and dependent (see Chapter 9). This keeps him safe from the murderous, jealous instincts of the father as adult male – an instinct that will be thwarted if his child remains infantile. This is also unconsciously picked up by the son who must remain babyish to his father's adult, to keep himself safe, too.

Unfortunately, such collusions and unconscious transactions also prevent the son from negotiating the Oedipal stage and, thus, he remains enmeshed with his mother.

Is it useful to reintegrate the absent father?

Yes – but it is difficult because complicated forces are at work in the family and in the marital relationship.

Absent fathers are common in clinical practice with disabled children, and it is usual to come across a family where the father has either left at an early stage in the family's life cycle or absents himself by working night shifts, for instance, or for long hours during the day. The effect of the disappearing father is to set up different realities in the worlds of the mother and the father of a dyslexic child. Shared decision-making is not possible, because of divergent impressions and reactions. This can fracture the parental relationship.

Usually, the parents separate into two camps – overprotective mother and hostile father – which are so safely opposite that there can be little chance of an accidental rapprochement. This may, of course, be an unconscious and useful way of rejecting the marital partnership. If, after negotiating this swamp of motivations, acting out and pay-offs, a counsellor can help to realign these relationships between mother and father, she might be able to reintegrate the father into his family.

This will bring the father back on the side of both his partner and child, supporting and defending them both. The normal marital partnership allows the child to separate, and the parents are able to enact the Oedipal drama to the psychological safety and benefit of the child.

The father's reintegration also reduces the terrifying influence of the mother. This gives a dyslexic child a strong male role figure in a world dominated by demanding female figures, whether anxious overprotective mother or critical female teacher.

The father can also provide a balancing, sensible, solid role for both mother and child – if he is acknowledged and empowered. Mostly, fathers simply do not know what their role is in the lives of these unhappy, disorientated people whom he often loves very much. 'We are often quick to blame the father for opting out, but further exploration sometimes reveals that the father often feels left out and frustrated, and has difficulty finding a way into the intense mother-and-child relationship' (Bungener and McCormack 1994, p. 368).

Generally speaking, father involvement is significantly related to later positive child outcome. When a father is happily and deeply involved in the life of his dyslexic child, that child will prosper (Flouri and Buchanan 2003).

Can a father become usefully engaged with his dyslexic child?

Yes – and to very good effect if it can be achieved.

Some fathers find that a child with a disability can bring about life-transforming experiences. For others, the experience causes relentless stress, disorientates their life goals and affects their work patterns. Bray et al. (1995) identify two main types of father in the families of disabled children: 'unconditional' and 'transforming'. Fathers who display unconditional love, give devotion to their children by just accepting whatever they do and patiently standing by them through all their endeavours. Fathers who display transforming love use transforming acts such as altering the house for their child or transforming the child himself and, in so doing, enhance both of their life opportunities.

How useful is spouse support of the father to the mother?

It is estimated that this is the most important role of fathers.

In giving practical and emotional spouse support to his wife, he becomes an important coping resource for mothers of disabled children. Relative to other forms of social support, Beresford (1994) considered it the most significant, and the most related to a successful outcome of care. Perceived support is also more important than its objective existence. Knowing that the father's support is forthcoming, and that he is cheerful and willing to help, contributes more to the mother's well-being than the actual tasks carried out.

Do fathers provide useful role models?

Yes – and, despite maternal help, some dyslexic children still feel more understood by their dyslexic fathers. They value his dyslexic viewpoint in supporting them: 'dyslexic parents can be a positive asset in providing role models and understanding to their dyslexic children' (Riddick 1996, p. 157). A dyslexic father can sometimes know just the right thing to say or do. He can sometimes empathize with his dyslexic child in a way that they both understand, and no one else in the family can.

What about critical fathers?
Fathers of dyslexic children can often be overstrict and highly critical of their dyslexic child. There are many negative effects of this type of parenting.

When coupled with the common situation of the overprotective mother, the effect of the overstrict father is to make the child both anxious and a more likely target of bullying. Other effects can be that the son develops ill-judged behaviour to prove himself (Gomez 1991). Since such a father is also less likely to indulge in horseplay and games with his son – which can insulate children from negative peer effects – the critical father exacerbates his son's already poor social cognition (Flouri and Buchanan 2003).

What about paternal horseplay with dyslexic children?
It is a very good thing. One of the sources of damage in maternal overprotection is that this horseplay is often stopped.

Popular boys have fathers who are physically playful and happy to play with them (Vanzetti and Duck 1996). In fact, recent research shows that fathers who playfight with their children produce children who are 'among the friendliest and most peaceful and popular in the playground. By contrast, children who are mollycoddled at home and discouraged from rough behaviour are much more likely to turn into bullies or their victims' (Durham 2003).

This paternal playfighting forces a child to confront how he relates to other people, and the rules of engagement are learned in a safe place with someone who models when and how to stop.

Do fathers protect their dyslexic children?
Not enough. In fact, some dyslexic children blame their father for not protecting them, either from bullying at school or engulfment by their mother. Some fathers can be oblivious to the betrayal felt by their children – sons or daughters – who think that their father – rather than their mother – should have protected them from harmful experiences.

Overprotective parenting of dyslexic children

How is overprotective parenting relevant to dyslexia?
Overprotection is commonly found in all types of disability – not just dyslexia – and is mostly associated with maternal behaviour.

It is true that in a normal, healthy family dynamic, mothers are 'experienced as more compromising and as fostering greater intimacy in comparison to fathers' (Honess et al. 1997, p. 367), particularly by boys. There is a point, however, when this turns into overprotection and enmeshment that are harmful for the psychological development of the child. There is clearly a risk that an overprotected child will collude in the crusade against their own independence and buy into the family's view of their helplessness.

Is overprotection common with dyslexic children?

Yes – definitely. Overprotective behaviour occurs frequently in the families of dyslexic children.

In fact, overprotection, usually by a mother of a son or, more rarely, by a father of a daughter, is found so commonly among dyslexics of all ages that it might also be considered a symptom of dyslexia – since it is more prevalent than mixed handedness or dyscalculia.

Linked to this overprotection is usually marital difficulty, including some very jealous and resentful husbands, and a background clamour of spiteful, unhappy siblings.

Gomez (1991) believes that overprotection originates in maternal compensation for an unsatisfactory marriage or because of unresolved, undeserved guilt when a child is sick or handicapped. This behaviour encourages neurosis but not psychosis and, significantly, as was noted in the previous chapter, is linked to bullying. 'Sons who become mother's boys suffer social disadvantage: they are disliked and despised by their peers through school onwards' (p. 49).

Whatever the reasons, it is always worth remembering that there are pay-offs for everyone in overprotection – it is never what it seems. It is one of the most rich, collusive patterns of family behaviour, and it is powered by a variety of conscious and unconscious reasons.

Is there a repressed and denied dislike of the dyslexic child?

Yes – and I would estimate that this is one of the main reasons.

Overprotection can be powered by latent and denied feelings of dislike, disappointment or even hatred that the mother or father feels towards an excruciatingly problematic dyslexic child. This incongruent reaction – which the child can pick up but not explain or discuss – has two effects. First, it can make him anxious and, secondly, the overprotection itself, by implicitly suggesting that he cannot manage alone, is disempowering and adds both to the increased probability of bullying at school and the encouragement of a victim self-image. Unfortunately, in this situation, the dyslexic child starts to show even more dependence, anxiety and neediness – the very behaviour that the mother, and particularly the father, may so dislike and cannot express.

Does the mother have a problem in separating from her child?

In some ways, yes, but the problem has many layers.

There is certainly a scenario where the child's dyslexia gives the mother an excuse to avoid separation. She uses overprotection to keep him enmeshed with her. In this case, the mother can find ways in which her dyslexic child is rewarded for remaining helpless and failed, since his success renders her redundant. Such mothers can resist help for their dyslexic child, or even sabotage it.

This situation is also made worse when the mother herself is dyslexic, since she may be acting out her own feelings of failure and, often, the inability of her own mother to help her. She can create her own fantasized ending to what she had wanted for herself. In such cases, Glaser (1995) believes that the relationship becomes explicitly abusive. The 'nature of this parent-child relationship may not continue to serve the child's best interests and needs, unless a change in the relationship is possible' (p. 73).

What is the role of the mother's own separation anxiety?

Maternal fear of separation and attachment problems will cause her to overprotect her dyslexic child because it is her own self as child that she sees in him. In some ways, he does not exist as a separate person from her.

Dyslexic mothers who have been badly abused by their own parents and at school resemble the abused, separation-afraid mothers described in the classic study by Bowlby (1991). Such mothers can be distrustful and highly sensitive to any type of separation, even the most commonplace, and can react with high levels of anxiety or anger. Bowlby's description of such mothers chimes in with my observation of the mothers of some dyslexic children, in that where the parent-child relationship becomes inverted the child is also expected to be grateful for such care and not notice the demands being made. He must conform to seeing the parent in whatever light she chooses, and the mother is often unaware of the pressure she is putting on her child while claiming to protect him.

Bowlby also observed that the overprotective parent could be intensely anxious about the availability of her own attachment figures. She is unconsciously 'inverting the normal parent-child relationship by requiring the child to be a parent figure and adopting the role of child for herself' (p. 305).

She seeks from her own child the loving care she either lost or never had. Not unexpectedly, the marital relations of the parents are usually very disturbed.

Is the mother's mother important?

She is, and one commonly missed feature of the overprotective mother of a dyslexic child is that she can be locked in a mutually ambivalent relationship with both her own mother and her child.

In this case, Bowlby (1991) describes how overprotective behaviour by the mother to the child comes from three sources.

These are: redirecting (displacing) anger, engendered initially by her own mother, against her own child; misattributing to the child the rejecting and/or demanding characteristics of her own mother, and being angry with the child accordingly; modelling angry behaviour towards the child on the angry behaviour exhibited by her own mother.

According to Bowlby, this type of mother can also have a rather passive husband who tends to opt out of his roles as husband and father. Sexual relations are likely to be sparse or absent.

Is overprotection the embodiment of the female 'tiger' role?
Absolutely.

In fact, this female characteristic practically powers the entire dyslexia industry.

As noted earlier, many mothers of dyslexic children become formidable warriors in defence of their dyslexic child, and it is not unusual for mothers of dyslexic children to feel that they are taking on the whole world – education authority, husband, other children, family members and teachers. She can also feel that she is the only one in the family to help the dyslexic child: 'as well as shouldering the major responsibility for helping their dyslexic child [mothers] also had to mediate between their husband and child or between their dyslexic child and their non-dyslexic brothers and sisters' (Riddick 1996, p. 166).

This gives such mothers the sense that they are battling the world alone; that their dyslexic child must rely on them since no one else is available. It is here, in my experience, that the maternal tiger quality emerges, and what started out as a mission becomes a crusade. In the ensuing battle for recognition and help, the child can become infantilized and dependent.

There is, in short, a thin line between the defence of a dyslexic child and his disempowerment through suffocatingly overprotective parenting. It is also very easy for mothers to lose sight of the fact that their child has qualities other than his dyslexia. Such mothers can acquire an alarming tunnel vision, pouring vast amounts of energy into their child's dyslexia so that they can see little else.

There can be complicated pay-offs in this situation, not least when it evolves within the context of an unsatisfactory marital relationship.

Can overprotection be a valid action against a hostile, jealous father?
Unfortunately, yes.

Mothers of a dyslexic child are often unsupported – if not discouraged – by the child's father. The mother then perceives her child as being left with only one supportive and understanding parent – herself. Such mothers may find themselves engaged in running battles with the dyslexic child's father, whose hostility to his son can be remarkable. For example, not at all uncommon is the family where the dyslexic father wants his son to get the help that he was denied and then resents his son for receiving the help that he did not. Such a father can also daily see and dislike in his child the unbearable reminder of his own failure as a child. Such fathers can show their dislike in both direct and underhand ways.

Other mothers, in open conflict with the father over what should be done about their child's dyslexia, are often exasperated with their husband who does not seem to understand fully the nature of his son's problem. I have no doubt that this 'lack of understanding' is often intentional. Parental politics – usually involving a jealous husband – start to intervene. What started as a simple maternal battle fuelled by instinct and anger eventually takes on complicated marital luggage.

Paternal jealousy of his son is a serious problem in dyslexic fathers. I have seen it so often. In the most extreme cases, the father makes the mother choose between him and their son who, in one family with whom I worked, was only 11 years old.

I have also seen remarkably infantile and jealous responses from fathers when their dyslexic son is first assessed and the psychologist praises the child for his performance. As the previously critical, but now relieved and proud, mother preens over the psychologist's remarks, I have, for example, seen one father elbow himself in front of his son; another who interrupted, shouting remarks such as 'I was good at this, too', 'I had problems with this, too', like a hem-tugging toddler; and another who scowled resentfully at his son throughout the whole discussion, his arms furiously crossed and his foot tapping in irritation.

In these situations, the brewing problems are clearly there to read, even as the mother walks happily out of the room, arm around her son's shoulder, with father left to follow – forgotten by them both.

Are there simpler reasons for overprotection, such as fear or transference?

Overprotection is ostensibly motivated by a fear that the child will come to harm.

Sometimes, a counsellor will wonder if this is a denied parental wish that the child will actually come to harm. Often, however, such protectiveness can be simple anxiety about letting the child go: a valid response to real need in the child. 'When a toddler first tries to walk and falls over, parents feel frightened and elated. Slowly they get used to the risks involved in all ordinary development. However, when a child is born with a disability 'that feeling of protectiveness lasts longer. There can be a very difficult path to keep between protecting the child in the environment and denying a child the dignity of the normal risks of exploration' (Sinason 1993, p. 34).

On a related issue, Barrett et al. (2002) also found that overprotective parenting of children with disabilities, such as OCD, was clearly a response to the child's distress, and should be interpreted as parents trying to cope with a very difficult child.

There might also be transference of the child's feelings of helplessness onto the parents, who act this out through excessive care. In the same way, a parent's lack of confidence in their child may be a parallel process of the child's own lack of confidence in himself. The transference process will be similar to that which occurs between teachers and dyslexic children (described in Chapter 3).

In short, the direction of effect of overprotection may not be that of the family on the dyslexic, but the dyslexic child – with all his fears and anxieties – on the family. Such families need considerable reassurance and support.

What happens in a parent-child alliance?
Overprotection of the dyslexic child may be acted out in a dysfunctional family through an alliance with one of his parents.

Minuchin (1974) first demonstrated how one parent could form an alliance with a child against the other parent. One important feature of this cross-generational coalition is that the parent's high emotional support for the child is in stark comparison with the marriage relationship and with the other parent-child relationships. When the child is favoured over a partner in the marriage, trouble starts.

In such a cross-generational alliance, both parents are unable to discipline the child effectively, and they place him in a power position equal to one of the parents. The authority of the other parent is undermined, and this can make the child anxious. Furthermore, the parent enticing the child into a coalition can use guilt mechanisms to keep the child in the emotional alliance, also putting the child into a conflict of loyalty – causing distress and further anxiety. The pushes and pulls for the child are horrible.

Mathijssen et al. (1998) usefully examined which dyad – mother-child, father-child and mother-father dyads – had the largest association with child pathology. They found that children with no positive relation with either parent showed significant levels of externalizing (violent acting-out) behaviour.

I do not find this to be the case with a dyslexic child – they will almost always have at least one parent on their side. This might explain why externalizing behaviour is much less linked with dyslexia than internalizing behaviour (anxiety), which is more associated with enmeshment. Interestingly, Mathijssen et al. also found that having one or two positive relationships was associated with less problem behaviour.

A further issue to consider is whether the child-parent coalition arises to protect the family integrity, that is, an unconscious decision by the mother to absorb the child's difficult behaviour. It is a question of the lesser of two evils. Mathijssen et al. (1998), in their study on problematic alliances, conceded: 'we could not rule out the possibility that some negative family relationships arose from the problem behaviour exhibited by the child rather than being the cause of it' (p. 486).

What are the effects of overprotection on the child?

It disempowers and disables them, often for life. 'Children who remain overprotected fail to overcome anxieties and are likely to develop a self-view of frailty' (Glaser 1995, p. 79). In these circumstances, as Etkin (1993) observes, '[parental] roles in *enduring* timidity cannot be overestimated' (p. 17, my italics).

Overprotection can also extinguish the child as an individual. 'The failure to respect the child's individuality interferes with the development of a sense of self. The child may be unable to leave the parent or feel too guilty to express his or her own wishes' (Glaser 1995, p. 79). This leads to dependence and a variety of social impairments, such as low self-esteem, social naivety and low social competence (Espelata et al. 2000, McFarlane et al. 1995).

Overprotection is particularly implicated in generating anxiety. With dyslexic children, who are anxious enough already, overprotection only adds to the problem. Barrett et al. (2002) review a number of studies on childhood anxiety disorders, such as separation anxiety and social phobia, and conclude that there is a strong association between maternal control, protection and childhood anxiety. Overprotective parents also encourage avoidance solutions to problems and are less likely to encourage pro-social solutions to ambiguous social situations. None of this will reduce, but will certainly add to, the dyslexic child's problems with peers and other relationships.

Overprotection is also unhelpful for any child, since the subtext of the behaviour is that the child cannot cope alone, or that he is helpless. This is particularly bad for dyslexics because they, more than most, need to find some ways of feeling in control of their life.

What particular counselling issues arise because of parental overprotection?

There are three broad areas.

First, overprotective parenting of dyslexic children is particularly frustrating for a counsellor since parents are often actively motivated to resist change in their child. Such parents can abruptly terminate their child's counselling when their son or daughter starts to become more independent. Parents can also unconsciously sabotage the counselling, such as by getting the date wrong, 'accidentally' arranging other activities at that time or being late.

I recall a particularly frustrating case with a 12-year-old dyslexic girl whose mother always had a work 'crisis' on Friday – her daughter's counselling evening – so that they were either late or did not attend. Her daughter, newly confident, eventually decided to come to her counselling sessions by bus. The mother then started to dock her daughter's pocket money for an imaginative range of infractions. So, my client then started a Saturday job to get her own money to pay the fares but needed a lift to start the job while she built up funds. Her mother then developed more 'crises', this time on Saturdays, that ultimately cost her daughter her job through unpunctuality. The daughter gave up her job and gave up her counselling. I never saw her again.

I have colleagues who believe that counselling can only, at best, be supportive when parents are sufficiently toxic to sabotage all their best efforts to achieve therapeutic change in a child or adolescent client. I think that they have a point.

Second, maternal overprotection will also generate extremely powerful transference between counsellors and dyslexic clients of all ages. Apart from the straightforward invitation to the counsellor to enter into another overprotective alliance, this transference can also carry the approach/avoidance conflicts of someone who is addicted to overprotection but fears engulfment.

Such a client can force the counselling relationship to spin its wheels while he shifts repetitively between seducing, and withdrawing from, the counsellor. In my experience, some respectful – if robust – counsellor congruence can usually move things forward and, in the process, model the type of empowering, congruent relationship that the client will not have had with his mother (see Chapter 12).

Third, the effect of overprotective parenting is also physically present in the presenting childlike appearance (little-girl hair styles and T-bar shoes; messy *Just William* boys) and demeanour (wistful, sad, 'lost child in a big world') of dyslexic adult clients, and passive or cutesy behaviour in some dyslexic children. Adult clients may also be locked into relationships where they are encouraged to remain childlike by a strongly parenting, protective partner. This, more than anything, creates the Peter Pan dyslexic.

This 'uncooked' feature of the dyslexic personality is as unacknowledged in the psychological literature on dyslexia as it is central to the counselling experience with dyslexic clients. I shall discuss this in more detail in Chapter 9.

Positive family support for a dyslexic child

How important is family support?
It is crucial.

There is a respectable research tradition known as 'resilience' literature, which examines the protective influence of the parent-child relationship on child problem behaviour (e.g. Rutter 1975).

One conclusion of this work is that, even when children are experiencing peer-relationship problems, the quality of their relationship with their parents can help to offset some of the adverse effects of peer rejection (Vanzetti and Duck 1996). Reinforcing this perspective for dyslexic children, Reynolds and Gregg (2002), in their study on dyslexic college students, found that the difference between high and low stress levels in the students was predicted by the degree of parental support: 'The most extraordinary finding of the study was the significance of perceived parental support in reducing emotional distress in college students with learning disabilities ... A positive family environment also contributed to low stress levels in college students with learning disabilities' (p. 1).

What family characteristics are helpful to a dyslexic child?
Warmth

Dyslexic children like structure so they tend to thrive with well-boundaried parents, in a secure relationship where there is good parental supervision and family cohesion (Rutter 1975, Emery 1982). None of this would be half as effective, however, without emotional warmth. This is the magic ingredient. A warm, supportive relationship with one or both parents will provide security for the dyslexic child and then 'many children at risk develop normally, particularly if given a reasonably adequate environment' (Masten et al. 1988, p. 746).

Furthermore, emotional warmth from parents has the opposite effect to overprotection. McFarlane et al. (1995), for example, found that, whereas overprotection led to low self-esteem and low social competence, emotional warmth led to good problem-solving skills and good impulse control. Warm, sensitive, responsive parenting also plays a protective role in high-risk situations by making children feel safe: 'children develop a sense of being in control when their parents are responsive' (Maccoby 1980, p. 286).

Encouragement

Some parents of dyslexic children worry that if they make allowance for their child's difficulties then they will destroy his ability to lead a normal life. This is fine as long as the parents explain to their child that what they are giving is encouragement rather than a heartless lack of empathy. In short, they are not ignoring his disability, but equipping him to cope with his disability. It is an investment for the future.

It is, however, a thin line to walk: 'Many of the most capable adults with disabilities admit to this dilemma. They know that some of their talents are due to their parents' refusal to accept the disability. However, they also consider there was an emotional price to pay' (Sinason 1993, p. 37).

Optimism

Beresford (1994), in his article on the resources used by parents in the care of a disabled child, maintained that optimism was an important resource. The parents' belief in a positive future was transmitted to their child and enabled them all to deal with any problems that came their way. Work by Veerman (1995) and Kappers and Veerman (1995), on dyslexic adolescents, found that even negative events could be reframed as positive by well-functioning families. Importantly, the more optimistic the family, the lower the reading retardation in the children.

SECTION FOUR
EFFECT

Introduction

A dyslexic woman writes about her experience of being dyslexic:

'Much of the debate about dyslexia at present seems to be focused on what a wonderful thing it is. It helps to know that some people with dyslexia have succeeded against the odds. I'm not bitter, I'm one of them. If it helps the massive problem of low self-esteem of many dyslexics, then so much the better. But somewhere in the clamour of good tidings, some of the reality of the situation is being lost.

So what is my point? I find it irritating to be told that I should celebrate my dyslexia. My peers read what I have written and find it immature. My spelling problems are not usually bad enough to seriously impair meaning, but bad spelling conveys an illusion of carelessness, or worse, stupidity. I am sick of being dyslexic, I am sick of having to battle with words, and the persistent cry to look on the bright side is nothing short of maddening.

Dyslexia affects everything I do; it means that, when I come home from work, I am too tired to cope with text-based media, and the idea of curling up with a book is almost comical. I have been consistently unable to learn to drive, and most employers reject application forms which contain spelling mistakes, or explanations that these result from the applicant's dyslexia.

When I write a cheque, I am dyslexic. When I fill in a form, I am dyslexic, when I put my shoes on, I am dyslexic. I know that. You know that because I told you. The innocent bystander sees a slow, clumsy woman, and I often see her too.

There is also a bigger issue. To constantly champion the view that dyslexia is the best thing that can happen to a person is to distract from the real problems it causes. It ignores the everyday frustrations of living with the thing which damages the self-esteem of the dyslexic. If we think that everyone else is delighting in their non-lateral thought processes, being inventive, then the isolation we feel is deepened.

It is really hard to cope with the feeling that these other people are in the same boat as we are, and yet seem to manage without apparently experiencing the same difficulties. However much we may achieve in our chosen fields, there is the ever-present assumption that our literacy is somehow lacking. Sympathy from others is not helpful, what we need is support, real solutions to our very real problems. We all really do suffer from dyslexia. Few of us can spare the time in our disordered existences to revel in our marvellous gift.

Of course, there is a positive side to dyslexia. But to suggest all we need is specialist teaching to improve our spelling or reading is to belittle the problem. Such teaching is vital, but it is not a panacea allowing us to experience the world with a special and unique perspective. Living with dyslexia is like wading upstream, frequently out of our depth, throughout life. It seems unhelpful to be so gloomy, but it is the truth. I am truly grateful for all the energy and enthusiasm that goes into helping to understand and ameliorate the condition. But however good things get dyslexia remains with us as an unwelcome irritation and, at times, as a real disability. All I ask is that you don't patronise us, don't pat us on the head and tell us we're lucky really. We're not. I'm not.'

(adapted from Pearson 2001, p. 33)

CHAPTER 7

The psychological and social effects of dyslexia

Summary

In order to understand the psychological and social effects of dyslexia, it is necessary to keep in mind three broad caveats.

First, dyslexic behaviour is assumed to be the secondary effect of the primary cognitive deficits in reading, but complications can occur when these secondary effects turn into primary ones and go on to affect reading through a 'loop' of failure. The different effects can get hard to disentangle. For example, reading leads to failure, failure to anxiety and anxiety impairs the reading ability of a dyslexic.

Second, there are a number of mediating variables that cloud the effects of pure dyslexia on behaviour and academic performance, in particular ADHD.

Third, 'reading disability' must not be equated with 'dyslexia'. Reading disability is a much wider category that includes children whose reading failure is linked to non-dyslexic reasons, such as low IQ and socio-economic adversity. Unfortunately, 'much of the research has focused on children with a range of reading disabilities and not on children with specific reading difficulties' (Riddick 1996, p. 44). It is important not to confuse the effects of one with the other.

Research on reading problems

What do we know of the effects of *general* reading disability?

We know that it is a significant source of social disruption and a monstrous waste of ability.

Maughan (1995), in a review of studies on reading disabilities, identifies the effects as depression, anxiety, low self-esteem, dysfunctional attributions,

155

poor achievement motivation, inattentiveness, disruptive behaviour, aggression and delinquency. Other work suggests that the majority of children with severe reading disability also suffer from emotional disturbance and that 15%–20% of problems in the areas of reading and learning are linked to emotional difficulties (Hales 1994). Riddick (1996) also found that children with reading disabilities are more likely to have behavioural or emotional difficulties.

The direction of effect remains a problem in interpreting these results. Do behavioural difficulties lead to reading disabilities or vice versa? If they are also linked with highly adverse socio-economic circumstances, reading problems must be considered an associated, rather than the main, effect.

What do we know of the effects of *specific* reading disability in dyslexia?
The research results suggest that the effects are overwhelmingly negative and that dyslexia is a 'severely disabling condition' (Cooper 1999, p. 190).

The British Psychological Society's (BPS) report on dyslexia (1999) even goes so far as to suggest that emotional and behavioural difficulties could be taken as a diagnosis of dyslexia in their own right: particularly in relation to school absence.

Do the social and emotional effects of dyslexia vary over time?
Yes.

Dyslexia is a developmental disorder so its effects will change and develop too. Cumulative experiences, maturation and coping strategies all make their mark. Riddick (1996) found that some problems had even significantly decreased by adulthood suggesting that they were closely related to children's experiences in school. Hales (1994) specifically researched the development of dyslexic problems by age group. He found that very young dyslexic children exhibited tension and frustration, middle-school children had high anxiety and low motivation and, in secondary school, dyslexics wanted to keep in the background at all costs. Hales also found distinctive effects in adults that contrasted with those of young- and middle-school-age children, and McLoughlin (2002) reported specific problems in employment for adult dyslexics.

Strangely, no research on adult dyslexics examines sexual or relationship problems, although, in my work with dyslexic clients of both sexes and at all ages, these are not insignificant areas of difficulty. Intuitively, given the social and interpersonal difficulties of dyslexics, this must be a rich area of enquiry. Again, my position is that this has to do with the infantilizing of dyslexics (see Chapter 9).

What do we know about the effects of dyslexia on girls?

While externalizing disorders are more common in dyslexic males, internalizing disorders, such as depression and withdrawal, comprise almost the entire effect for females: 'for girls, a specific association exists between [reading disability] and internalising symptomatology' (Willcutt and Pennington 2000, p. 1046).

In adulthood, reading-disabled women and girls were still scoring much higher than controls on measures of anxiety and depression. The drop in their confidence and optimism started to plunge dramatically during the middle-school years (Hales 1994). Riddick (1996) speculates that a significant factor may be the amount of 'self-blame, sensitivity to criticism or expectations of others' (p. 46), and learning-disabled, adolescent girls were particularly vulnerable to adjustment problems.

Generally, there is little research of any depth on women or girls. This is because, until recently, dyslexia was assumed to have a 4:1 male bias (see Chapter 1). Now that we know the proportions are more equal, it is to be hoped that the female response to dyslexia will be better researched.

What are the broad indications of existing research on the effects of dyslexia?

Dyslexia, stress and anxiety are correlated.

My own experiences would support this position. I have never yet met a dyslexic who has not been under stress for most of his life, or has not manifested some variant of anxiety-related disorder. If it is not the stress of pressure – either to avoid failure or find success – it is that of boredom: of shoehorning a gallon of intellect and ability into pint pots of menial jobs and low expectations.

This stress and anxiety are the direct and indirect responses to actual and anticipated failure, fear, frustration, suppressed anger and the erosion of confidence. Coping with these feelings – literally finding ways of staying sane and cheerful – lead, I propose, to two broad categories of psychological effect on dyslexic clients: inner- and outer-directed. Inner-directed, or 'internalizing', effects include stress, depression and anxiety and, on balance, are those 'most widely associated with learning disabilities' (Grigorenko 2001, p. 112). The outer-directed, or 'externalizing', effects, for which the linking evidence to dyslexia is more mixed, include conduct disorders, crime and suicide. All effects are complicated by the presence of ADHD.

The inner-directed effects of dyslexia

Stress

Is dyslexia linked to stress?

All dyslexics have some form of stress-related disorder. There is no such person as a stress-free dyslexic. Stress rides in the slipstream of dyslexia.

The counsellor can usefully approach the nature of dyslexic stress from the perspectives of (1) post-traumatic stress disorder (PTSD) and (2) the theory of 'daily hassles'.

How do dyslexics acquire PTSD?

Most dyslexic children do not realize that they have a problem until some new and traumatic incident enters their lives.

This can be the sudden exclusion from their peer group, the shocking, intense anger of a teacher or parent, or the physical thump of a bully. It can also be the sudden shock of realizing something unidentifiable is terribly wrong – a feeling that compares to the cold horror experienced at the news of a loved one's death or the confirmation of a fatal illness.

These events sear into the memory and retain their potency well into adult life.

One client recalled how, one day – without warning or explanation – she was separated from her friends and placed in a lonely, alien classroom of strangely behaved children and given infantile games, only to be immediately spurned by her old friends in all subsequent play times. Another remembers the exact details of location and weather on the day he received the first of many group chants of 'spastic'. A man in his fifties still has nightmares about the bulging eyes of a teacher who, long ago, leapt forward at him, mouth inches from his face, to yell that he was a 'silly, stupid, lazy, idle little git', even while he struggled to produce the best work he could.

The literature on dyslexic experience is full of these memories – but the consistent feature for many dyslexic clients is their suddenness. Clients record how things happened 'out of the blue' and how – suddenly – the world changed irrevocably for the worse.

What is also frequently observed is how such incidents mark the difference between one life and the next – pre- and post-dyslexia – an experience which compares to that of abused children who often see the first abusive act as marking off the final time in their life when they felt safe.

The explicit suddenness of these events means that, in one moment, the world is safe and predictable and, in the next, it is dangerous and random. In these instances, the dyslexic is traumatized as surely as if he were crushed in a car accident or hit by an unseen assailant. His life may then be marked by all the classic symptoms of post-traumatic stress disorder (PTSD).

There are two types of PTSD: Type 1 (an acute, single-impact traumatic event) and Type II, or 'Complex', PTSD (the product of a series of traumatic events or prolonged exposure to a stress or stressors). Dyslexic children, in my experience, can have both types at once. The psychological research on PTSD is immense: one review accessed over 3,000 computerized citations for the acronym PTSD. There are a few excellent recent reviews (Perrin et al. 2000, Stallard et al. 1999, Rose 2002), which also include the DSM IV Criteria for PTSD.

What are the behavioural effects of PTSD?

Victims of PTSD re-experience traumas through repetitive and intrusive thoughts. These are unbidden and random but occur mainly in quiet times or when falling asleep.

Small reminders trigger off vivid recollections, the experience changing with age and maturity. For example, while adults may have visual flashbacks, very young children do not and are more likely to show dissociative phenomena, numbing or traumatic amnesia. Some adult dyslexics can be affected by the smell of a pencil. Some will even avoid driving past schools.

PTSD also has considerable co-morbidity, including a lifetime link with major depression (48%), alcohol or drug abuse (65%), generalized anxiety disorder (16%) and panic disorder (11%). Panic attacks, hyper-vigilance and anxiety are common (Scott and Stradlin 2000).

There is no obvious pattern to how long the effects of PTSD last. Yule et al. (2000) found that a quarter of some trauma survivors had not recovered after five years, and a third after eight years. Around 59% of sufferers warranted a lifetime diagnosis of PTSD.

What are the psychological effects of PTSD?

The central effect is the dramatic rewriting of a person's script.

The world is no longer safe. 'Within an instant, the social world becomes a dangerous place, one in which people are potential threats to your safety' (Goleman 1995, p. 202). I see this so often in dyslexic clients: their hyper-vigilance, reactivity and constant anxiety that something terrible will happen.

Another significant effect involves flashbacks to the traumatic experience. In this respect, it is notable that there are frequent references in the literature to dyslexic people slipping rapidly into past experiences when faced with stress-producing situations (see Miles and Varma 1995, Riddick et al. 1999).

This effect is also much worse if the trauma occurred when the person felt totally helpless – as often happens with a young child isolated in a school environment, far from home and help: 'The element of helplessness is what makes a given event *subjectively* overwhelming' (Goleman 1995, p. 204).

What is 'Complex' (or Type II) PTSD?

This occurs when the survivor has had to adapt to the effects of long-term abuse, and it is found in survivors of prolonged trauma.

It is especially relevant to dyslexics, many of whom have endured years of bullying by teachers, peers, parents and siblings. Rigby (2002), for example, quotes a Swedish study where victims of workplace bullying have had to be treated in a Swedish rehabilitation clinic for PTSD. Their character had undergone drastic changes as the result of this long-term, severe victimization (Leymann and Gustaffson 1996).

The specific effects of Complex PTSD trauma include the immobilizing, dissociated effects witnessed in victims of child sexual abuse. I have observed this effect in severely traumatized dyslexics, some as young as nine.

At particular risk, are conscientious, intelligent dyslexics who are driven to succeed despite excessive bullying and critical teacher or parent pressure. Their anxious fear of work leads to a nightmare sequence of inability to concentrate, further anxiety, lack of sleep, inability to concentrate and so on. I have known such dyslexic clients to become almost catatonic, referred to doctors and therapists after being found rocking, staring at the wall for hours on end, dissociated and shut down.

Dissociation is a severe response but, in some ways, it is also a sensible, adaptive answer to extreme anxiety and stress. Rose (2002) considers it an entirely logical defence.

Unfortunately, long-term stress can set up a pattern where a disassociated response is learned, particularly where the trauma is 'chronic and invasive and from which physical escape is not possible' (Walker et al. 1999, p. 366).

What are the physical effects of PTSD?

PTSD induces permanent physical changes in the brain and in the chemical responsiveness of the body (see Scott and Stradlin 2000 and Goleman 1995).

Of the many brain effects of trauma, the most marked is damage to the amygdala through the implanting of trigger memories. The traumatic experiences 'become memories emblazoned in the emotional circuitry' (Goleman 1995, p. 201). Another brain effect involves decreased hippocampal function from the effects of excessive stress hormones such as glucocorticoid. Decreased hippocampal function leads to behavioural inhibition and hyper-responsiveness. In chronic PTSD, there is an eventual decrease of glucocorticoid production and the body slowly becomes depleted.

Overall, 'exposure to an aversive experience lays down powerful memory traces that are difficult to extinguish, stored in a circuit in which the amygdala plays a basic central role, but that has thalamic, hippocampal and cortical components' (quoted in Rose 2002, p. 69). Glaser (2000), in a review of the physical effects of child abuse, concluded that the effects of PTSD were so serious that children with PTSD risk 'an impairment in their cognitive functioning' (p. 109).

Are dyslexics especially vulnerable to PTSD?

I think that they are.

For example, the effects of PTSD in traumatized children are also those commonly evident in dyslexic children, including 'dissociative reactions, difficulties with aspects of executive function and educational under-achievement' (op. cit., p. 107). Furthermore, both dyslexic children and PTSD sufferers demonstrate problems in memory and concentration.

The significance of this research is that it prompts two questions. Does the brain organization of dyslexic children make them more susceptible to a PTSD response to stress? Does the direction of PTSD exacerbate pre-existing tendencies in the dyslexia syndrome?

In this respect, the study by Perrin et al. (2000) is interesting. He describes how children affected by PTSD report difficulties in concentration, especially in schoolwork, and memory problems both in mastering new material and in retaining previously learned skills. Moradi et al. (1999) found that PTSD patients reported problems in memory, concentration, attention and sequencing/planning. They found that 77.8% of the PTSD subjects had memory problems (compared with 13.6% in controls), a proportion that is similar to that found in dyslexics.

What is also significant in Moradi's study is that the groups with the worst PTSD were also the worst readers, with the worst memory, with no link to depression and *with no difference on verbal IQ* (my italics). In other words, those worst affected by PTSD had clear dyslexic characteristics.

Tsui (1990) also found that PTSD was related to academic performance and assumed the PTSD affected the academic performance rather than the academic performance preceding the PTSD.

The net effect of this is to suggest that the counsellor might well consider PTSD to be a specific stress risk for dyslexic clients.

It also invites two interesting questions. First, are the detrimental psychological effects seen in dyslexics due to their dyslexia or the stress they have experienced? Is the effect of stress exacerbated in dyslexics because of their idiosyncratic brain organization?

Is PTSD ever cured?
Never entirely.

PTSD leaves permanent physical changes in the brain, and some victims of PTSD will carry the effects of their trauma all their lives, even to the extent of permanent personality change. They 'may never be the same biologically' (Goleman 1995, p. 204), and it has to be accepted that life for them has changed forever.

Sufferers from PTSD can become a different person and, 'in contrast to most other emotional disorders, they suffer an abrupt discontinuity of identity. Close relatives and friends become acutely aware of this change' (Scott and Stradlin 2003, p. 72). There is usually a split autobiography so that the safe world up to the trauma is lost. For the sufferer, whatever the therapy they use, there will also always be a waiting twinge of fear. 'Emotional learning is lifelong' (Goleman 1995, p. 214).

This is a hard burden to bear for a sufferer who acquires PTSD as the result of a natural disaster. How much worse it must be if the victim of PTSD knows that their suffering was avoidable.

Dyslexics who incur PTSD through their school experiences must be very, very angry that this type of institutionalized abuse has caused such enormous and permanent psychological damage.

What are the protective factors against PTSD?
The child's personality and his family – particularly his mother.

Regarding the child's personality, Stallard et al. (1999) observe: 'The child's subjective appraisal of the situation appears to be an important mediating factor and may explain why some children can be significantly affected by objectively minor traumas' (p. 1075).

As for family effects, Rutter (1975) showed that it was not the event but how a child's family functioned afterwards that influenced the child's long-term adjustment. The mother's initial reaction was very important. If her distress was extreme, it influenced the child's later distress, not least because it deprived her child of a caretaker for his own distress. On the other hand, calm, coping maternal reaction cooled the burn of trauma before it could cause deeper damage.

What is important to remember is that PTSD does not have to be the inevitable response to terrible and unexpected events: 'the majority of individuals exposed to a trauma do not develop the disorder' (Perrin et al. 2000, p. 277). DSM IV prevalence rates go between 3% and 58% of exposure responses. Furthermore, PTSD 'is certainly less prevalent than would be expected given that traumatic events affect anything from 40% to 70% of the population' (op. cit., p. 277).

Protective factors are, therefore, most important, and some dyslexic clients, given the same apparent traumatic stress, will develop psychopathology, while others will not.

What is the counselling response to PTSD?

PTSD is a serious mental health condition, as bad as any major psychiatric disorder, and, as Rose (2002) emphasizes, the formation of the therapeutic bond is essential.

PTSD responds well to Cognitive Behavioural Therapy (CBT), and this is the treatment of choice. In CBT, the client's perception of loss of control, as well as all the automatic thoughts of helplessness, can be challenged and a sense of control retaught (see Chapter 12).

There are some therapists who favour the importance of narrative rehearsal; of recreating the initial trauma in the safety of a secure therapeutic relationship. They restructure the 'story', and shift the client's role in it from 'victim' to 'survivor' and, thence, to 'thriver' roles.

Narrative therapy and CBT must, however, be carefully managed with a dyslexic client who might have severe problems with sequencing. Usefully, memories of the PTSD are usually stored in visual, crude, preverbal form that dyslexic clients can access more easily than others. For this reason, art therapy can be a valuable adjunct.

One problem with PTSD is that the client will often operate a powerful denial that can lead to a unique and disruptive transference. Victims may deny the condition or find it hard to talk about. Another problem is that many PTSD sufferers also feel cut off from others. In both these instances, group work can be especially useful, particularly if such clients feel more at ease with other traumatized victims. It is certainly my experience that many victims of bullying are liberated by hearing similar experiences from others.

Rose (2002) reviews a useful approach to PTSD counselling that utilizes the idea that trauma memories of the event are sorted at two levels. There are verbally accessible memories (VAMs), which are superficial, conscious and contain details and feelings about the event. There are also situationally accessible memories (SAMs), which are located at an unconscious level without verbal access but are triggered automatically when the context is similar to the trauma. VAMs are best accessed through the counselling relationship and SAMs by CBT. VAMs should be accessed before SAMs – the counsellor before CBT – otherwise anger, fear or shame will block the retrieval of the habituated responses.

What is the theory of 'daily hassle' stress?

This stress is almost the complete opposite of PTSD. It is also more perva-sive, to the extent that stress research has identified that small, wearing, demanding incidents – 'daily hassles' – are even more perilous in the stress lexicon than major life events.

Daily hassles are not seen in trivial terms (Lu 1991). The earliest research conceptualized them as 'salient and harmful or threatening to the endors-er's well-being' (Lazarus 1984, p. 375). The other main characteristic about these insidious and persistent 'hassles' is that they are endlessly present in the sufferer's life. They are the psychological equivalent of living perma-nently in a cloud of small, biting mosquitoes. Significantly, the drift of such research has found that minor daily stressors provide a powerful prediction of psychological distress, and they 'outperform life events' as predictors of both anxiety and stress (Chamberlain and Zika 1990, p. 47).

Furthermore, they are not simply the downstream effects of major life events but independent predictors of mental health outcome so that, com-pared to life-events, daily hassles are 'better predictors of symptom development, overall health status and energy levels' (McNamara 2000, p. 12).

Do daily hassles cause stress to dyslexics?

Yes. I would say that small daily inconveniences cause more stress to dyslex-ics than anything else.

Like the frustrating dodging of pedestrians which slows our progress on a busy street, or the endless tiny adjustments our body makes on a long train journey, these daily hassles are wearing beyond belief. Even 50 years ago, the Danish neurologist Knud Hermann, in one of the first texts on dyslexia ('word blindness'), noted: 'It is exceedingly difficult for the normal person to picture all the social difficulties which word blindness can cause. Even when his condition is only moderately severe, the word-blind person is aware of it daily and in innumerable ways. His difficulties extend from trivialities, which are of little practical importance but are embarrassing, to serious occupational disabilities' (Hermann 1959, p. 148).

Morgan and Klein (2000) observe that adults who have only minor dyslexia are placed under extra stress through the constant effort needed to perform ordinary, daily tasks, from reading instructions on a packet to working out what people are saying.

To a dyslexic, the effect of missing a bus, for the tenth time in a month, through lateness and misreading of the timetable might be more stressful than being on that bus when it crashes into a bridge.

Daily hassles also make you ill. Meade et al. (2001) found that the fre-quency of negative life events was associated with greater illness among 12-to 14-year-olds.

Are daily hassles general or particular?
They are always relevant to a particular group.

Chamberlain and Zika (1990), in a review of this literature, concluded that concerns were appropriate to age, occupation, the social visibility of the hassle and the person's retrospective dysfunction. Much as you would expect, the elderly were hassled over health, young mothers over meals and students over work. Overall, differences in concerns 'are relevant to the personal and social situations of individuals' (op. cit., p. 470). This only serves to emphasize how important it is for the counsellor to see the world through dyslexic eyes. What is a hassle to a dyslexic may not be the slightest problem for you.

My experience is also that the degree to which an apparently innocuous event becomes a daily hassle will increase with the severity of the client's dyslexia, and his short-term memory problems in particular.

What common causes of daily stress are also associated with dyslexia?
When junior children are asked to rank the most stressful things that they can think of, at least 12 of the 16 stressors – such as getting lost, being left alone, being ridiculed in class, tests and examinations, breaking or losing things, being different, performing in public – are all associated with the dyslexic experience (Winkley 1996). With dyslexics, these same stressors retain their potency well into adulthood and – because of the power of early trauma – have the means to disrupt dyslexics all their life.

Is there a 'final straw' with daily hassles?
Yes. Whereas PTSD has a sudden and dramatic effect, daily hassles have the 'straw on the camel's back' effect.

Like a malignancy, daily hassles build up insidiously and can suddenly break through the psychological skin when coping mechanisms critically overload and fail. Sandberg et al. (2001) observe that 'different symptoms often begin at different times, [and] ... there may be a considerable time gap between the first appearance of symptoms and the first evidence of significant social impairment resulting from disorder' (p. 524).

While not everyone will respond in this way – after all, as Sandberg et al. observe, there are far more life events than disorder onsets – the study did identify the characteristics of those individuals most at risk. Vulnerable individuals had 'one carrying long-term threat' and had an 'accumulation of acute life events, together with associated chronic psychosocial adversity, and genetic risk' (p. 531). These are all characteristics associated with dyslexia, and I have no doubt that many dyslexics are extremely vulnerable to the 'last straw' of stress. For a counsellor, this research also provides a caution regarding any 'innocuous' presenting reason for a dyslexic client's visit.

Depression

What is the evidence on depression among dyslexics?
Not a lot, unfortunately.

There is no doubt that some dyslexics, some of the time, feel depressed, but there is not much hard evidence on the specific link between dyslexia and depression. Like an emotional quark, some dyslexic depression clearly exists, but it has defied accurate measurement of its true nature, not least because the research does not distinguish between low mood and clinical depression, nor use gradations of severity in self-reports of depression.

There are other problems:

Existing research is not clear in its conclusions

In her review of published research on all learning disabilities and depression, Heath (2001) examines evidence for a link but finds that 'a critical analysis of the literature' fails to support evidence that 'children and adolescents with learning disability are at greater risk for depression' (p. 4). She found that the research was minimal, often overly diverse and plagued by methodological problems, making even very basic generalizations impossible.

Also, much of the work was on general reading disability, and the results were not clear-cut.

Mixed samples

Research that examines the link between reading disability and internalizing symptoms, such as depression (e.g. Willcutt and Pennington 2000), usually includes children with a variety of disabilities rather than just dyslexia. Many of these children with reading disability had other reasons for their depression – such as very adverse home circumstances.

Mediating variables

When research does suggest a direct relationship between reading difficulty – specific or general – and depression, there are usually mediating variables (Rutter 1975). Of these, the most confounding variable is ADHD and its further links with conduct disorder. (This important point is discussed in more detail later.) Duane (1991), for example, reported a threefold increase in psychiatric diagnoses in children with dyslexia and depression but most also had conduct disorder. As Fawcett (1995) observes of this rather muddled type of research; 'Of course, it is difficult to establish whether this is a cause, an effect or simply correlated with dyslexia' (p. 14).

Definition of depression

Research on depression in dyslexics is further compromised by the identification of what constitutes 'depression' in dyslexic children. For example, research has indicated that parent, teacher and peer reports of children's depression may conflict with the child's own report (Heath 2001). Although Heath concludes: 'the self-report of the child must take precedence since depression is an internalized disorder' (p. 31), not all researchers are this careful.

This is even more of a problem with dyslexics in whom it is easy to infer depression. The natural dyslexic demeanour, including a rather flat expression and slow, non-reactive responses, that might be read as symptomatic of early depression in a non-dyslexic, are present in normal, non-depressed dyslexic behaviour (also, see Chapter 9).

This problem was illustrated in work by Boetsch et al. (1996), who found that teachers and parents reported depression in dyslexic children that, on the basis of the children's self-reports of depressive symptomatology, was not present.

Correlation or cause?

Most of the evidence on dyslexia and depression is correlative rather than causative. To confuse matters further, the correlations move in both directions. For example, learning disabilities are commonly observed in depressed individuals, and depressive disorders elevated in youths with learning disabilities (Grigorenko 2001). We do not know exactly why this is the case.

Additionally, Grigorenko observes from research that between 14% and 32% of youth with learning disabilities are depressed. Yet this must mean that between 86% and 78% of youths with learning disabilities are not depressed at all. They may be stressed and they may be anxious – most dyslexics are – but they are not *depressed*, which is a completely different affliction altogether. So what is the cause of depression in that minority of reading-disabled youth – since reading disability alone is not an adequate explanation?

The missing variable

In the habitual focus on simple reading failure as a cause of dyslexic depression, other potentially causative variables are ignored. Certainly, it is not helpful simply to blame depression on reading difficulties – since many children with reading disability are clearly not depressed.

What is ignored is the role of relationship failure and social isolation. This is a pity since what is important about the evidence on depression in *all* children is that the main mediating variable is almost always a problem with relationships. Depressed children are those who are rejected or isolated by their peers, and who often have 'deficits in social skills and interpersonal relationships' (Kennedy et al. 1989, p. 562). Since relational problems are endemic among dyslexic children, it is likely – research methodologies notwithstanding – that it is the most socially unskilled and isolated dyslexic children and adults who are most likely to be those who experience depression.

Anxiety and fear

Is there more evidence of anxiety in dyslexics?
Yes, there is clear evidence of anxiety disorders among those with learning disabilities and – specifically – dyslexics (Grigorenko 2001), although there exist the same caveats about research design and direction of effect as with depression.

Far more research is available on anxiety than depression probably because anxiety disorders in general are the most prevalent disorder for all children and adolescents: around 20% of adolescents are affected. 'Anxiety is a significant problem among children and adolescents being neither uncommon nor necessarily harmless' (Legrand et al. 1999, p. 954).

Importantly, it is largely a response to outside stimuli. Although both family and genetic influences are implicated, anxiety: 'is almost entirely attributable to environmental influences unique to each individual' (op. cit., p. 953).

Anxiety is not an innocuous disorder, even at a sub-clinical level, and what is not often appreciated is that anxiety can occur in response to subliminal stressors (Kemp-Wheeler and Hill 1987). This may be why panic attacks can seem to arise for no obvious reasons. I also believe that subliminal response might account for why some traumatized dyslexics have to endure a malevolent form of free-floating anxiety that roars out of nowhere in any situation involving change or literacy which, in most of the modern world, is everywhere.

Anxiety can present in a stunning variety of ways, including irritability, restlessness, poor concentration, incoherence even to the degree of being unable to say a word, fear of going mad or being rooted to the spot. Physical symptoms include dizziness, faintness, sweating, tremor, tension in neck, chest or abdomen, nausea, shortness of breath, diarrhoea, increased urination, palpitations, hyperventilation. It even leads to spasms, fits, tachycardia, insomnia and altered states of consciousness (Gomez 1991).

I have seen most of these symptoms in dyslexic clients at one time or another. Panic attacks are the most dramatic, and fear of going mad the saddest.

Anxiety is also linked with alcoholism, and over 60% of alcoholics, mainly men, start drinking because of anxiety symptoms. In this respect, I have certainly encountered a remarkable degree of alcohol and drug-related anxiety conditions in both dyslexic men and women. In this respect, I would estimate that, as a group, they are significantly more likely to use drink and drugs to cope with their anxiety than non-dyslexics are.

Of the specific research on dyslexia, these are useful points for a counsellor:

What is normal anxiety?

It is dangerous to respond to the intuitive assumption that dyslexics will present with this or that internalizing disorder and to lose sight of the fact that anyone of that age might present with a similar symptom.

This does not just apply to dyslexics. It is a characteristic of counselling that the mere fact that someone has presented for therapy invites us to misread normality for pathology. Sometimes, we need to keep a clear head about whether we are seeing a problematic symptom or talking up a natural characteristic that may be utterly unremarkable for the client's age or circumstances.

For example, I see many dyslexic children who are anxious and fearful as a result of bullying and who report frightening dreams involving attacks by sharks and wolves. I also see dyslexic children who exhibit other fears that are normal in child development, and it would be careless – if easy – to make the wrong associations.

The literature on fear and anxiety in children frequently cautions us on this. Ollendick et al. (2002), in their review of research on this issue, emphasize the normality of fear and anxiety during different stages of a child's development. Gomez (1991) reminds us: 'Everyone is anxious some of the time – survival depends upon alertness to danger' (p. 68).

Equally, we must distinguish between a rational human response to a real threat, as opposed to the irrational, neurotic and often learned response of excessive anxiety that has become an end in itself.

This is particularly relevant for dyslexics who may be experiencing a very real threat to themselves. There is anxiety, and there is rational fear. We should decide 'whether the nature of the problem is actually unrealistic anxiety as opposed to fear and stress regarding real threats such as bullying, violence and abandonment' (Dadds and Barrett 2001, p. 1003).

What are the common causes of anxiety in childhood?

There are a number of writers who provide lists of anxieties specific to children (e.g. Winkley 1996). In these lists, fear of isolation and abandonment are common and understandable. Two sources of more complex ideas are suggested by Winnicott (1965) and Jacobs (1986). In both these texts, I am struck by how almost every one of these childhood anxieties are particularized in the dyslexic condition.

Winnicott, for example, lists these basic anxieties in children:

- going to pieces
- falling for ever
- having no relationship to the body
- having no orientation
- complete isolation because of there being no means of communication

Jacobs adds to this

- not understanding
- not knowing
- being disorientated in new circumstances
- fear of the notion of emptiness or a vacuum

Jacobs believes that these anxieties are dispelled by the creative illusion of the breast (these are very early anxieties revisited by an older child).This theory might cast some light on the infantilized and mother-bound tendency of dyslexics, discussed in more detail in Chapters 6, 8 and 9.

What is excessive anxiety?

The DSM IV definition of excessive anxiety or phobia is when a client's reactions are way out of proportion to the demands of the situation, cannot be explained or reasoned away, are beyond voluntary control or lead to an avoidance of the feared situation. Other important signs are that such fears persist over an extended period of time, are unadaptive or are not age- or stage-specific.

Excessive anxiety occurs a lot in dyslexics, and it is a serious and disabling condition that distresses and frightens the client. It is overwhelmingly the presenting reason for referral either by the dyslexic or his doctor.

Anxiety often leads to panic attacks in both dyslexic children and adults, and some of the panic attacks can occur in the counselling session. These can arise when there is an unexpected retrieval of traumatic memories, or may be sparked by some innocuous event or noise. It can also, as noted above, occur for no obvious reason. I would advise any counsellor working with dyslexic clients to know how to act in the event of a panic attack since the effects can be appalling and, in severe cases, imitate epileptic seizure.

Both adult and child dyslexics experience excessive anxiety in uncontained, unsafe and unsupported circumstances. This is why it surges out of control in periods of change and transition: from school to university, university to job, in promotion or moving house. Any fear of abandonment or loss – particularly of relationships – tends to trigger uncontrolled anxiety in dyslexics, bringing back old memories of isolation in childhood, with dramatic psychological effect.

Is there a link in dyslexia between levels of anxiety and intelligence?
Yes – and not in the expected direction.

One of the most significant findings in the research by Hales (1994) on the behavioural aspects of dyslexia was that there was an inverse relationship between IQ and anxiety in dyslexic children. Low-IQ dyslexic children from middle-school years upwards tended to have higher levels of anxiety. Hales identified the intelligent use of coping strategies as a factor protecting the higher-IQ sample.

Do physical and psychosomatic symptoms of anxiety affect dyslexics?
Yes – but the evidence is sparse.

My experience is that a small minority of dyslexic children will have masked their anxiety to the extent that only psychosomatic symptoms will give a clue to their problems. Porter and Rourke (1985), for example, also found that 10% of a sample of learning-disabled children had somatic problems, such as migraines or stomach upsets, despite scoring normally on an inventory of social and emotional functioning.

Do dyslexic children suffer from bed-wetting (enuresis)?
Again, this is not the subject of much research, but I would say that bed-wetting in dyslexic children is common, usually as they start to have problems in school.

Miles (1993) writes of a dyslexic child who, at age eight, was 'still bed-wetting and full of nervous twitches' (p. 144), another wet the bed until age nine. On an anecdotal basis, I believe that enuresis is linked to dyslexia, and I was interested to read a recent review (Von Gontard 1998) which noted that enuresis was associated with 'delayed motor and speech milestones' (p. 443), both of which are associated with dyslexia.

I found no studies on dyslexia and enuresis, but I would guess that it is associated with about 30% of dyslexic children – some of it very severe, including total soaking of the bed, every night, for months on end. This causes stress both from the act of wetting itself and also from the reactions of others, including teasing by peers and siblings and ill-disguised parental irritation. It is just one more of the 'daily hassles' to which I referred earlier.

Again, it is essential to know what is common and normal. Rutter (1975) observes that it is a 'very common problem in the school child' (p. 290) and, at seven years, one child in five still wets his bed occasionally and, at ten years, one in fourteen does so. It reduces largely by adolescence to only one child in 33.

A certain amount of enuresis in children has a purely physiological origin due to delay in the development of the biological brain mechanism needed for bladder control. There is also a genetic link, so it runs in families. Day-wetting is principally a physical condition, but night-wetting less so.

What interests the counsellor is the important psychological element to enuresis.

Rutter (1975) estimates that about a quarter to a third of enuretic children have emotional or behavioural difficulties – a rate well above that in the general population.

Von Gontard also reports that the associated rate of psychiatric disorders in enuresis was in the range of 15%-30%, significantly higher than controls. In paediatric settings the rate was 29% and in child psychiatric hospitals 70%. Even infrequent wetting of one to six episodes a year was linked to anxiety.

Von Gontard, does not, however, make a clear distinction between the physical and psychological causes. He concludes that there is a biological predisposition that is activated during stress. In other words, those without this predisposition will demonstrate stress in other ways. He found that about 20% of enuretics get dry with specific encouragement. Of the other measures, alarm treatment (a moisture-sensitive electrical pad that wakes the child by buzzer or vibration) remains the most effective. Dryness was attained by alarm in 66% of cases, and 51% remained dry after five months.

Significantly for the therapist, the success rate for verbal psychotherapies was only 21%, and 11% on follow up. Pharmacological treatment was associated with an even lower success rate and a higher relapse rate than alarm treatment.

Do dyslexics experience obsessive-compulsive disorder (OCD)?

Strictly speaking, this is not a disorder linked directly to dyslexia. It is only linked through the anxiety route.

If a dyslexic child is predisposed to OCD, and he becomes anxious, then the OCD will flare up. In over 20 years of counselling, I have seen just a handful of dyslexic children with OCD, but the symptoms can be acutely distressing to witness. I recall one dyslexic child whose work anxieties were linked to obsessions about evil. His endless hand washing in very hot water, followed by furious scrubbing to dry them, left his hands like raw meat.

They were so sore that he had to hold them up in the air in front of him, like a surgeon. Medication made an immediate difference to him in a few days and a dramatic difference in a few weeks.

This is an anxiety-related disorder that originates in childhood, and at least half of the adults who get OCD already had it as children (Heyman 1997).

It is not common, and only affects around 2% of all children and adolescents. Shafran (2001) found, of children referred for an anxiety disorder, only 18% had OCD as their only diagnosis. OCD is, however, extremely serious, presenting, in its own right, as a cause of suicide.

The obsessions and compulsions are repetitive compulsive acts that the person feels driven to perform according to certain rules. The purpose of the action is to prevent a dreaded event or to reduce distress – which is excessive. Compulsive acts include washing, repeating, checking, ordering and counting. Obsessive concerns include family catastrophes, contamination and sexual or religious preoccupations. With adults, the most common features are checking, symmetry, ordering, cleanliness, washing and hoarding. Obsessive touching is the most common in children.

OCD is considered to be part of a spectrum that includes Body Dysmorphic Disorder, Tourette's syndrome and eating disorders.

OCD is probably the most acutely distressing of all anxiety disorders. It is highly disabling, associated with chronic psychiatric co-morbidity and long-term social impairment. The sufferers are in an almost unending state of unbearable torment.

Counsellors would be wise to give this presenting disorder a wide berth. It is a medical disorder, and general counselling alone is very unlikely to be effective. Heyman (1997), in a review of OCD for the *British Medical Journal*, observes that, while it is a 'favourite candidate for psychodynamic interpretations, the mounting evidence is for a neuropsychiatric basis' (p. 44) to guide treatments.

The best treatment has been found to be with drugs, such as Prozac and Seroxat, and cognitive behavioural treatments (CBT), instead of or alongside medication (Heyman 1997, Shafran 2001).

CBT treatment includes exposure, response prevention and relaxation training. A recent research development also suggests that OCD might be linked to autoimmune disorder, with antibiotic treatment showing good results.

The average age of onset of this terrible disorder is 10.3 years, with most sufferers starting it before reaching their eighteenth birthday. Although it is not closely associated with the onset of dyslexic symptoms, these will exacerbate it.

There are good specialist units for OCD including that at the Maudsley Hospital, London.

Is anxiety a protective factor for dyslexic children?
Yes. Being anxious keeps dyslexic children out of trouble.

Anxious children are much less likely to be linked with any sort of externalizing or problem behaviour. All their negative affect goes inwards rather
than outwards. Pine et al. (2000), for example, found that conduct disorder
was linked with low anxiety, and high anxiety and an inhibited tempera-
ment were negatively associated with conduct disorders. They concluded
that clinicians need not be worried about severe behavioural problems
among children with social phobia.

Anxious children also have a lower risk for delinquency. More recently,
Elliott and Thomas (2003) reviewed a research project tracking 12,000 people over 30 years. The 'highly significant' findings indicated that, whereas
badly behaved children were more likely to turn to crime, be unemployed,
unhappy or dissatisfied in later life, children who demonstrated high levels
of internalizing behaviour, who were often worried, cried a lot and were
fussy and fearful 'had a tendency to develop into successful adults'.

The externalizing effects of dyslexia

Conduct disorder

Are there higher incidences of conduct disorder in dyslexic children?
On the surface, it looks like this could be the case.

There is, for example, a great deal of academic research on conduct disorder, and much on the link between conduct disorder and general
reading problems.

Hill (2002), for example, reviewed evidence that children with reading
problems exhibit more frequent emotional and behavioural difficulties
than children without reading problems. He found evidence for high rates
of reading problems and general academic failure in samples of conduct-
disordered or delinquent children. Children with reading deficits were
nearly five times more likely to exhibit antisocial behaviours than were children in the general population.

Individuals with reading disability are also significantly more likely than
individuals without reading disability to meet criteria for attention deficit
hyperactivity disorder, oppositional defiant disorder, conduct disorder,
overanxious disorder and depression. One review concluded that reading
disability is associated with 'significant elevations on all measures of internalising and externalising symptoms' (Willcutt and Pennington 2000, p.
1045).

On closer examination, however, the evidence linking conduct disorder
to dyslexia, specifically, is not clear-cut:

Cause and effect are easily muddled

This includes two possible areas of confusion. First, reading disabilities are not the same as dyslexia. Second, conduct disorder that is linked to any reading disability may also be mediated by wider socio-economic and family problems, as well as the independent presence of ADHD.

Correct identification of dyslexia is missing from the available studies

It is the discrepancy between IQ and reading ability that hints at the presence of dyslexia, and this is not included in most studies of reading disability and conduct disorder. This is a point that Farrell et al. (1999) make in their review of the educational attainments of pupils with behavioural disorder. Clinicians 'should establish whether there is a significant discrepancy between a child's cognitive ability and academic attainment' (p. 50) in reaching conclusions about treatment. In fact, using such discrepancy measurements in their study, Farrell et al. found that only 12.3% of the Emotional and Behavioural Difficulties (EBD) children in their sample specifically had dyslexia.

Types of conduct disorder may differ with reading disability

There is also the suggestion that the type of conduct disorders associated with dyslexia are not as serious as those associated with general reading disability. Riddick (1996) notes that the behavioural problems of dyslexics mainly took the form of inattentiveness and restlessness, while the more extreme behavioural difficulties, commonly seen as conduct disorders, were far less frequent. The suggestion is that, where the reading disability is principally a dyslexic one, problems largely follow the disorder rather than precede it and are well attacked through literacy and social-skills training.

Farrell et al. (1999) found that those pupils in their sample who were accurately identified with only dyslexia were relatively easy to treat, with literacy teaching quickly producing changes in self-esteem and behaviour.

It is also true that many dyslexics survive conduct disorders without long-term harm, when dyslexia is the main difficulty rather than the more complicated factors of socio-economic deprivation or links with ADHD. Matty (1997) noted 'it is true that a surprising number of well-adjusted and successful dyslexics admit to periods of involvement, in varying degrees, with delinquent behaviour' (p. 8).

Dyslexia and crime

Is there a link between general reading disability and crime?
Yes.

Different studies have found a link, and there is undoubted evidence of much higher literacy problems in prisoners than in the general population. For example, Svensson et al. (2001), noting that the connection between reading disability and juvenile delinquency 'is well established' (p. 62) went on to find that, among adult prisoners, the prevalence of reading disability and behaviour problems was higher than in the general population.

In the UK, 60–70% of the prison population (of 65,000) have literacy levels so low that they are ineligible for 96% of all jobs.

Seeman (2002) also reviews American evidence that 95% of juveniles had more than average learning difficulties at the time of their arrest, and that up to 92.8% of young offenders in New York were illiterate in the basic subjects of English and mathematics. She cites an article in the *New York Times* that three out of four juvenile delinquents had learning problems.

Is there a link between dyslexia and criminal behaviour?
Not necessarily. Here, too, the link is too tenuous: 'dyslexia on it own is insufficient as an explanation of criminal behaviour, as the number of dyslexics who turn to crime is relatively small' (Miles 2001, p. 58).

Again, the problem is the width of definition. Dyslexia is not the only type of reading disability, and confusing dyslexia with other reading problems does not help to clarify this issue. Over-generalized statements such as that by Lundberg (1995) – 'The incidence of dyslexia among criminal groups seems to be very high, although the causal factors are far from certain' (p. 47) – contribute little to our understanding of the links between criminality and dyslexia.

Nonetheless, this link is hotly debated: 'Today the relationship between dyslexia and anti-social or criminal behaviour is arguably one of the most controversial in the field of dyslexia' (Kirk and Reid 2001, p. 77), and specialist dyslexia journals and conferences have discussed the issue at length (Miles 2001).

On the one hand, there is definitely some respectable evidence that the prison rates of dyslexia are relatively high. Turner (2000a), for example, found that 17.5% of the inmates in Feltham Prison 'met stringent criteria for dyslexia' (p. 5), while Kirk and Reid (2001) found that 31% of a near-random sample of probationers was found to be dyslexic. These rates compare to general estimates of dyslexia in the population of up to 10%.

On the other hand, some research disputes this. One recent study on institutionalised juvenile delinquents concluded: 'The high prevalence of reading and writing disabilities seems primarily to be related to social and cultural factors, home backgrounds, limited school attendance and poor self-esteem rather than to constitutional problems of a dyslexic nature' (Svensson et al. 2001, p. 62).

Is there help for dyslexic prisoners?
Yes – and it is very effective.

The Dyspel Pilot Project, which provided diagnoses and specialist tuition to dyslexic offenders, found that less than 5% of those diagnosed had had their dyslexia identified at school. Many were serious truants or sent to EBD schools with their dyslexia never having been diagnosed. 'Most told of very distressing memories of school including frequent public humiliation in front of their peers, and they described violent outbursts in response to frustration at not learning and being mocked, humiliated or called stupid' (Morgan and Klein 2000, p. 60).

Many prison inmates badly wanted to learn to read but many were intimidated, or unaware of support for them: 'Several spoke of standing outside colleges, too frightened to go in, certain they would be told they were too stupid to get on a course' (op. cit., p. 60).

Where literacy is easily available to prisoners, it is eagerly taken up.

For example, a project set up in September 1998 jointly by the BDA and the Pentonville Prison's Education Coordinator funded six computers and reading tuition. They were concerned whether dyslexic men with poor self-esteem and an embittered, cynical attitude towards education would want to come forward. The response was, however, very enthusiastic, and soon there was a waiting list. 'Students comment that, for the first time in their lives, they feel in control of their learning – leading to a boost in self-confidence and self-esteem. There are now plans to take the course into 13 other prisons' (Meridian 2002).

The PALS Project – a partnership between the Dyslexia Institute and the Nottinghamshire Probation Service – has had similar success with referral, assessment and teaching for dyslexic offenders (Apiafi 2001). The striking success of teaching literacy in prison was also the subject of a detailed report in *The Sunday Times* (23 February 2003).

The acquisition of literacy is clearly an effective antidote to re-offending among prisoners.

Studies in the USA, for example, show a 25% reduction in re-offending, by remediating problems of dyslexia in prisoners, and it is notable that the Director-General of the Prison Service in the United Kingdom has made a commitment to reduce the low levels of literacy in prison by 15% by 2005 (Meridian 2002), in order to reduce recidivism rates.

Social-skills instruction among dyslexic prisoners can also help. Breir (1994) showed that psychosocial training drastically reduced the chances of criminal relapse.

Why is dyslexia linked with crime?
There are a number of suggested reasons.

Alm and Andersen (1997), for example, believe that dyslexics turn away from a world that is 'inconsistent and difficult to handle' (p. 247). Acting out and revenge are understandable. Looking at the same point from another angle, it also may be that crime provides a source of money and self-respect for dyslexics who are usually marginalized in the world of conventional work. In this respect, crime becomes both a coping strategy and a useful ego-defence for a resourceful dyslexic.

The secondary effects of dyslexia also cause problems when dyslexics badly misread many social situations and get arrested. More specifically, dyslexics get into trouble when signing documents they cannot read or are involved in legal processes that they do not understand and cannot negotiate without confusion.

Morgan (1997), a probation officer, supports this latter view in a disturbing review of the ways in which a dyslexic can seriously disadvantage himself when caught up in the legal system. He mentions instances where dyslexics have become confused about times and dates, forgotten the order of events and unwittingly incriminated themselves by signing statements that they cannot read and which may not be a true account of what they intended to say.

Disorganization means that the correct day for a court appearance may be missed, and dyslexics may also not return to court at a later date because they forget and, anyway, will not be able to read court details on appearance or their offences on a charge sheet. Legal aid means filling in a form but, not only will they have problems understanding what the form requires, dyslexics will also be filling it in under stressful conditions, which, as we noted in Chapter 3, causes further difficulty

On the face of it, it is astonishing that the number of dyslexics who turn to crime, or unwittingly get incriminated, is as small as it is.

Attention Deficit Hyperactivity Disorder (ADHD)

Does ADHD increase the chances of a dyslexic having conduct disorder?

Yes.

On this issue, however, it is important to remember that dyslexic children are often inattentive due to the boredom and difficulty of being in school. This is not ADHD – it may simply be ADD (Attention Deficit Disorder) or just a natural squirminess and distractibility that are linked to being dyslexic and not to the more serious and physical condition of ADHD. Real ADHD is much more serious. It is a genetic and physiological disorder linked to brain function, and is often the main precipitator of severe behavioural problems in dyslexics who have both disorders.

The conduct disorder in ADHD comes from poor adaptive communication skills – which dyslexics also have – but which are mediated in ADHD through disruption, breaking of social norms, and aggressive, oppositional and hyperactive behaviour (Clark et al. 2002). One study, for example, found that children with hyperactivity problems find it difficult to gain acceptance by their peers, and their behavioural problems are maintained and can grow as a result of this rejection (Deater-Deckard 2001). Terwogt (2002) also found that friends would help sad children, but angry children were avoided and did not attract altruistic behaviour.

What is important is that we cannot assume that dyslexia alone leads to conduct problems, or that conduct problems are inevitable in dyslexia.

It is much more likely that dyslexia, when mediated by ADHD (or serious social-skills problems that are also linked to ADHD), leads to conduct problems but, when ADHD is removed, dyslexia is significantly less likely to be associated with conduct disorder. In fact, this uncomplicated form of dyslexia is more likely to be associated with internalizing, depressive, anxious or fearful symptoms (Willcutt and Pennington 2000, Grigorenko 2001).

Are dyslexics with ADHD more likely to commit crime?
Yes. There is some evidence that it is the link with ADHD that increases the chance of a dyslexic being in prison.

The dyslexia may be mediated by any acting-out, aggression or conduct disorder linked to hyperactivity. Babinski et al. (1999), for example, showed that hyperactivity, impulsivity and early conduct problems independently, as well as jointly, predicted a greater likelihood of having an arrest record: 'the symptoms of hyperactivity-impulsivity, but not inattention, contribute to the risk for criminal involvement over and beyond the risk associated with early conduct problems alone' (p. 347).

Interestingly, the study by Babinski et al. supported other research in finding that attention problems in childhood alone – which are associated more with straightforward dyslexia and not dyslexia/ADHD – do not seem to lead to later criminal activity.

Is it possible to counsel dyslexic children with ADHD?
Generally speaking, it is not a good idea.

Counselling alone is not best placed to help children with this distressing disorder, and it is almost impossible to operate in one-to-one counselling with ADHD children since they have a limited attention span, cannot keep still and find it hard to focus on feelings.

Counsellors must also establish, first, if true ADHD is present, as opposed to ADD or general inattentiveness. The first step, therefore, is to refer the child to a specialist paediatric psychiatrist because, if ADHD is present, the condition needs first to be controlled through pharmacological means. Prescribed drugs can markedly improve cognitive functioning, reading and spelling and have a significant positive effect on behaviour. Only when the medication is in place can therapy usefully proceed.

There is a good review of psychiatric and paediatric practice in ADHD treatment by Salmon and Kemp (2002). What is useful about this is that it also shows the proportion of paediatric specialists who use therapeutic techniques such as social-skills training (37%), cognitive therapies (38%), behaviour modification (81%) and parent training (58%), emphases that reflect best practice in ADHD treatments.

Suicide

Is dyslexia a cause of suicide?

Yes – but the exact route to suicide, and the numbers of dyslexic people who decide to kill themselves, are unknown.

Why a person attempts suicide is a complex issue, but there are some clear links between suicide and the circumstances linked to dyslexia, such as bullying, school failure, isolation, pressure to achieve academically, peer rejection and the impaired expression of feelings of frustration, depression, guilt and hostility (Thompson and Rudolph 1996, Harrington et al. 1994).

Other studies conclude more directly that: 'children with learning disabilities or other learning difficulties that cause constant frustration are more likely to attempt suicide [and] gifted children may attempt suicide because their advanced intellectual ability makes relating to children their own age difficult' (Thompson and Rudolph 1996, p. 446).

Suicide among dyslexics is often referred to but not in any detail. Peer (2002) put a note on the BDA forum asking whether parents and teachers had come across any stories of dyslexic children or adults who had committed suicide. Within two days, she had received six stories. Dyslexia affects children's whole lives, she observes, and 'these stories are heart breaking and should make all of us sit up and think ... we are dealing with human beings who are often fragile and vulnerable and for whom the ramifications of failure are enormous' (p. 32).

Riddick (1996) also described how children wanted to kill themselves as a direct consequence of the problems they were encountering because of their dyslexia. One mother said of her son: 'He wanted to be dead, there was nothing for him. He wanted his tie so he could hang himself' (p. 107).

Notably, Winkley (1996) observes that the number of attempted suicides increases during the school term and decreases during school holidays. It is also found that the number of attempts increases in May and June, just before the GCSE examinations. Children as young as ten have tried to kill themselves because of school pressures in tests and examinations, although, in most case of child suicide, depression is a predisposing factor (National Children's Bureau Factsheet 1996).

What is poignant, of course, is that dyslexic children who commit suicide rarely leave notes, because they cannot write.

What are the signs of suicidal tendency?

A depressed or suicidal child may be extremely quiet and withdrawn or highly active and agitated. Depression may also be masked by overactivity, gaiety or acting-out behaviour.

Personal loss, events that damage self-esteem or traumatic life crises can precipitate suicide. Winkley (1996) also notes the significance of 'last straw' events – often involving bullying and rejection – that usually follow on long-term stress. The decision to die is often impulsive.

Chronic sleeplessness, loss of appetite, withdrawal or any extreme behavioural change can also be taken as warning signs. Depression and severe mood disorder are important indicators, particularly if accompanied by worsening feelings of hopelessness, worthlessness or guilt. Risk of suicide remains for some time after episodes of mood disorder. Children with depression remain at high risk of suicide for protracted periods of time (Fisher et al. 1996).

What are the facts about suicide?

It is worth noting that suicide is quite rare.

In 1994, in the UK, five boys and two girls aged ten to 14 years and 65 males and 12 females aged 15 to 19 died as a result of suicide or self-inflicted injury. Parasuicide (self-harm) is much more common.

It has been suggested that 19,000 young people aged from ten to 14 are referred annually to hospital following parasuicidal self-poisoning or self-injury. Some 2,000 are between ten and 14, and mostly girls. Women are especially vulnerable to suicide attempt, and parasuicide occurs two or three times more often in females than males. Winkley (1996) reports that one in every 100 young women between 15 and 19 makes a suicide attempt. By contrast, actual suicide is a more male behavioural response.

The usual methods of parasuicide are poisoning and drug overdose. Hanging, jumping, drowning, shooting, drug overdose or inhalation of car fumes is the usual means of completed suicide. Men use more aggressive methods, such as hanging, girls favour overdosing, commonly with paracetamol. There is evidence of increased suicide among young men (19-24 years old), which increased by 78% between 1980 and 1990.

How do counsellors work with dyslexics and suicide?

Consideration of suicide by any client, particularly when details of the suicide are being rehearsed, is an unambiguous expression of extreme distress that must always be taken seriously by a counsellor.

The contemplation of suicide in a dyslexic client may also be a metaphor for wanting to escape when no other options are available. This is a common feeling among dyslexics who cannot escape from parental pressure, school failure and bullying, from both sides. Counselling may well defuse the problem and find some solutions.

Sometimes, however, the counsellor may have to take urgent, practical steps to avert a tragedy, including a rapid professional referral or contacting the client's doctor. Discussion in supervision, if there is time, may be needed to determine how far the counsellor wants to be proactive outside the normal counselling role, including, in the case of a child, contacting parents and school. Every counsellor will have their own professional opinion on what to do.

My default position is always to act. I will have been clear to my client at the beginning of counselling that I will discuss all possible options with them if I fear for their safety, but I will, in the end, take action.

Dyslexia – whatever its effects – is not worth dying for.

CHAPTER 8

Isolation

Summary

Unsought and unwanted isolation is a wretched feeling, and it taps into the most basic human fear of abandonment.

Notably, of stressful events imagined by junior children, loss and feeling lost were seen as the most stressful of all (Winkley 1996). Rowe (1984) refers to isolation as 'torture' (p. 369) and that the one thing that affects even the strongest characters is being isolated from all human contact. The longer the person is kept in isolation, the more serious and long-lasting the effects are. Tillich (1952) observes how any human most fears isolation: 'the despair of emptiness and meaninglessness' (p. 51), and Erich Fromm (2000) considered isolation the primary source of anxiety.

Isolation is one of the worst effects of being dyslexic, and is the principal cause of both adaptive and maladaptive coping strategies. Some dyslexics spend their entire lives isolated from others.

Those dyslexics who escape isolation – who are well integrated socially – have far fewer problems. Difficulty with reading is much less of a problem than being unable to form relationships. Those dyslexics who *only* have problems with reading do not have a higher frequency of internalizing symptoms than controls (Rourke and Fuerst 1996). Difficulty with reading is just failure, and people learn how to cope with failure and may even benefit from it.

Difficulty with relationships leads to loneliness, and this is far, far worse.

Isolation and dyslexia

How do dyslexics become isolated?
Dyslexics become isolated through a number of routes:

- Outward communication is faulty. Their own language-processing difficulties cause speech to logjam inside them, and their non-verbal
behaviour, which is an important adjunct to speech, contains disturbing
transmission errors. In the most severe cases of dyslexia, outward communication is almost nullified so that the dyslexic can present – totally
wrongly – as completely unresponsive or even autistic. It is as if all the
colours and passions of a great and vivid painting are trapped behind a
piece of plain, white card.
- Inward communication is faulty. Dyslexics find it hard to process incoming speech from other people. Information-processing delays and
cognitive problems mean that dyslexics take longer to receive and
understand what others say. In addition, dyslexics find it hard to read
non-verbal behaviour. They make the wrong interpretations of how
other people behave and then, unfortunately, act on it.
- Problems in literacy mean that the dyslexic child is separated within the
class or is withdrawn for 'remedial work', so he fails to integrate properly with his age group.

This generally poor communication with others means that dyslexics
have deficient 'social cognition' or 'theory of mind'. This is the ability to
decode human behaviour and intention. High social cognition is directly
related to popularity and the ability to make friends, whereas low social
cognition is linked to rejection and bullying. The presence of ADHD just
makes this worse.

These problems make dyslexics anxious and depressed, and depression,
in itself, is a sufficient cause for rejection by others. Depressed children are
universally rejected by their peers.

The net effect is that dyslexics, from an early age, start the process of
being 'othered'. This characteristic threads through the dyslexic experience
and is considered to be a central feature of dyslexic isolation (Pollak 1999).

Indeed, dyslexics often report feeling different from others at a very
early age. For example, an Israeli study found that dyslexic boys had significantly higher levels of loneliness than their non-dyslexic peers, and they
had 'high expectations of being lonely – in the future, in general, and in
new situations in particular' (Tur-Kaspa et al. 1998, p. 54).

I would suggest that this sense of feeling different from everyone else, of
being the eternal wallflower at the great human party, is the most common
reason for dyslexic clients to seek counselling. It is certainly the one unify-
ing source of pain.

Do dyslexic isolation problems start with parents?
My experience would lead me to say no.

I accept that there is an argument that the dyslexic communication deficiency might lead to attachment problems with parents, but I do not think that it is as simple as that. If anything, the problem, as I noted in Chapter 6, lies in an overly close relationship with parents, particularly the mother. Dyslexics are less likely to be isolated in this relationship than destructively enmeshed.

Often, dyslexic children have relatively normal relationships with their parents and – since there is not an autistic dimension to the dyslexic communication problem and they are capable of great warmth and responsiveness – the parent-dyslexic child relationship often adapts well to the child's deficiencies. The parent-dyslexic child relationship is no less inherently dysfunctional than, say, a parent with a blind or deaf child.

Even in dyslexic children who have flat facial expression or severe language problems, the relationship with their parents can be affectionate and close, if a little oddly expressed. Where problems are mediated by the depression of a dyslexic mother, the attachment problems will follow those of the depression rather than the dyslexia.

Do dyslexic isolation problems start with siblings?
Most possibly.

As I noted in Chapter 5, excessive closeness of the dyslexic child with his mother in particular sets up problems with his siblings. This can then lead to poor social cognition and inadequate training in relationships with other children, ending in unsatisfactory peer relationships at school.

Do dyslexic isolation problems start in peer relationships?
Yes. The dyslexic's relational problems frequently have their roots in peer problems at school.

Furthermore, it is universally reported by parents that dyslexic problems start when their child goes to school. This is when parents report that they 'lose' their normal child. As Leach (1994) observes: 'Many aspects of development depend on the mutual aid of peer interaction – pleasant and unpleasant' (p. 156), and it is not overstating the case to say that to be accepted or rejected by one's peer group can determine a happy or unhappy childhood. Peers are important to children; up to 70% of child friendships remain solid and happy over a year. Furthermore, it is normal for children to spend a lot of time with peers. Children of 7–11 years spend over 40% of their time with friends. If you have no friends, this amounts to an awful lot of time alone or – rather – being lonely (Vanzetti and Duck 1996).

Peers also interact as equals. Their relationship is more symmetrical and less hierarchical than with adults. This is its value to growing up. There is no imposed power, as with an adult and child, so conflict must be resolved between the children. Piaget (1932) argued that children get benefits from peers that they do not get from adults.

Unfortunately, children also have many inventive ways of hurting and rejecting each other, including stopping interaction, preventing friendships, exercising control, domination, and aggression (various forms) or invoking a third party to do or say something hurtful. 'Taken together, [these studies] point to a remarkable array of social relational weapons that boys and girls use against one another, with physical aggression being the tip of the iceberg' (Deater-Deckard 2001, p. 566).

Externalizing and hyperactive children have the worst time of it since their wild, aggressive and ill-judged behaviours both invite and guarantee isolation. They are also great playthings in their own right when they react interestingly to peer provocation.

As I described in Chapter 3, dyslexic children suffer from all these hurtful manifestations of peer rejection, and depression and emotional difficulties mainly occur in those dyslexic children who have the poorest social skills and the most marked aspects of the 'clumsy child syndrome' (Heath 2001, Kavale and Forness 1994).

Peer rejection sets up problems in relationships throughout the dyslexic's entire life, leading to a range of psychological problems in adulthood. Bullying has a particularly toxic effect on all types of relationships. For example, it is my experience that many men who have difficulties in relationships with women had experienced bullying or harassment at school.

What is the main vehicle for relationship problems in dyslexic people?
Poor social skills and deeply flawed social cognition.

These are unquestionably the main causes of the peer-relationship problems that isolate dyslexics. In fact, a meta-analysis of 152 studies on dyslexics showed that 75% of children and students with specific learning difficulties had social-skills deficits that distinguished them from comparison groups (Kavale and Forness 1994).

These problems not only prevent good communication with others but can actively get dyslexics into trouble with other people. 'Complaints that the dyslexic is often inappropriate in his language or comments are not confined to school and can equally lead to trouble and misunderstandings at home with parents, with siblings and with the extended family' (Thomson 1995b, p. 38).

Understanding specifically how these problems come about gives counsellors a more concrete way of helping dyslexic clients as well as preparing them for how these difficulties will impact on the counselling, one-to-one relationship. After all, the problems that dyslexics have in communicating with others, they will also have with you.

Isolation through non-verbal skills

Are non-verbal skills important in communication?
Some would argue that they *are* communication.

Hargie et al. (1994), for example, asserting that 'the potency of the non-verbal aspects of behaviour cannot be underestimated' (p. 61), reminds us that verbal communication between people is relatively uncommon. We only speak for a total of ten to 11 minutes daily, in bursts that average about 2.5 seconds. Non-verbal communication, by contrast, has five times more effect than verbal communication and, when verbal and non-verbal styles conflict, the verbal styles are virtually disregarded. In social situations, 'much of the information we are transmitting and receiving is being conveyed via the non-verbal channel' (op. cit., p. 36).

Children and adolescents, in particular, pay more attention to visual components, so children who are poor at giving and interpreting non-verbal signals are doubly disadvantaged. It is a paradox of child communication that those who most long to communicate, and who are most in need of non-verbal skills, are those who are the most deficient in them. This group includes not only dyslexics but also children who are chronically ill or handicapped (Meijer et al. 2000).

How do dyslexics demonstrate poor non-verbal skills?
In a rich variety of inept and socially startling ways.

This may be directly linked to the severity of the dyslexia, but it is not in any way linked to intelligence. In fact, for reasons I cannot fathom, the gifted dyslexic can be among the worst of all at expressing and decoding non-verbal behaviour.

On the in-coming channel, dyslexics can miss subtle social cues, decode them wrongly or make inaccurate social inferences. They can also mangle out-going non-verbal communication to the degree that the people they interact with receive transmissions that are all over the place. This can leave people feeling inexplicably uncomfortable, or concluding – entirely inaccurately – that the dyslexic person is upset, bored, cold or angry with them. In short, interaction with a dyslexic can feel unrewarding and unsatisfying. It can be awkward, uneasy, jangling and very hard work.

There are obviously degrees of this, but it is not unusual for a dyslexic to be coded as antisocial and odd: one to be avoided.

Why do other people not look beyond this dyslexic demeanour?
In social-psychological terms, human beings are 'cognitive misers' or 'cognitively economical' (Fiske and Taylor 1984). They are rarely motivated to

engage in the mental activity necessary to make a detailed evaluation of others.

People will not spend time wondering if what they are seeing is exactly what a dyslexic is thinking. It is the nature of human biology to make a quick cognitive judgement and rapidly assign what is seen to a stereotype. Stereotypes facilitate communication because they are processed quickly. They 'streamline cognition and increase the intelligibility of an otherwise dauntingly complex social world. For many of us, this temptation to think categorically about others is irresistible' (Macrae and Bodenhausen 2001, p. 251).

It is simplistic to see this as just a judgement. This is the way of human relating, and it speeds up interactions in a social species. It is also a survival mechanism from the time when speed of reaction could make the difference between staying alive or not.

Unfortunately for the dyslexic, the trait first perceived by others affects the interpretation of those given later. We tend to form overly simplistic pictures of people and assume that they are highly consistent. A happy mood, for example, encourages us to see more positive things in that person and, since all good things are assumed to go together, there is a halo effect.

By the same reasoning, people who present on first meeting as cold, awkward or depressed, are seen as trouble. They will be avoided, because a happy, relaxed mood is precious and needs to be protected. Erratic behaviour is the most worrying behaviour of all, and a person exhibiting it is particularly liable to be avoided. This is, again, a survival mechanism, in that such behaviour is commonly associated with danger and madness.

Unfortunately, dyslexic behaviour can present as both depressed and erratic. Even their happy side can have a manic side – particularly when they flick from a smile to an intense stare as they struggle to process information.

Specifically, how do dyslexics create problems in non-verbal communication?

It is often hard to tell, so it is common in the dyslexic literature to refer to the poor communication skills of the dyslexic in a rather received and unspecific way.

This is not particularly helpful, so I have, therefore, attempted to analyse why and how the dyslexic's poor social and verbal skills might come about. I offer the following suggestions:

Non-conforming behaviour

Dyslexics can find it hard to work out the norms in a social group since these are often transmitted too subtly for dyslexics to pick up. Unfortunately, this can be read as group non-conformity and 'anyone who fails to conform is placed under pressure to do so and, if he continues in his non-conforming behaviour, he is rejected' (Argyle 1994, p. 169).

A deviant becomes the object of group attention while the group tries to neutralize him and persuade him to change his behaviour. Mockery is often included as a device to bring the deviant to heel, which is damaging in its own way. Eventually, the group gives up: 'deviation is often greeted with surprise, non-verbal signals of disapproval, verbal attempts at influence and finally by rejection and exclusion from the group' (op. cit., p. 170).

Poor social synchrony

There will be no proper interaction between people unless their movements mesh together in a synchronized and coordinated manner. Synchrony makes interaction smooth and satisfying, and is a core feature of intimacy and friendship quality (Hughes and Dunn 2002). If two people are getting on well, they mirror each other, but incongruence in synchrony is experienced as uncomfortable.

Dyslexics, however, give a great deal of incongruent and scrambled physical signals – an unconscious and worrying mixture of dominant and submissive, happy and sad that makes others feel unsafe and anxious. The dyslexic tendency to get behind because of processing difficulties also sets whole conversations out of rhythm.

Dyslexic rates of physical synchrony are also slow. Bodily movements between communicating people are usually finely coordinated at fractions of a second in a 'gestural dance'. They normally synchronize at one eighth of a second. For a dyslexic or dyspraxic, this is too fast, so they are always physically out of synch when interacting with a non-dyslexic.

Incongruence is the bane of a dyslexic's life. If they do not get it from others, they are unwittingly conveying it themselves.

Unfamiliarity

As Duck (1988) observes: 'We all have a preference for the familiar over the unfamiliar' (p. 12). This is based not only on our need for inclusion, but 'our concerns that we be members of a community of equals' (p. 12). People like others who are similar to them. Unfortunately, disliking people because they are different is a stronger psychological drive than liking people because they are similar. This is known as the 'repulsion hypothesis' (Argyle 1994) and is a powerful human survival instinct.

Lack of touch

Poor peer relationships mean that you are touched less, but tactile exploration is of crucial importance in the behavioural development of young adults. Best friends twine around each other, and members of a group pat, hit, cuddle, grapple and grab at each other.

Isolated children are not touched, and this damages them. Unfortunately, their desperation to be touched, to get any contact at all, can often lead dyslexics into unwise invasions of personal space that lead to even more communication problems (see 'Isolation through kinaesthetics', below).

Transmission of ambiguous information

Relating is also an attempt to gather information about people. Human beings are social animals, and we are thirsty for information about each other. Non-verbal and verbal skills tell us a lot about people, and reading this information is, no doubt, a sharp survival tool. It once enabled humans to read very quickly what their reaction should be in the next ten seconds, and those who read fast and accurately stayed around to contribute to the human gene pool.

Through the same historical mechanism, people who convey information clearly, who are expressive in face and body, are likely to make people feel more at ease, and those who cannot, or who do not, convey information easily will make us uneasy and anxious.

Dyslexics transmit ambiguous, or not enough, information and so make others feel strangely 'starved', edgy and uncomfortable.

Contagion of dampening reactions

There is a lot of evidence for emotional contagion; that is, we catch each other's emotion by some primitive mechanism of copying and feedback. There is a high facial correlation between two good interactors, and they process very fast. This is not just transference but an ancient social skill.

People who are facially expressive can 'turn on' the expressive behaviour of others. The corollary, of course, is that facial inexpressiveness dampens that of others, and they themselves become less expressive. This continues with other interactions, so an inexpressive reaction from one person can have a ripple effect on others. This is why an inexpressive or depressed persona can be a real dampener on a social group – hence the term 'wet blanket' – and is also why depressed children are more likely to be rejected or isolated by their peers than those who are fearful.

Depression flattens facial reaction while fear, at least, animates it, and there is more fun to be had over the emotional prodding of a frightened child since the group can catch the facial dance of fear. Depressed children just underreact and go away (Kennedy et al. 1989). By these means, the inexpressive dyslexic child – and the depressed dyslexic child in particular – will be rejected since they are, in effect, toxic to the group's energy and fun.

Inappropriate use of gestures

We move parts of our body while we speak – continuously. These movements are iconic; that is, they resemble what the voice is talking about. Gestures are also part of speaking, including head nods. Gestures, importantly, also reflect emotional states, and, when he is emotionally aroused, a person produces diffuse, pointless bodily movements and touches himself, often on the face by scratching and forehead wiping. Active gesturing, therefore, indicates arousal, so the other person will be aroused and expectant too.

Hyperactive dyslexics are like this most of the time, and they are hard to be with. It can be wearing when you talk to someone who never stops moving, since the listener is in a constant state of expectant arousal. It is also tiring because the movements really mean nothing, go nowhere, and so are not easy to read.

Leakage

If we try to conceal our true feelings, leakage occurs in less well-controlled parts of the body; for example, clenching hands or a shaky voice. This leakage subtly indicates incongruence, making the observer feel quite on edge. Many dyslexics have these types of behaviour, whether from the unextinguished primitive reflexes of dyspraxia, genuine social anxiety or because of hyperactive tendencies. Anybody interacting with them will feel as if they are on a caffeine rush. I can find a 15-minute session with a slightly hyperactive or dyspraxic dyslexic to be more wearing than a one hour session with anyone else, since the constant overactiveness sets up synchrony in me. It is very contagious.

Mixed signals of dominance and submission

An unsmiling face can be used to indicate dominance, and being stared at by a stranger can make us feel uncomfortable, not only because of his dominance cues but also because of the lack of information conveyed. It generates unpleasant physiological arousal since it can indicate incipient attack.

A long direct gaze – which dyslexics use a lot as they concentrate on what you are saying – is also a classic signal of dominance but usually goes with an upright posture and low voice pitch. When it is teamed with the high pitch of anxiety and the drooping posture of dyspraxic weakness, this is difficult for the listener to file.

Some dyslexics also try to smile when they are uncomfortable in an attempt to help along a difficult situation. Smiling, they learn, is a useful defence, and a powerful default position to assume in times of social danger.

Unfortunately, excessive smiling can be a mixed signal. The anxious smile that dyslexics use to get themselves out of trouble is little more than bared teeth, and is used by all primates to convey fear and submission. This expression may have evolved into human laughter and smiling, but when it goes wrong it conveys the opposite, and the smile's recipient rarely knows how to respond appropriately.

Difficulty in reading and conveying facial expressions

The facial expression has an important evolutionary role in care-taking and relating. We are a social species. It is for this reason that there are six main facial expressions – happiness, surprise, fear, sadness, anger, disgust/contempt – all of which have evolutionary and survival uses.

Reading faces is essential for the development of attachment behaviours, and the absence of facial expression has been found to destroy relationships in primates. In the rare cases of very severe dyslexia, where symptoms can easily mimic autism, problems in reading faces may also have affected the dyslexic child's bonding with his parents. If both a dyslexic mother and dyslexic child have problems in reading facial expression, I would surmise that an attachment problem might arise. There appears to be no research on this.

Reading facial expression is also critical to the development of social responsiveness, such as in understanding the feelings of friends, but dyslexics are less accurate in reading facial expressions than non-dyslexics (Robinson and Whiting 2001).

Dyslexics can also have very flat expressions of facial emotion – sometimes disconcertingly so. They also need to concentrate hard, most of the time, and it is difficult to concentrate and smile at the same time.

Gaze

Gaze is central to communication. It is a powerful social signal from the first mother and baby mutual gaze at three to four weeks. Getting gaze right is crucial, and the conventions of gaze are subtle and important. For example, when two people are talking they look at each other between 25% and 75% of the time, but they look nearly twice as much while listening than while talking.

Small flickering changes in gaze can give very different messages. Leaking gaze to right or left shows boredom, widening the eyes denotes acknowledgement, facial expression changes around the eyes can 'look daggers', but when occurring with a lowered head can convey sexual attraction. A fixed, wide-eyed gaze and downturned mouth – that dyslexics commonly use when concentrating – can, however, also convey 'get me out of here'.

Gaze usefully opens up a channel, so that another's non-verbal signs can be read. It also communicates to the other person that you are attending to them and that they are important. The correct gaze can help people to like and trust each other more.

Gaze also indicates that something is about to start – whether flirting or a game of football – and can be an invitation to join in.

Dyslexics are not good at judging gaze correctly. As noted earlier, one unfortunate effect of the blank dyslexic expression of concentration is that it makes their gaze alarming to see and confusing to read. With other dyslexics, their social anxiety can lead to a peculiar sideways or flicking gaze with people they do not know. This overly short gaze also causes problems since the recipient feels both unimportant and disliked. Further communication – through the unspoken conventions of gaze – are shut down, and the bewildered dyslexic never quite understands why.

Unattractive characteristics

Physically attractive people are consistently judged more favourably on almost every dimension (Argyle 1994). This effectively handicaps those more messy or untidy dyslexics, the eccentric dressers and all dyspraxic dyslexics. When dyslexics concentrate hard on what people say, they can also appear surly and pugnacious.

Poor listening

Dyslexics have problems with the basic skill of listening well to others, and, as noted above, their listening skills – such as concentration and gaze – can be bizarre. Nodding and tilting of the head – which indicate interest or convey an invitation to another to carry on talking – are also difficult for dyslexics. They can find head movements difficult, and so hold their heads very still. This can be because some have stiff neck muscles through immature reflexes. For other dyslexics, it is a feature of social cognition that they have never grasped.

Isolation through language problems

What are the dyslexic's language problems?

Although they are not mutually exclusive, the dyslexic language communication problems can be broadly grouped into two problem areas: (1) conversation and information processing and (2) articulacy, speech and delivery.

Why do dyslexics have problems in conversation and information processing?
There are a number of reasons.

Dyslexics may simply be inexperienced at conversation, and so cannot sustain a conversation unless others do all the work for them. Low confidence also makes matters worse, and speaking in front of others can be a terrifying experience for dyslexics. Dyslexics do not always understand why things go wrong in conversations with others. This, in itself, leads to additional social anxiety for dyslexics who cannot predict whether their conversation will cause mockery or incomprehension from others. It can be simpler to say nothing, so nothing gets said to them.

It is easy to see why the first meeting with a counsellor can be nerve-wracking for dyslexics, and I suspect that counsellors will not see the vast majority of language-disabled dyslexics – which is a pity because these are the ones who are most in need of help. For similar reasons, a counsellor may also find a dyslexic client rather taciturn. A good counselling relationship can, however, encourage the articulacy that lies beneath, and such clients can become astonishingly expressive.

A dyslexic's reaction to others' speech is also compromised if they have a long information-processing lag. This works in two ways. First, the dyslexic has to hear, retain, unpack and then react to any incoming conversational information. By the time one sentence has been digested and the dyslexic is ready to respond, other speakers have moved several sentences down the line. This does not allow the to-and-fro of chat which bonds a social group. In addition, if there is any interruption, the dyslexic's short-term memory can fail, so all information is lost. Even a simple question can derail a dyslexic in conversation.

While all this difficult negotiation of the conversational dance is going on, the dyslexic can often have a rather off-putting look, not unlike someone trying to understand a foreign language. It is this very typical dyslexic expression – immobilized face, slightly open mouth, rigid stance, slight frown, head jutting forwards, a peering and panicked expression – that can dislocate a conversational exchange. Having a conversation with someone who does this all the time is disquieting for the other person.

What sort of problems with articulacy, speech and delivery do dyslexics have?
Dyslexia does not always affect oral skills but, when it does, it can cause difficulties in converting thoughts and ideas into spoken words.

The main problems are:

Hesitant method of delivery
Many of the normal dyslexic verbal mannerisms mimic the speech patterns

of unassertive and unconfident people. These will include hesitation, over-long pauses, sudden jerky delivery, mumbling, looking down, jumbling the order of words and failing to make eye contact while talking.

Dyslexics also use unfinished or trailing sentences, many 'ums' and 'ers', repetitive panicky noises as they try to find the next word, apologies (lots and lots of apologies), and self-critical statements ('I'm probably wrong', 'I know this is stupid'). Some of these mannerisms are based in the dyslexic condition while others are used as stalling tactics.

The listener and, clearly, the counsellor, must disentangle the physical (long pauses, mumbling) from the psychosocial (shortness of breath, self-critical statements). Unfortunately, these 'self-deprecating words and mannerisms may have become automatic and habitual' (Bartlett and Moody 2000, p. 161).

Answering questions is also a problem for dyslexics since they believe that a quick answer is called for. The advantages of waiting and looking thoughtful is something they discover although sometimes, especially when attached to a question like 'Cup of tea?', such a tactic can cancel out any positive effect.

Sequencing

Dyslexics have problems with all types of sequence. Human speech, however, requires delicate and subtle patterns of sequence, including breaks and interactions. Dyslexics can quickly lose the sequence in conversation and give up. They have a well-oiled ability, honed during years of incomprehensible lessons at school, of putting on an attentive expression and, psychologically, going walkabout.

Memory

Conversation requires that you take account of more than just the last utterance; you are influenced by all of them, but the last three are the most important. A poor memory makes this difficult, and you can lose the way. A counsellor who normally avoids responding to client queries of 'What was I just talking about?' may need to revise this position with dyslexics.

Finding the words

Stuttering is not a commonly observed problem in dyslexics. What is much more common is that some dyslexics can't get their words out quickly enough. Others, particularly children, do not wait for them to do so, and the conversation steams on down the line with the dyslexic always running to catch up. This pressure then leads to further difficulty in accessing words.

The main gift a counsellor can give to a dyslexic is time to get his words out. This will relax him and make him communicate far better in the long run, since he will not be anxious. Building in a time lag in conversations with dyslexics is important. Content, too, can be muddled as a dyslexic client loses the narrative thread or forgets what they were saying. Some therapies would experience such 'forgetting' as a defence. For dyslexics it is just the way they are.

Missing what is said

Poor processing skills lead to dyslexics only hearing half, if anything, of what is being said. Of what is actually heard, selective perception may lead to the negative part being retained. A counsellor cannot always assume that her communication with a dyslexic is either getting over to him, or being heard by him. Without knowing quite why, the counsellor will pick up that there has been a serious breakdown in communication.

Voice and speech patterns

Voices elicit stereotyped personality traits. For example, a depressed person speaks slowly, at a low and falling pitch. Dyslexics can speak like this when they are really quite happy. Unfortunately, the other person will read low mood into this delivery. Another trait of an anxious, introverted dyslexic can be that of an extrovert, who speaks loudly and with fewer pauses. Dyslexics can also flak you with rapid unending speech that, on closer attention, has little understandable direction and much off-target content.

Isolation through kinaesthetics

How do dyslexics manage space (kinaesthetics)?
Dyslexics have strange spatial awareness and can often stand too close.

They can also make inappropriate invasions of personal space as they try to concentrate fully on what is said. Sometimes they stand too far away, and at odd angles, speaking at you from 45 degrees. This can lead to a strong urge to circle around them or lean forward to bring yourself into their eye line. Otherwise, you have to speak to their ear.

Distances between people are such that we move closer to people whom we like, and proximity is a cue for liking – if it is accepted. We seek just the right degree of proximity. The wrong type jangles. If personal space is invaded, it indicates a claim to higher intimacy than we want, while standing too far away suggests aloofness and coldness.

Sometimes, aggressive kinaesthetics is the problem with dyslexic adults. This includes pacing while talking, standing too close to listen, or leaning forward into the other person's bodyline. They can make sharp or flailing gestures with their hands, while glaring at the listener and making an over-loud, emphatic delivery.

Their patterns of touching can also be slightly out of synch – either too much or too little. Touch is governed by strict rules on which parts of the body touch is permitted, by whom, and in what contexts (at a party or on the tube). It is permitted for close relationships but, since some dyslexics have never had close relationships with anyone (the problem is worse if he has a dyslexic mother who had no good experience of touch herself), they can find any touch or closeness difficult.

Isolation through lack of social cognition

What is social cognition?
It is the ability to understand people by reading what they are thinking or feeling, and judging their possible responses.

Social cognition involves more than just labelling a social response from emotional cues such as facial expression and posture. It is the ability to look at a social context and then predict and explain the behaviour and feelings of others. Social cognition encompasses a variety of concepts such as 'theory of mind', 'internal working models of relationships', 'mentalizing', 'attribution' and 'empathy'. All these concepts have respectable research traditions showing that social cognitive processes, of whatever construct, have direct consequences for social competence and positive social relationships. This form of social intelligence is correlated positively with peer acceptance (Czeschlik and Rost 1995).

In short, those with good social cognition are popular. They read others very well indeed, and are socially competent. They have repertoires of social knowledge, a positive outlook, an open and congenial style, offer assistance spontaneously to others, refrain from aggression, have high levels of sociable behaviour and are responsive.

By contrast, those who fail to acquire social cognition will be unpopular and disadvantaged (Hollin 1993). They lack social skills, overlook social signals – such as bored, irritated looks – and make wrong interpretations of social situations, including inappropriate attributions of hostility. They cannot think through a social situation and do not have the performance skills to communicate their needs and intentions to other people (Spence 1987, Slaughter et al. 2002).

Do dyslexics have good social cognition?
Generally, no. For reasons that are not fully understood, many dyslexics are very poor at social cognition.

One theory is that dyslexics, with slow information processing and a blind spot for abstraction and subtlety, do not read social situations well. The subsequent social failure leads to rejection, so any further chance of learning social cognition is denied them. Their own lack of social skills prevents them from getting 'reinforcing outcomes from interaction with others' (Kennedy et al. 1989, p. 562).

The skill is stillborn or, more optimistically (see Cognitive Behavioural Therapy in Chapter 12), goes dormant.

There is also some evidence, noted in Section 3, that problems in social cognition arise because of dysfunction in the dyslexic child's relationships with his parents and siblings that are then exacerbated in disastrous peer relationships at school. Poor social cognition has also been noted in those with language disabilities, which many dyslexics also have (Cohen et al. 1998).

Interestingly, it may also be the dyslexic's inability to access eye contact – through anxiety, social awkwardness or avoidance by others – that is to blame. Skuse (2003) found evidence that low eye contact led to low social cognition through an understimulation of an important neural pathway in the brain that is responsible for the processing of social information.

On the basis of this evidence, it would seem that dyslexic social cognition is glued to a depressing downward spiral whereby low eye contact leads to poor social cognition that makes relating to other people difficult that leads to reduced eye contact – and so on.

Clearly, the dyslexic's problems with social cognition may also cause problems in the therapeutic relationship, and a counsellor may find working with a dyslexic client a little challenging at times. The counsellor and her dyslexic client may well have problems reading each other. In this respect, at least, the dyslexic is on home territory.

Is social-cognitive-skills training effective?

Yes – very much so. I shall return to this in more detail in Chapter 12, but it is obvious that training in social-cognitive skills is a fast route to peer acceptance and elimination of many of the social-skills problems that underlie the dyslexic problems with relationships.

Dyslexics can be coached in social-cognitive skills, and this is an effective form of treatment (Humfress et al. 2002). Whitney et al. (1994) found that such training with special-needs children led to the children reporting themselves more confident and happier.

Isolation through victim behaviour

Is victim behaviour common in dyslexics?

Yes. In fact, my experience is that this is one of the most common forms of maladaptive behaviour among dyslexic adults and children. Whether from bullying or learned helplessness, it is evident in over 80% of referrals.

A child who is abused 'internalizes both sides of the abusive relationship, learning the roles of both abuser and abused' (Cooper 1999, p. 218).

In this way, a significant number of dyslexic people learn how to be victims from how other people have treated them. They go on to have problems relating to others because they are entrenched in this victim behaviour that, in turn, encourages others to treat them badly.

Why does the dyslexic adopt victim behaviour?
It is chosen, learned, and then becomes useful.

It can, for example, bestow power on a dyslexic person that may not have been achieved in other contexts. Being a victim can also enable a relationship with others where no other is on offer. It can produce a lot of attention, even though it may be negative attention. These are all seductive outcomes for a lonely and isolated person.

In this role, dyslexics can invite other people – both children and adults – into a triangular relationship of 'persecutor' or 'rescuer' to their 'victim'. Anyone who accepts this invitation from the person in victim mode not only tacitly accepts the self-estimate of the person as a victim but will also find themselves acting to support it.

Like all learned, maladaptive behaviour, it repeats itself in different situations with similar patterns.

For example, if, despite all a school's best efforts, a dyslexic girl is somehow always being picked on, and her mother does not examine her daughter's role in these situations but responds habitually with protective, sympathetic attention, she is providing fertile ground for victim behaviour to develop in her daughter. Teachers who find themselves tempted to rail against certain children whose behaviour is always somehow designed (which it is) to annoy them, need to be wary of what is going on, since it may be that they are being drawn into the persecutor role.

There is a pay-off for the victim, in both these situations. Victim behaviour can draw attention away from failure. It can lead to increased attention from adults. By allowing all blame to reside in others, it can remove the need to take personal responsibility for work and self.

It is also common to find that a particular manifestation of victim behaviour has happened before. For example, one dyslexic girl regularly saw me because all the other girls excluded her by ganging up on her. I discovered that a similar pattern had occurred in all three of her previous schools, and with her sisters. Her parents, teachers, dinner ladies – a whole cohort – would comfort her. Digging more deeply, however, I found that she was constantly setting up irritating situations with other girls. This led to the desired effects – exclusion, victimization, adult attention and excuses for work avoidance.

Much of this process is unconscious, but it can be extremely powerful because the victim is getting a significant pay-off for this behaviour. If the other person also gets pay-offs for being a 'persecutor' or 'rescuer' because of their own psychology or background, all parties collude with each other. What is interesting, in my experience, is how all the parties to this beguiling, but deeply toxic, triangle manage to find each other.

What is learned helplessness?
This is a variation of victim behaviour, but in a more passive and serious form. It is more linked with depression.

It occurs in dyslexic people who have acquired an attitude that they no longer have any control over their lives. Learned helplessness is an external attribution, connected to anxiety and failure. It is a term coined by Seligman (1975), who assembled impressive evidence that, when placed in situations where outcomes are unaffected by their behaviour, people become passive and apathetic. They gradually withdraw and lose motivation.

Pumphrey and Reason (1991) noted that learned helplessness occurs naturally among those with reading difficulties.

Isolation through the latency stage

How is the latency stage relevant to relationship problems?
I think that it is highly significant that the age at which all the dyslexic child's problems start – seven-12 years – is also the exact stage – in psychoanalytic terms – that the child enters the 'latency' (Freud 1905) and 'age of industry' (Erickson 1968) stages.

Both theories stress that successful negotiation of the social tasks of this stage is crucial for social and sexual self-confidence in the growing child.

Seven years is the age at which dyslexic problems become apparent, the disabling social effects begin and the child's difficulties 'cause concern to both parents and teachers' (Povey and Todd 1993, p. 193). Between the ages of eight and 11, the dyslexic child can be clearly distinguished from the non-dyslexic child by his literacy and behavioural difficulties. 'The 8-11-year age group is, in fact, the peak period for 'dyslexic referrals' to the specialist agencies such as the School Psychological Service' (op. cit., p. 193). In short, the latency stage is that at which dyslexics have their first and most intense difficulties.

How is the latency stage important in social relationships?
Both Erickson (1968) and Freud (1905) emphasize that this is the age at which children move away from the narcissism of the oral and anal stages into the world of socialization, peer-group acceptance and strong self-concept.

At the latency stage, the child normally becomes preoccupied with developmental skills, activity and same-sex friendship. Energy is directed outwards to skills in social relationships and social play because strong drives are relatively dormant. This should be the age of hobbies, sports and same-sex friendships.

What are the effects of problems in the latency stage?
Principally, the ability to form good social relationships.

Jacobs (1986), for example, specifically identifies problems at the latency stage as perilous to the child's effective social development. When things go wrong with this stage, then the effects include:

- a negative self-concept
- feelings of inadequacy related to learning
- feelings of inferiority in establishing social relationships
- conflicts over values
- a confused sex-role identity
- unwillingness to face new challenges
- a lack of initiative
- dependency

In short, the child will develop all the normal character traits of a failed and damaged dyslexic. This theoretical approach to dyslexic isolation also explains other aspects of dyslexic behaviour and personality: the childlike nature of many dyslexics, their self-absorption, their enmeshment with home and their apparently irrational desire to return to education.

Also, when he is either traumatized during, or locked into, a stage of psychoanalytic development, a child does not pass easily to the next stage – and may even regress to the previous one. This notion would suggest that a dyslexic child who has had problems at the latency stage might not only regress to an earlier stage (remaining over-enmeshed with family and mother) but also be unable to move on to the genital stage of sexual development thereby retaining an infantile rather than adult sexuality. I shall return to this last point in the next chapter.

Jacobs (1986) specifically links poor transmission through the latency stage with neurotic behaviours in adults. In this respect, I am struck by how much Argyle's depiction of communication problems in neurotic adults resembles those in some severely dyslexic adults. Neurotics are socially isolated people with fewer friends, and may engage in 'queer destructive social techniques'. They are usually 'bad conversationalists', talk too fast and nervously or indistinctly, or 'lose control of the quality of their speech'. Their utterances are slow, and they make many speech errors. 'Others are very silent, showing little interest in others, speaking very briefly and in a slow and rather monotonous voice, rarely taking over the conversation, sitting very still and rigid and assuming a dull fixed expression' (Argyle 1967, pp. 238–39).

Dyslexia, neurosis and the latency stage may well be linked. The joint problem, however, fetches up in the same place: isolation.

Misinterpreting dyslexic isolation

Can dyslexic isolation be cloaked?
Yes – by modesty, self-deprecation and 'good' behaviour.

Modesty can be a good behavioural substitute for isolation, particularly as it is valued in children by both teachers and other children. Being self-aggrandizing is not perceived positively, and immodesty or showing-off can often lead to negative social evaluation. Intelligent dyslexic children pick this difference up quite quickly, and – particularly for girls – it is easy for them to invite us to misinterpret modesty both because it is socially valued and because it makes their real lack of confidence invisible.

Teachers can easily read quiet, self-deprecating behaviour in a dyslexic as modesty, instead of withdrawal or low self-confidence. Counsellors, too, can read understated behaviour as a sign of socially skilled self-deprecation rather than straightforward adapted behaviour.

The dyslexic is also constantly wary of social rebuff, and modesty can be a fast track to social acceptance, manipulating the fact that 'a self-deprecating presentation of the self can lead to enhanced social evaluation' (Banerjee 2000, p. 499).

Modesty and self-deprecation are useful learned responses. They provide a smokescreen which can continue into adult life as a coping strategy and a deflector screen. These behaviours can also be used by dyslexic children to hide problems from parents.

Is isolation the same as 'lonely' or 'alone'
No. While it is true that isolation can make many dyslexic children lonely, it can also make other dyslexic people self-contained and happy to be alone.

In some ways, it may be said that their isolation has led dyslexics to confront and extinguish the fears of existential isolation in a way that the non-dyslexic may never do. Dyslexic isolation can become a healthy choice in a mature personality. It may even be an integral and essential part of the dyslexic experience.

It is, therefore, important not to assume that dyslexic children or adults are lonely when they are alone. We should also distinguish between 'lonely' and 'solitary', the latter referring to people who do not enjoy groups.

There is a sizeable minority of dyslexic people who enjoy being alone and have no problems with it. Anecdotally, I would say that this is when the dyslexia is severe, and is associated with either very high intelligence or marked creative/artistic skills. Some of the artistic group are entirely comfortable in their own world, totally immersed in picking up visual cues that re-emerge later – sometimes many years later – in stunning painting and sculpture.

Smyth and Anderson (2000) found that it is also important not to see solitude as loneliness even in clumsy or dyspraxic children: 'there may be different routes to solitude, even in children with coordination difficulties' (p. 370). Qualter and Munn (2002) also found that a child who operated outside of a peer group was not necessarily noxious to the group or the object of bullying by it. In fact, such a child moved in and out of the group as it suited him.

Neither does spending time alone indicate a lack of social network. Asendorpf (1993) asserts that there are many different types of solitude in childhood, including social isolation which is a freely chosen withdrawal from others. Some children also need space to be alone, and to have this choice respected. There is 'a higher risk of making unsociable children shy by trying to make them more sociable' (op. cit., p. 1079).

What is important is what the child wants and needs.

For example, Asendorpf's notion of social isolation contrasts with that of social rejection. A child in the first group is happy to be separate from the group, but a child in the other is not, because he is forcibly excluded from the group. Rejection from the group is not a problem if you do not care whether you are in the group anyway, 'It is loneliness and *not* rejection that co-occurs with emotional problems' (Qualter and Munn 2002, p. 233).

On balance, it is important to establish what isolation means to the individual dyslexic person. Do they feel pain or comfort in solitude? Not to respect this difference is to introduce yet one more example of incongruence into their lives.

CHAPTER 9

Survival strategies and dyslexia

Summary

This chapter reviews those psychological survival strategies used by dyslexics to help them to cope with the social and emotional fall-out of dyslexia. This is very much a therapeutic rather than a purely psychological viewpoint, and balances the biological and literacy-based research that can sometimes see dyslexic people as 'broken learning machines' (Hales 1994, p. 172).

Self-esteem and dyslexia

How does self-esteem feature in dyslexia?
It has been consistently suggested that dyslexic people have lower self-esteem than non-dyslexic controls.

It is not surprising, therefore, that counsellors are presented with the task of improving dyslexic self-esteem, setting up a programme to enhance self-esteem (Humphrey 2002) or 'strengthening an individual's self-concept' (Hay 2000, p. 345). There is a suggestion that there is a self-esteem bucket per dyslexic person that needs filling up.

My own experience, however, is that the notion of self-esteem is easy to conceptualize but, like mercury, extremely slippery and elusive when you try to get to grips with it. There is also powerful, emerging research that challenges the notion that the pursuit of a simple, unilateral notion of 'self-esteem' is useful or beneficial to either the individual or to society as a whole (Appleyard 2002). Consequently, I think that dyslexic self-esteem is complicated and, as an idea, it is worth unpicking.

Do dyslexics have lower self-esteem than non-dyslexics?
At first sight it would seem so, but hard evidence is lacking.

If one removes the research biases of design and interviewer artefact, there is not a lot there except anecdote and impressions. The evidence on low self-esteem is based on 'experiences recounted' (Riddick et al. 1999, p. 230), the 'barrage of anecdotal evidence from teachers and practitioners' (Humphrey 2002, p. 30), the case studies of eight dyslexic adolescents (Edwards 1994) and the fact that 22 dyslexic children were 'disappointed, frustrated, ashamed, fed up, sad, depressed, angry and embarrassed by their difficulties' (Riddick 1996, p. 129).

Barrett and Jones (1996) just assert that it would be naive to assume that dyslexics would have a good self-esteem given their learning difficulties.

Are there associated bodies of evidence?
Yes. There are inferential relationships.

For example, dyslexic children are often bullied and 'there is a strong relationship between feelings of poor self-esteem and bullying behaviour. The relationship was particularly strong among children with special-educational needs' (O'Moore and Hillery 1992, p. 64). There is also evidence that low self-concept and academic achievement are correlated, although the causal direction is not clear (see Chapter 3).

All that this shows, however, is that, when they fail at school or are bullied, some aspects of dyslexic children's self-concept can become 'low'. Inferences and generalization beyond this are unjustified.

Do special schools enhance dyslexic self-esteem?
Yes. This is because they focus on academic performance without the problems of mainstream school, and dyslexics learn to read and write very well.

It is the resultant academic success that contributes to huge increases in self-esteem. Thomson and Hartley (1980), for example, found that the main source of low self-esteem in dyslexic children had been their mainstream school environment. Those who had been to a specialist school for some years had increased their social self-esteem from 32% on entry to 84% on leaving. Academic self-esteem went from 45% on entry to 77% on leaving. Humphrey (2002) reviews other research that concluded 'children with special needs in segregated units tend to have a more positive sense of self than those educated in mainstream schools' (p. 30).

Is dyslexic self-esteem a single unity?
No – although I have to say that I would find the notion of self-esteem as a single unity easier to work with. In reality, it does not hold up to scrutiny.

Self-esteem can have many different facets. It can include concepts of control, optimism, self-image, self-talk and internalized role models. Thus, which part of their self-esteem is low for a particular client? Dyslexic children, for example, can have strikingly high ambitions for themselves alongside their literacy anxieties.

Coopersmith (1967) found that children assess their own success on a variety of criteria: power (the ability to influence and control others), significance (the acceptance, attention and affection of others), virtue (adherence to moral and ethical standards) and competence (successful performance in meeting demand for achievements).

Each of these areas can be subdivided, so that a child may see himself as a success in sport or science but not in academic performance. The approval of key people is also important at each stage. This is why father, teacher or peer approval are so central in establishing self-esteems at different ages, and why different areas of possible success for a dyslexic can buffer literacy failure.

In this respect, I am interested in the recent work by Mearns (1999) on the notion of 'configurations'. He sees these as 'a number of elements which form a coherent pattern ... within the Self' (p. 126), and believes that there is a 'complex family of parts' (p. 126) in any individual.

Using Mearns' analogy, dyslexics might have parts labelled 'victim at school', 'poor little boy', 'class dunce'. These can exist alongside 'best swimmer', 'great artist', 'brilliant mathematician', 'funny boy in class', and so on: 'It is not any one configuration within the client's Self which is important but the whole constellation of the configurations and the dynamics which define their inter-relationship. It is this dynamic integration which will result in an overall picture that reflects the person's Self' (p. 127).

In this context, it is interesting that recent research on modern dyslexics by DePonio (2001) found that dyslexic students had quite different levels of self-esteem related to friendship compared to that of academic performance. In the area of friendship, a high proportion of dyslexics regarded themselves as important members of their class, and thought their friends thought they had good ideas. Nonetheless, in the academic areas, half indicated that they were slow in finishing work and half admitted that they were nervous when the teacher called on them. The confidence experienced amongst family and close friends was not mirrored in class. Pupils recognized their own strengths and abilities, yet there was reluctance to apply this to academic performance.

Finally, dyslexics do not restrict their own self-esteem configuration as much as non-dyslexics do so for them. Researchers are fond of focusing on those parts of dyslexia that Mearns defined as the part that is labelled 'not for growth' (p. 127).

Is dyslexic self-esteem judged fairly?
No. It is, for most of us, the equivalent of our self-esteem being assessed on whether we can sing an aria or not.

Normally, we choose the areas in which we wish to compete, and we judge ourselves against high standards in those areas. For dyslexic children, the territory of literacy has been chosen for them, and they are being asked to succeed in an area for which they are not equipped. Once out of this area, or in parallel to it, a dyslexic person can succeed perfectly well. Some other, independent value of self-esteem can be established. The two areas do not have to cancel each other out. They can co-exist.

Does poor esteem in literacy contaminate everything else?

Of course it can, but it doesn't have to, and a counsellor can easily help here through a classic supportive therapeutic relationship or more direct use of CBT methods. Above all, a counsellor must not collude in unreasonable limitations imposed on a dyslexic child or adult.

I think that this 'oil-slick' view of 'low dyslexic self-esteem' – that it contaminates everything – is too easily assumed by parents, schools and the dyslexics themselves. This is what turns a problem into a disaster. The suggestion that 'it is only dyslexia' and 'yes, you have some problems – now how will you cope?' is far more useful than perpetuation of the 'poor me' and 'ain't it awful' approach, which is far too prevalent in dyslexic literature. This attitude adds to the weight of the problem rather than lightening or extinguishing it

Is 'poor self-esteem' a strategic psychological choice by a dyslexic client?

I think it is.

It is a basic tenet of counselling that children develop coping strategies when they are very young that not only fail to work when they are adults but eventually start to trip them up. These early strategies are carried forward unconsciously into adult life where they remain as unexamined handicaps. In this respect, a counsellor of a dyslexic client may wish to ask whether it has become useful for her client to adopt the working strategy of 'low self-esteem'.

My experience is that aspects of 'low self-esteem' may have complicated pay-offs in the life of a dyslexic client that may be hard to extinguish without reframing whole life systems, including significant relationships. I have, for example, commonly encountered, among my more honest clients, acknowledgement that variants of the 'I'm so thin/fat/stupid/unattractive/thick' dyslexic self-image can be used to charming and devastating effect with the opposite sex, or to annoy family members in satisfying passive-aggressive ways.

What improves self-esteem in dyslexics?

Literacy.

Most of all, dyslexics just want to learn to read and write, and all the evidence suggests that literacy, alone, improves self-esteem. Nothing else is as important. Additionally, when I ask dyslexic clients how they would know that their self-esteem had improved, their answer usually revolves around reduced anxiety levels and an improved sense of control. Certainly, when dyslexic clients find some control over their anxiety through classic therapeutic process and/or the direct help of cognitive-behavioural techniques, it is this that makes them feel so much better generally.

Would getting rid of dyslexia itself help?
Dyslexics would very much like to get rid of the effects of their dyslexia – the worst of which are poor literacy, relationship problems and anxiety.

It is absolutely essential to note, however, that many dyslexic people do not see improvements in their self-esteem arising from losing their dyslexia. It may seem an odd thing to say, but it is important to have respect for a dyslexic person's dyslexia. After all, their dyslexia is a significant part of who they are. Once we demonize their dyslexia, we demonize them.

For example, I once did an exercise in guided imagery with a group of ten- to 13-year-old dyslexic children in which they were invited to exchange anything they owned for anything they wanted. It was an important learning moment for me when I found that only two in this group of over 30 children wanted to give up their dyslexia. If we respect dyslexia for what it is, and the advantages and experiences it can bestow, we are automatically respecting the dyslexic person just as they are. Being accepted for who we are is also an important component in good self-esteem.

The infantilized dyslexic

Are dyslexics generally mature or immature for their age?
Immature – and strangely 'uncooked'.

In this respect, I find it interesting that so many of my dyslexic clients invite me into a maternal transference. They can present very often as childlike – in manner, dress and speech patterns. I also find it interesting that writers and researchers on the dyslexic adult should feel the need to say that the adult dyslexic is not a *dyslexic child grown up* (McLoughlin et al. 2002, Patton and Holloway 1992).

I think that such writers are missing the point. There is a case that dyslexic adults are very much grown-up children, and this can become an important issue both in counselling them as individuals and in working with their families. For example, I recently had a telephone call from the mother of a dyslexic to arrange counselling for him. She had not consulted with her son, who was in his twenties and married with a child. She found nothing odd about her request.

In terms of the Transactional Analysis (TA) drivers, the dyslexic child and adult, more than any other client group I encounter, has internalized the instruction 'Don't grow up'.

How do dyslexics internalize the notion that they should not grow up?
I suggest that there are a number of reasons: personal, familial and social.

All action in support of dyslexics is by non-dyslexics

This alone sends the message that dyslexics cannot look after themselves. They are not trusted to be out on their own. They need minders. Dyslexics do not represent themselves, and all the support and action for dyslexics is from non-dyslexics. Dyslexics themselves also have no group identity or political consciousness. A comparable political situation would have been for men to have led all the political action for the feminist movement while the women looked on in a rather uninterested and passive way. Most dyslexic adults have little interest in what is done on their behalf, and no idea whatsoever of what the dyslexia establishment is doing 'for them'. Generally, they carry on in their own, very individual way to make sense of the experiences they encounter.

Dyslexic self-protest is locked into the pre-literate stage

Should dyslexics wish to protest on their own behalf, they do not have the printed media available to them because of their disability. Their main symbol of protest has to be verbal. Since they also have speech and language difficulties, even that route is impaired.

Dyslexics are locked into the protest mechanisms of the toddler stage; that is, imperfect verbal protest and no literacy. This toddler protest occurs in the context of a big 'mummy' dyslexic world peopled by a powerful army of dyslexic researchers, campaigners and angry overprotective mothers. Just as no toddler has power, so can the dyslexic fear that they have no power in this wider world. This is probably why most dyslexics just let the dyslexia world get on with it.

As a counsellor, I would ask why the dyslexic person is such a tiny cog in the vast, and often cumbersome, production that would not exist without him. If he were the driver – think Richard Branson and the many other dyslexic millionaires – would it not run better and more efficiently? Furthermore, just why are people involved with a cause where the main recipients are marginalized both in and out of it? What is their stake in this?

I sense that if the dyslexic majority were to organize politically and demand the literacy that should have been theirs half a century ago, then the dyslexic establishment would find it very difficult – like a toddler challenging a parent.

Dyslexia is the only adult disability defined entirely by school

The origin of the dyslexic's problems lies in learning to read and write. These are school-related problems and, by definition, child-based. There is no other disability that is only defined through the failure to acquire a child's skill.

Without school and literacy, there would be no dyslexic disability. In pre-literate times, dyslexic adults would have been valued for their contribution to grown-up activities such as building and engineering. It is highly likely that they would have been the great leaders, military strategists and admired members of society.

Dyslexics have no adult role in modern society. Without any obvious signs of disability, they are more impaired from making an adult contribution than those who are deaf, blind or in wheelchairs. Dyslexia is a childlike disability, even when you are an adult. As a disability it is not even grown-up.

The female of the species is deadlier than the male

A dyslexic boy or girl – particularly a boy – creates his identity through surviving the attentions of powerful women. As Park (1995) suggests, 'All boys confront the same problem: how to feel strong in the presence of an all-powerful and demanding mother' (p. 5), but the dyslexic often has two such women to contend with. On the one hand, there is the protective, fierce mother and, on the other, the critical, powerful woman who teaches him. He can have two lionesses to manage – one at home from whom he must defend himself against engulfment, and one at school from whom he must defend himself against annihilation.

Childish behaviour, which elicits maternal reaction, becomes a survival mechanism at both home and school. The female teacher might not respond to a more grown-up response and, if he shows signs of independence, his mother might abandon him to more isolation, of which he has plenty, or – perhaps worse – an envious, hostile father, waiting in the wings. Like a mouse surrounded by three large attentive cats, staying very small and very still is a sensible option.

That I find no reference to the emasculation and castration fears of the dyslexic male is also a function of the other main effect of this powerful feminine influence – the desexualization of the dyslexic (see below).

Mummy stays powerful if the dyslexic child stays helpless

Women discover themselves through their dyslexic children. Women who would not have dreamed of arguing with a traffic warden before their child was diagnosed as dyslexic, learn to take on local authorities, barristers and school organizations. They confront and manipulate head teachers and tribunals, lobby MPs and go on radio and television to fight for their children.

Mothers of dyslexic children are the unsung heroes of the dyslexia world. Yet, there is another side to this. What happens if their dyslexic child no longer needs them? Where does their identity go? Does an independent, enabled dyslexic child mean that they have to forgo that powerful identity? What do they do with their new self? There is a real danger that women might have a stake in keeping their disabled child both a child and disabled. The child, sensing this, can sabotage his recovery.

A troubled child can save a buckled marriage

A very common scenario in dyslexic family therapy is the child who causes problems so that his parents have to unite to solve them. The parents collude in this because, without the dyslexic child continuing to be a problem, their marital problems would have to be faced. All parties are in on this happy collusion but, at the centre, is the child – or rather a troubled child. An untroubled child would not hold the centre, which threatens the home and marriage with disaster.

By being a problem, the child is a solution. This is a worry for any child, but for a dyslexic child who fears isolation, and abhors change, it is more so. The dyslexic child can use both his childishness and his dyslexia in this situation. Some dyslexic adults are still locked into this role well into their twenties and thirties.

Where is daddy?

The absent father prevents his son from making a satisfactory transition of the Oedipal stage, leaving the dyslexic boy locked into an early, unconscious sexual liaison with his mother.

'What he needs is someone to help him deal with the terror which she can provoke so that he can gain a glimpse of how she really is – most likely a woman trying to do the best she can in difficult circumstances. Only the presence of an attentive father, or a father-substitute, willing to expose his strengths and weaknesses, someone who will listen to him and talk with him can neutralise the boy's anxiety about intimacy with her' (Park 1995, p. 5).

It is also the case that the father often envies this small, dyslexic, male interloper who steals so much time and energy from his wife. If the father is not dyslexic, and secretly thinks his son is just stupid, he alienates his son by criticism and scorn. If the father is dyslexic, his son is competing with him for what he needs, and has grown up with himself; the protection and safety of a powerful woman – his mother/wife.

Commonly, a dyslexic son has to compete with a jealous adult man who does not act like a father because he was not fathered himself. The son is, thus, under-fathered and starved of male influence, which further emasculates him and perpetuates the family norm of paternal-absence (Biddulph 1998). Generations of dyslexic sons have decided that it is safer not to grow up. This way, at least, their mothers will protect them.

Clearly, it is not just the genetic components of dyslexia that are inherited but a whole swathe of behavioural effects, too.

The only time that this does not occur is with a dyslexic father with an unsympathetic non-dyslexic wife. The father is then protective of his son, understands him and often has a superb, close relationship with him. Such children are very well adjusted, since the mother is protective – but not too much so – and the father is engaged and kind. Such dyslexic children embody dyslexia's best features, and they cope very well indeed – often better than non-dyslexic boys. They are also much more adult and independent in their relationships and lifestyle.

Inadequate transition of the latency stage

The problems with dyslexia coincide with the latency stage of development. The failed transition of the latency stage prevents the safe passage of the dyslexic child to adolescent sexuality – the genital stage – or forces his regression to the narcissistic aspects of the pre-latent oral and anal stages, including a more infantile sexuality.

Regression to, or marooning in, the pre-latent stage means returning to the intimate and dependent family relationship of the young child. This stage is usually left when, in the latency stage, the child moves to a more social relationship with the rest of the world.

Locked into this earlier stage, and unable to move forward into adolescent sexuality, the dyslexic can remain eternally narcissistic and childlike. He may also remain pre-sexual, avoiding – even in manhood – the company of women who might be sexually attracted to him.

Frequently, he discovers, in his twenties and thirties, the gang of male friends that the latency stage denied to him ten years earlier. So tenacious and protective is this group, that it is often only the determined attention of a strong, older, rather motherly and bossy woman who prises him away. Almost with relief, the dyslexic returns to the enveloping female cocoon he knows so very well.

'But he is so creative and artistic', or 'get on with your colouring'

Dyslexics are praised for their artistic and creative ability. While it may be true, this attitude can also seem like one big consolation prize for missing the payout of literacy. It compares to the dyslexic in the remedial class who is given colouring-in to occupy him because he is seen as too thick to learn how to read. Colouring and creativity are symbolic of the infant school; of the children who cannot yet read.

The emphasis on the dyslexic's creativity and 'gift' also compares to the early social stereotypes of blacks who – lacking political status or education – were portrayed as happy children; their main asset being a 'natural sense of rhythm'. Dyslexics also lacks political status and education, and their main asset is considered to be their 'gift' of creativity.

Dyslexic sexuality

Of dyslexics in this country, 80% of them are aged 16 or over. This means that the majority of dyslexic people in this country are adult dyslexics. The overwhelming image of dyslexia, however, is associated with childhood. I believe that this generates a powerful impetus in the dyslexia field for dyslexics to remain pre-sexual.

Sex is for adults. If you have been eternally encouraged to remain child-like, or you have no adult role models and no peer group with which to try out a sexual and romantic relationship, what happens about sex? If, as a dyslexic, you also have problems reading interpersonal cues, how can you know if someone finds you attractive? If you have no confidence because of those hundreds of thousands of negative introjects over your lifetime, how on earth do you find the confidence to approach a woman?

One attractive, but very diffident, dyslexic student client once observed to me that, even if a woman was transmitting on all channels that she fancied him, he would never notice. Even if he did notice, a dyslexic has then got to get past his lack of confidence, his pre-genital childlike mannerisms and his nervousness about women, all of which are well-fostered in childhood. The temptation to find a woman just like his mother must be overwhelming – although this can give rise to serious complications around sexuality.

Certainly, sex and intimacy very often cause problems for a dyslexic. When women have only symbolized mothering, annihilation and engulf-ment, and there has been little or no adolescent sexual experimentation, then all sexual relationships are a minefield.

I don't know how many dyslexics are cross-dressers, but I bet the number is not small – for all the reasons given above, but also because it is known to reduce anxiety. I would also guess that problems with intimacy, impotence and anxious attachment occur a lot with dyslexics, and that dyslexic homo-sexuals are relatively more sexually adjusted than heterosexuals.

With dyslexic females, the problem does not seem to exist. They have often had the advantage of being largely ignored by both parents, so they have been able to find their own way to adulthood. I do not offer a representative sample, but adult female dyslexics seem to have a far more robust and happy sexuality with a taste for creative, unselfconscious experimentation.

Given that sex is a form of communication, and communication is a central problem with dyslexics, it is an interesting question why there is almost no research on sex and dyslexia, or any commentary on the nature and resolution of sexual problems in dyslexics. Both semantically and socially, sex is hidden in dyslexia.

Work published by dyslexics is presented in a patronizing and childish way

When work by dyslexic writers is published in dyslexia journals, it is often unedited and presented with all its spelling mistakes, whereas non-dyslexic writers will have the usual editorial corrections. The effect of this is to make dyslexic writers appear childish and incompetent. The dyslexic author, Davis (1997), whose book is an account of the experience of being dyslexic, is published in the large print associated with young children's reading books.

Coping strategies: balancing out the negative

Can dyslexics survive their negative experiences?
Yes – and this is not unusual. Many children who have had challenging experiences find strategies to cope.

Rutter (1985), for example, writing about the effects of adversity on children, showed that, while some children succumb, many others develop resilience in the face of adversity: 'The notion of effective and ineffective coping is a very plausible one' (p. 359).

Cowie and Dawkins (2002), in a study on psychotherapeutic intervention with children, found that: 'Most young people appear to cope with the difficulties that they encounter. They may be sad, angry, upset or disappointed, but they are not overwhelmed by the ups and downs of life' (p. 23).

The same is true of dyslexics – both children and adults.

Is there acknowledgement of the dyslexic's ability to cope?
Not really. Dyslexia literature and research does not dwell on this aspect of the dyslexic character, a tendency that colludes with the view that dyslexics can only be disabled or infantile.

Pumphrey and Reason (1991) are two of the few writers in this field who note the wider picture. For example, they quote research on the negative effects of dyslexia that showed linguistic/cognitive factors to account for 42% of the variance but the social-emotional factor for only 27%. They advise researchers: 'do not make blanket assumptions about social and emotional influences' (p. 69).

Porter and Rourke (1985) also showed that, while 25% of dyslexics had a depressive/anxious profile, 15% were aggressive and the largest number – over 50% – showed no disturbance at all.

A similar study by Speece et al. (1985) found that one-third of learning-disabled children demonstrated completely normal profiles in social-emotional functioning, while Ackerman et al. (1986) found that a significant proportion of learning-disabled pupils were regarded as popular with their peers in after-school interests. DePonio (2001) found that, of the dyslexics studied, only a few fell into the category regarded as a serious indicator of low self-concept.

Rourke (1988) also questioned the inevitability of learning difficulties leading to anxiety, low self-esteem and further difficulties, and Riddick (1996) reviewed research studies which 'underline the point that it is important not to assume that all children with dyslexia will automatically have social or emotional difficulties' (p. 33).

Finally, the recent report by the British Psychological Society's working party on dyslexia concludes that 'adverse emotional consequences [of dyslexia] are not inevitable'. Much depends on 'individual coping strategies' and the degree to which the dyslexic's school and home can 'cushion' their difficulties (BPS 1999, p. 43).

Many dyslexics cope perfectly well. They use strategies to do so. These are unlikely to be the dyslexics who reach counsellors, but counsellors can usefully examine how the adjusted dyslexics cope, and what they are doing to stay on an even keel.

Do dyslexics develop coping strategies?

Yes. Everyone can develop coping strategies – even children with serious chronic disorders (Wallender and Varni 1998), and a dyslexic is no exception. Their greater creativity and problem-solving skills also make them well-equipped to help themselves.

'Dyslexic people learn to accommodate to a greater or lesser degree depending on their own personality and the type of support they have received from both home and school. Individuals will experience difficulties throughout their lives and the majority learn to develop strategies to enable them to cope most of the time' (BDA 2003).

Morgan and Klein (2000), reporting on dyslexic adults, found that their difficulties 'no longer impede their ability to conduct their daily lives ... [they] have overcome many of the more obvious symptoms' (p. 63).

What coping strategies do dyslexics commonly use?
The main coping strategies are:

Social support and encouragement

Social support buffers hardship; and encouragement, in particular, is priceless to a dyslexic. Such support is the most powerful indicator of how well people will survive stressful experiences, and social support has a direct buffering effect on stress reactions (Vanzetti and Duck 1996).

Riddick (1996) found that a relationship with an adult who believed in, and encouraged, a dyslexic child made a huge difference to their self-esteem. Sometimes, just teaching a dyslexic child to ask for help can be the most sensible and empowering think an adult can do.

Effort

There is some evidence that struggle strengthens people. Wood (1983) has built an entire therapy around this assumption: 'The increase in self-respect will be directly proportional to the degree of difficulty and the amount of vigour and determination that we apply to the task' (p. 6) (see also Chapter 2).

Parental modelling

Our reaction to fear and stress is affected by how we saw our parents react to similar situations. Phobias, for example, can appear through direct observational learning from, and modelling on, parents (Rachman 1977).

Dyslexic children who see a dyslexic parent cope, or who are encouraged by their parents to deal courageously and sensibly with their dyslexia, will acquire the same attitude. This parental reaction will also be taken as the model when other problems appear. The degree to which parents see something as 'no big deal – we'll sort this out' or 'omigod, it's a disaster' will be internalized by their child. Harrington (1995) found that 'parental reactions to disaster are very important in mediating the psychological impact on children' (p. 120).

Modelling of coping behaviour by significant others – such as teacher or a therapist – is also effective, as well as knowing that powerful media role models are dyslexic, too (see Appendix F).

Perception of threat

There are two stages in response to a threat – whether it is a car approaching too fast or a teacher advancing with a reading book.

First, is the situation a threat? Second, can I cope and deal with this threat?

An over-anxious person 'tends to overestimate danger and underestimate coping resources' (Trower et al. 1988). An anxious person also shows 'selective abstraction' – the tendency to be hypersensitive to the threatening aspects of the situation and ignore the positive or benign aspects.

This is a fertile basis for counselling, particularly therapeutic models that aim to challenge and extinguish automatic and catastrophizing thoughts. Such models are particularly effective with those dyslexics who tend to read threat into all unknown situations (see Chapter 5).

Determination and persistence

The notion of determination and stubborn refusal to give up pervades many of the personal interviews I have conducted with dyslexic clients and adults. When I ask 'What has dyslexia given you?', they almost always reflect on their ability to struggle, cope, survive and 'stay in there'. Parents often observe this characteristic in their dyslexic child.

Weekes (1997), for example, quotes a mother on her dyslexic child who, although he was clumsy, poorly coordinated and had problems with reading and spelling, also had 'a dogged determination' (p. 58), which always got him through.

In this context, I was interested to read a research report in *The Sunday Times* (24 November 2002) on the 'Kevin' syndrome. It seems that young adults in their twenties are increasingly behaving like confused and insecure adolescents, and having problems adjusting to adult life: 'having been praised highly during their school years, the realization that they are nobody special comes as a shock'. Many dyslexic teenagers who leave school have had many years to internalize the common view of others that they are 'nobody special', and have had to find ways to cope with the idea. This may account for why many dyslexic students are so valued at university and have such a remarkable reputation for hard work. I do not meet many dyslexic 'Kevins'.

The strengthening power of adversity

Early stresses can make us strong. This is a characteristic that is often observed in therapy: 'the steely courage that sometimes accompanies early damage' (Martin 2001, p. 10). This effect of adversity was originally investigated by Selye (1956), who found that previous experiences can toughen people or 'inoculate' them against further stress.

It is now commonly observed that all abused children – whether dyslexic or not – are typified by 'ego-resiliency, ego-over control, and self-esteem' (Glaser 2000, p. 105). Ego-control, in particular, can be useful since 'it is probably more feasible to encourage children to develop strategies of gaining control over their actions ... self-organisation by the child needs to be encouraged and fostered by those intervening' (p. 110).

The importance of perceived control

This is a most important coping mechanism, since it can change attitudes to a potential stressor. Encouraging a view that a person has the power to change the way they live their lives – that they can choose to do things differently – is probably the most significant step forward for anyone with a disability.

Dyslexic adults often reach this conclusion on their own. Encouraging it in dyslexic children is a perfect way forward: 'You have dyslexia. It is going to be tough, but let's look at ways of dealing with it'. Taking control can also mean avoiding stressful situations, such as applying for the wrong type of job (see Chapter 10). In one recent study, dyslexic students had developed coping strategies that sensibly and parsimoniously 'involved not allowing themselves to be put in a situation where they might appear to fail' (McDougall et al. 2002, p. 2).

Extroversion and humour

Morgan and Klein (2000) refer to the dyslexic use of humour as a coping strategy. 'Many dyslexic people learn to use their charm and good verbal skills to "talk their way out of trouble"' (p. 71). Others use humour to soften the effects of doing things wrong or forgetting to do things. The class clown at school is a very common dyslexic school role. Making people laugh distracts them from your failure. Dyslexic adults also use humour to avoid embarrassment in reading or mispronunciation.

A mixture

The reality is that dyslexics use more than one coping strategy, and, the more they use, the more buffered they are from the effects of their disability. There is some evidence that the new generation of younger dyslexics, who have multiple support, are faring far better than dyslexics did in the past.

Lane (2001), for example, found that parental understanding of dyslexic difficulties, coupled with formal assessment (see Chapter 10), may have enabled the children in her study to preserve their self-esteem. In fact, the children's locus of control became more internal over the year of study. 'This could be due to a number of factors, including their difficulties being formally recognised, being given specific remedial help, exposure to successful role models in the media and a recognition that some have areas [of skill] in the national curriculum' (p. 1).

McDougall (2001) found, too: 'Recent research presents a more optimistic picture of dyslexic children's experiences than earlier work, and suggests that the attitudes of others may be changing and that more support may be available to help children' (p. 7).

Do dyslexics find ways of coping with academic work?
Yes – and they have considerable experience and ingenuity in doing this.

'Compensated dyslexics' are those who have learnt to read and acquire basic skills by different routes.

Interest is one significant factor. Morgan and Klein (2000), for example, refer to highly successful dyslexic adults, in a range of fields, who are able to read at a much higher level in their own subject than general texts in a newspaper. Fink (1995) also found that her successful dyslexic adults sample had learned to read through a passionate interest in their chosen subject. Morgan and Klein (2000) record the advice of a dyslexic student: 'Find something you're interested in and the reading and writing will come from there' (p. 18).

The other main way in which such compensated dyslexic adults learn to read is through contextual clues.

Snowling (2000) refers to this compensation as a 'proficiency and deficiency' (p. 198). She observes that some dyslexic children have an ability to read words in sentences that are embedded in texts, and are better at it than non-dyslexics. In effect, they see sentences as patterns in context. This is also linked to the dyslexic ability to visualize whole situations at a glance. In this respect, dyslexics can use their innate abilities as a coping strategy, and to compensate for their phonological impairment.

Finally, it is worth noting that adult dyslexics can do very well indeed in academic and literary-based employment (McDougall 2001, Hellendoorn and Ruijsenaars 2000). Vogel and Adelman (1999), for example, found that teachers with dyslexia had a higher salary and more job satisfaction – despite the need for help with language-related tasks and more time to complete tasks.

Do dyslexics benefit from their experiences?
They do – and this is encapsulated in the relatively new research tradition of post-traumatic growth (PTG) (see Calhoun and Tedeschi 1999 and O'Leary et al. 1998).

I find this concept useful when looking at how dyslexics commonly emerge from their experiences with considerable wisdom and humour. On the basis that both failure and disappointment can be beneficial (Craib 1994), or Nietzsche's assertion that 'what does not kill us makes us stronger', it appears that people can emerge from psychological trauma in 'psychological credit'. As counsellors, we can fail 'to see the extent to which people can at times benefit in from some way from their experiences' (Linley and Joseph 2002, p. 14). This concept – post-traumatic growth – may even be more prevalent than post-traumatic stress.

What is post-traumatic growth?
It is the positive side-effect of human damage.

Linley and Joseph, for example, report that 30%–90% of survivors report some positive changes following trauma. Their relationships are enhanced in some ways, they feel increased compassion and altruism and 'have an increased sense of personal resiliency and strength, perhaps coupled with a greater acceptance of their vulnerabilities and limitations' (p. 15). These people are often aware of changes in life philosophy and find a fresh appreciation for each day. Importantly, the experience of growth can co-exist with that of distress.

How can a counsellor use the theory of post-traumatic growth?
Post-traumatic growth (PTG) can arise as a result of the rumination and restructuring that take place in the weeks, months and even years following a trauma.

It is a process of change that develops with self-knowledge and greater resilience. Focusing on the client's new, positive traits can help them to repair self-schemas damaged by the trauma or to challenge negative self-schemas that have arisen as a result of the trauma. This provides hope that the trauma has not just caused damage but might even have done some good, and 'there may even be the potential for positive gains arising from it' (Linley and Joseph 2002, p. 17).

Research on the social and psychological effects of dyslexia: a critique

In researching the topics discussed in this chapter, it became clear that research in this area is significantly impaired in a number of ways. There are, for example, certain fundamental assumptions about the effects of dyslexia, deeply entrenched in the dyslexia culture, which are also deeply entrenched in the research.

That these effects are both assumed and, therefore, 'discovered' by researchers in this field is an important and worrying issue in its own right. Thus, in examining the effects of dyslexia, it is useful to end both this chapter and section by casting an eye over the research from which these effects emerge. I would raise the following points:

- The research field that identifies the psychological and social effects of dyslexia is relatively young, sparse and has little of the rigour and test-retest validity of its older, sister areas in, say, clinical and cognitive psychology. Riddick (1996), for example, has criticized the lack of a systematic sampling policy in this field, and the unrepresentative sampling, often of white, middle-class children and parents. Qualitative research from seven or eight subjects is interesting but cannot be applied universally, and research on dyslexic women and girls is almost non-existent despite recent evidence that the number of dyslexic females is nearly equal to that of dyslexic males. There is, furthermore, no good research whatsoever on sexual or relational problems in dyslexic adults, issues that are burning for investigation.

- Much of the research appears to have a predetermined directional bias; for example, that the direct cause of a dyslexic's problem is their dyslexia and that the effects of dyslexia are all bad. Also, many studies start from the directional hypothesis that the effect of dyslexia is negative. Against the trend of all other psychological research, this field does not favour the null hypothesis. This means that no researcher really believes that there may be either no effect of dyslexia or that there might be a positive effect.

- This directional assumption leads to reportage that seems to have a few blind spots. For example, Riddick et al. (1999) report that around a dozen studies have shown that up to 25% of dyslexic samples met the criteria for serious anxiety disorder. Yet, the normal percentage of adolescents and children with serious anxiety disorder is around 20% representing 'the most prevalent psychiatric disorder in this age group' (Legrand et al. 1999, p. 953). Thus, the rate of serious anxiety in dyslexics does not appear to be significantly higher than non-dyslexics, unless dyslexics make up most of the entire seriously anxious adolescent population. Importantly, does this research not show that the vast majority of dyslexics – 75% – do not suffer from a major anxiety disorder? It would be useful to know what these dyslexics are like and what we can learn from them. The directional bias of such research reportage only focuses researchers on the research stereotype.

- If a reported experience by other people conflicts with the dyslexic's own reported experience, it is the non-dyslexic view that is given greater credence. As a counsellor, I find this troubling not least because it goes against the therapeutic assumption that the client is trustworthy and is the best source of information. The rejection of the dyslexic's reported experience is, I believe, part of the infantilizing of dyslexics (see Chapter 9), and also reveals assumptions of disability in dyslexics: that they don't know their own minds.

- There is a danger that dyslexia researchers are colluding with the socially defined negative view of dyslexia, which the dyslexic has also internalized. In other words, researchers may just be measuring their own bias coming back the other way. If, for example, a dyslexic manages to have no bad experiences, or just has a few specific bad experiences, or has only good experiences or finds ways of surviving very bad experiences intact, current researchers in this field would seem to be reluctant to uncover it or, if they did uncover it, to report it without bias. In some ways, this research bias compares to early research on women and blacks that had conspicuous blind spots about intelligence and ability.

Riddick (1996), in her seminal work on dyslexia, was clearly aware of these pitfalls. She observes: 'there is little research on the social and emotional consequences of dyslexia [but] *despite* the paucity of research, concerned clinicians and educationalists have consistently pointed to the devastating effects that dyslexia or specific learning disabilities can have on some children's lives ... this is a difficult and complex area to research' (p. 32, my italics).

Furthermore, there is nothing on a therapeutic or psychoanalytic perspective, or on issues of concern to dyslexics themselves.

In fact, nobody – it seems – has ever asked dyslexics what they would like to know about themselves. I wonder why.

SECTION FIVE
COUNSELLING

Introduction

While walking along a river bank, a counsellor sees a child drowning. Immediately, she dives in and saves a life. Once safely on dry land, the counsellor turns to see two more children in the same predicament and bravely dives in and saves two more lives. Exhausted but relieved, the counsellor sits down on the river bank when a passer-by approaches and comments: 'I've just watched you save three children's lives. That's fantastic, but could I make a suggestion? Have you ever considered going around the bend in the river upstream to see who might be pushing them in?' (adapted from Mackay 2002, quoted in Cowie and Dawkins 2002).

Counselling dyslexic clients will involve more than just the therapeutic process.

This is one branch of therapy that really benefits from some practical additional help from the counsellor to the client.

Some therapists might find this uncomfortable. Nevertheless, a counsellor working effectively with dyslexic clients needs to:

1. understand *what it means to be dyslexic*
2. be able to access *help with reading and writing*
3. know how to get an *assessment and diagnosis* of dyslexia and follow up the results
4. understand how *the counselling process* must adjust for the client's dyslexia

The most effective systems for dyslexic counselling combine all four areas.

One of these components without the other will provide counselling for dyslexic clients that is, at best, just 'good enough' and, at worst, is just 'not good enough at all'.

CHAPTER 10

Counselling practice with dyslexic clients

Summary

An effective counselling system for dyslexic clients combines assessment, literacy training and counselling. The evidence is that the best counselling provision for dyslexic clients makes an intelligent, integrated use of all these components.

Effective counselling systems for dyslexics

How do effective counselling systems work?

One part alone is always less effective than the whole.

For example, counselling work alone aimed at enhancing dyslexic self-esteem or stress reduction will have a limited effect. In fact, Pumphrey (1979) found that even direct literacy instruction of a dyslexic had more effect than counselling alone. There is also good evidence that many dyslexic problems can be solved through a focus on assessment, literacy and social-skills training, with counselling providing back-up support.

Lawrence (1971), for example, found that dyslexic children who received remedial help with reading showed a greater improvement when this was supplemented by a therapeutic approach aimed at enhancing self-esteem. Clients receiving reading instruction, alongside counselling or drama therapy, enjoyed greater success in reading and self-esteem than those who received reading help only.

The solutions are not proportional. Counselling alone will sort out 20% of the problems, whereas literacy training alone will sort out 80% (Kline and Kline 1973).

McLoughlin et al. (2002), for example, are clear that: 'Counselling is the logical extension of the assessment process' (p. 33). They add that those dyslexics who are most likely to emerge into adulthood with their egos intact are usually the ones who have received a combination of diagnosis, understanding and appropriate support.

What systems have used combined assessment and counselling to help dyslexics?
Mostly – those in the universities.

These provide some of the best support systems for dyslexic help and provision. For example, The Dyslexia Unit at the University of Wales, Bangor, provides assessment, counselling and study skills in one department. The emphasis is on creating coping strategies and support, particularly during critical periods for dyslexics such as course changes and examinations. The counsellor also provides specific help with organization and practical problems (Miles and Gilroy 1986).

This multilayered approach to dyslexic counselling is integral to the whole process since it addresses both practical and emotional problems.

Are there voluntary projects?
There are many informal projects set up by motivated individuals that support dyslexics in and out of the main system.

The common characteristic is that they address both the emotional and literacy problems of dyslexic adults and children. I have already referred in Chapter 7 to the different programmes providing help for dyslexic inmates in prisons, such as the Dyspel programmes. The PALS (Positive Action through Learning Support) is a similar system, working with probation officers and employment offices for referral, assessment and teaching of dyslexic offenders There is also Link into Learning. This teaches adult-based literacy programmes. In addition to the more traditional 'bottom up' approach to literacy normally taught to children, Link into Learning uses an intensive 'top down' system that utilizes dyslexic adults' existing learning strategies. Other psychological problems of the students are picked up along the way.

Springboard For Children is a literacy charity working in south London, supporting 130 children in six schools around Peckham, with a teaching staff of 26 teachers and volunteers. It gives high standards of individual support for dyslexic children in all the schools in its area, and was founded by a committee of local residents who set it up and trained as dyslexia teachers. The Harris City Technology College was established in 1997, specifically to attract dyslexic children. The college designs its whole teaching to foster the skills and bypass the difficulties of dyslexics, particularly those who are well motivated with supportive parents. There are universities, too, as noted above, who have identified dyslexia as niche markets.

Many offer screening, counselling and special teaching for dyslexics. These are considered to be areas of excellence.

Are there any counsellors who have dyslexia?
I have no exact idea because the information is not available.

My response to an advertisement in the British Association of Counselling and Psychotherapy (BACP) journal (Summer 2002) yielded 28 replies from dyslexic counsellors that, if typical, suggests that there are not many. Certain inferences can be made from statistics about the numbers of people working in counselling and psychotherapy. In 2002, BACP had 19,836 individual members of whom 4,111 were accredited (20.7%). Of the individual members, 83% were female and 17% male. There are also 140,000 volunteer counsellors in the UK, giving a total estimate of 250,000 people using 'counselling skills' in their line of work in the UK.

On the higher estimate of 10% of the population being dyslexic, this suggests that there are around 400 accredited counsellors in the UK who are dyslexic. My experience talking to dyslexic counsellors is that they find the paperwork for accreditation an almost impossible hurdle, so I would estimate that the real number is less than half this. Finding a non-accredited dyslexic counsellor member of BACP is more probable. On previous assumptions – there are around 1600–1800 in the UK.

The overall indication is that there is very little chance that a dyslexic client will find an accredited dyslexic counsellor by chance. It is even less likely that any dyslexic client will find any dyslexic counsellor who operates in their area. It would be helpful if dyslexic counsellors could form a sub-group – as their abilities and understanding of dyslexia would be valuable.

Counselling for dyslexics in primary care

Is dyslexia understood in primary care?
Not really – considering that dyslexia is one of the most prevalent, heritable and disabling conditions in this country.

Cooke (2001), in her observations on dyslexia provision, records her disappointment that 'even now and despite the accumulated evidence over many years' (p. 51) 28% of clinical professionals are unable to recognize what are considered typical cases of dyslexia. This compares to the fact that, in an episode of the quiz show *The Weakest Link* (January 2002), a contestant given the symptoms of dyslexia and asked to describe the condition answered correctly without hesitation. It seems that the public understanding of dyslexia has not quite trickled into the professional, where there is still some residual resistance. A dyslexic's mother, university, counsellor or

teacher are still more likely to recognize dyslexia than primary-care professionals.

Do dyslexics use primary care for help?

They must do, but the referral procedures do not record dyslexia.

In this respect, I remember attending an informal workshop given by a
child psychiatrist who estimated that the majority of his child referrals for
conduct disorder and depression had unidentified learning and reading
difficulties. He despaired at the fact that questions about literacy were not
asked, as a matter of procedure, for all the psychiatric referrals of children,
since treatment for this was so much easier when the reading difficulty was
identified.

There is nothing available that tells us how many dyslexics appear –
either in GP surgeries or in psychiatric clinics – with primary or secondary
symptoms of illiteracy.

The response from the British Dyslexia Association to my question
about NHS referrals of dyslexics was: 'Dyslexia is largely ignored by the
NHS as it is the province of educational rather than clinical psychologists.
GP funding allows for referral for dyslexia assessment, but GPs are not usually informed as to whom they should refer on. Most parents and
individuals have to arrange private assessments.'

Some indication of numbers can be gleaned from American studies of
psychiatric referrals of dyslexic students. Mattison (2001), for example,
found that, of the 141 behaviourally disturbed students referred for consul-
tation to the school psychiatrist because of ongoing behaviour problems
despite specialized school intervention, over 75% were identified as learning-disabled.

The British Dyslexia Association has published a booklet on dyslexia
specifically for doctors, nurses and other health workers (BDA 1996). This
is an excellent primer for the presenting symptoms and treatment of
dyslexic patients, including the different processes of assessment and referral. It is certainly recommended reading for anyone who might meet a
dyslexic in primary-care settings.

Are GPs a useful area for dyslexic referrals?

Yes. This is because GPs are still a first stop for parents worried about their
child's behavioural problems at school. Garralda and Bailey (1986) found
that work with children occupies about a third to a quarter of a doctor's time.
The authors' review of research in four developing countries indicated that,
of children attending primary-care facilities, 10%–29% were found to be disturbed, and it is a fair assumption that a significant number of them would
have been disturbed because of learning problems – including dyslexia.

Is there counselling provision for dyslexics in GP surgeries?

Yes – more so than in any other area of the NHS.

Importantly, new evidence from BACP demonstrates that there is an extremely robust counselling presence located alongside GPs in their practices (Jenkins 2002, Mellor-Clark 2000). Between 1992 and 1998, the provision of counselling in primary care had grown from 31% to 51% of all GP practices, and is now regarded as very effective (Reid 2001). In 50% of GP practices, counsellors work as members of the primary healthcare team (PHCT). Of these, 87% are women averaging 48 years of age, with about six years' experience as a primary-care counsellor.

Usefully, these counsellors employ a variety of psychotherapeutic treatments (Jenkins 2002) so many would be well suited to help with the effects of dyslexia: 47% of the 1,031 counsellors used CBT alone or in combination with other treatments, 60% psychotherapy alone or in combination and 79% person-centred alone or in combination.

Problems of a psychosocial nature now compose the second largest presenting symptom cluster for primary-care counsellors.

Counselling adults with dyslexia

Are there specific issues to consider in counselling adult dyslexic clients?

Yes – in a broad sense, there are.

Adult dyslexics are already damaged by their experiences; however, it is important to remember that they have survived those experiences. They are not children, and problems of work and literacy replace the child's problems of school and literacy. It is, however, the child in the dyslexic adult who was damaged, and response to that damage resides in adult life choices (Huges and Dawson 1995).

In this respect, dyslexics are no different from any adult clients in that the key to understanding their problems lies in discovering what coping strategies – conscious and unconscious, adaptive and maladaptive – have been internalized and carried forward from childhood to adulthood.

Counselling dyslexic adults is, therefore, informed to a major extent by an understanding of the dyslexic child's experiences with school, peers and all types of parental reaction. After all, as the International Adult Literacy Survey found recently, over 60% of learning-disabled adults reported that their childhood problems still persisted into adult life (Fawcett 2003).

The one common area that arises regularly with dyslexic adults is, however, employment.

Do dyslexic adults have problems at work?

Yes – but, on balance, I would say that dyslexic employees at work are far more protected and supported than dyslexic children at school.

Specific problems are mentioned below, but one important issue a counsellor can examine when a dyslexic adult is having work problems is whether he is transferring his attitudes and perceptions of school onto the work situation. By doing so, dyslexics can become blind to the rights and options available to them and assiduously give power away to employers in the same way they were forced to with teachers. The transference between teacher and employer can be significant, and dyslexic adults can find it instructive when a counsellor draws attention to it.

The reality is that employers are often very helpful to dyslexics – after all, 10% of them are dyslexic themselves – and robust legal measures now exist to support disabled people at work (Marchington-Yeoman and Cooper 2002).

The BDA, recognizing the importance of informed employers to dyslexic employees, devoted the year 2003-2004 to 'dyslexia-wise' employment matters, including campaigns linked to major companies (such as the Ford Motor Company) and the publication of advice booklets for employers (for more details, see the BDA website given in Appendix C).

There are also some specialist books recently published that look directly at how a dyslexic can cope with all sorts of work problems (Bartlett and Moody 2000, McLoughlin 2002, Morgan and Klein 2000).

Importantly, it is at work that a number of adult dyslexics are first diagnosed.

Does literacy continue to cause problems in employment?

Yes – and the problems of literacy in employment will become more acute in the future.

As Fawcett (2003) observes, levels of literacy that sufficed 30 years ago are no longer adequate and 'higher levels of literacy are demanded in employment than ever before in the history of the UK' (p. 99). Furthermore, for the dyslexic, problems with literacy and language start well before the job itself.

These hurdles include filling in the application form, the first day at work (getting lost), interviews (speaking, listening and instant response) and promotion (more complex reading and writing). Other pitfalls are order forms, expenses claims forms, record forms, performance reports, financial data, planning in sequences, payslips, tax forms and diaries. Life becomes easier with seniority, since either a secretary appears, or delegation can be exploited, but many dyslexics still avoid promotion because they do not want to go on training courses.

Should a dyslexic employee disclose their dyslexia or not?

There are good reasons either way.

The Disability Code of Practice 1995 goes some way to help here, giving the dyslexic a chance not to tell if not directly asked. If a dyslexic is asked directly and denies his dyslexia, the employer cannot then be held accountable later for not providing help.

The Code requires the employer to make reasonable provision (see Appendix E) but, in my experience, some employers can be very helpful indeed, including buying specialist software, tape recorders for meetings and visual planning packages for dyslexic employees. With a little explanation, many co-workers can be encouraged to moderate the pressure on a dyslexic by, for example, giving slow, clear instruction and not talking too fast.

If a dyslexic does not disclose their disability, then they can get into all sorts of trouble because there is no good explanation when things go wrong. Disorganization and poor memory can lead to disasters that can look like incompetence, carelessness or an inability to do the job. This is not helpful to either the career prospects of the dyslexic employee or his stress levels. As Reid and Kirk (2001) observed, the problems for dyslexic adults are three-fold: finding employment, maintaining employment and enjoying employment.

Some dyslexic clients have simply had too much abuse and embarrassment about their dyslexia to discuss it freely, but, if there is no disclosure, the employer cannot be blamed for not understanding or helping. The counsellor will recognize that this situation is fertile ground for setting up scripts for failure ('see, I'm not good enough') and being a victim ('see, no one helps me').

There is almost no information about disclosure of dyslexia at work in the UK, but, in the USA, one study found that only 20% of the working dyslexic participants had disclosed their learning disability (Greenbaum et al. 1996). Concern about disclosure of dyslexia is rife in all adult dyslexics, and is probably valid. Furthermore, if discrimination did occur after disclosure, it is questionable whether those who had lost so much confidence at school, who have a rational fear of all large and powerful organizations and who operate alone, would want to take legal action in their own defence.

Is there practical support for dyslexics at work?

It depends.

Regarding literacy support – learning to read and write – there is not very much support for any dyslexic adult – working or not. A recent review of the provision in basic skills training for adults found that only 2% of adults in the greatest need were receiving basic skills support in England and Wales

(Brooks et al. 2001), and fewer than 250,000 of the 7 million illiterate adults were taking up education. Of these, 48% had less than functional literacy.

Regarding practical support, there is much more available. The texts referred to earlier are very good indeed for all sorts of information – both legal and practical. Appendix E gives more detail on the Disability Discrimination Act.

A dyslexic client might consider enrolling with local BDA befrienders who support workers and those on training courses (see the BDA website in Appendix C). Some of the best support and understanding come from trade unions. UNISON, the Public Services Union, for example, supports 130,000 dyslexic members and works with the BDA to provide practical support. USDAW, the shop and retail workers union, makes its education-al training services accessible to dyslexic people and often represents dyslexic members whose disability has got them into trouble at work.

The Guaranteed Interview Scheme is also helpful. This guarantees an invitation to the next stage of the selection process to anyone with a disabil-ity whose application meets the minimum criteria for a post. This enables dyslexics to get to the interview stage – even if the application form is not up to scratch. It doesn't guarantee a job, but it helps to get past the stum-bling blocks of judged text and scrambled telephone calls.

American employers run workplace literacy assessment and training programmes (Perin 1997), but, at present, the only general support for dyslexic employees comes from Employee Assistance Programmes (EAPs) that provide counselling support for employees in some companies.

Ongoing, daily practical support is not the counsellors' role, but what might help would be to refer clients to mentors and life coaches to support daily work problems. Mentoring services are available at local colleges and through some local authorities. Life coaches are appointed privately.

How do dyslexics make the right career choice?

With difficulty – and there are obstacles and pitfalls galore.

Dyslexics can choose careers, or exclude others, because they make incorrect assumptions about what is required, or underestimate their own abilities. Choosing a wrong career – whether one that is too easy or one that is too hard – may, however, be a coping strategy. For example, picking a safe goal (beauty therapist rather than nurse) can keep self-esteem intact. Similarly, choosing an impossible career (proofreader) gives a dyslexic a good excuse for staying safe in the warm nest of underestimation.

There is often a respectable proportion of dyslexic adults who want to train as teachers. They are usually motivated by a desire to use the insights they have gained in order to help dyslexic children in a more empathic way than they experienced. Dyslexics do make good teachers, and commonly provide lively, multisensory classroom experiences. They compensate for their dyslexia with double-wrapped organization and well-honed coping strategies. Unfortunately, most teaching courses do not admit dyslexic trainees (Singleton 1999).

Surprisingly, the Army caters very well for dyslexics, and dyslexic advisers are based in all 35 Army Information Offices and are transported worldwide to teach dyslexic soldiers.

Every job has its up- and downsides for dyslexics. For example, the dyslexic's abilities in intuitive problem-solving and lateral thinking make him good at science, engineering, medicine, nursing, social work and teaching, and some dyslexics can manage to do well in apparently dyslexia-unfriendly subjects such as law, public services and journalism (Rawson 1996). Unfortunately, problems with organization, direction, sequencing, time-keeping, deadlines, articulation and spelling can cause difficulties. There will always be problems digesting large amounts of text.

Dyslexic idiosyncrasies can get in the way in the most unpredictable ways. In one unusual case, quoted by Miles (1993), one dyslexic who reckoned that bell ringing had to be an ideal choice (flexible hours and no writing), was forced to give it up because he could not remember the ring change sequences.

It is obvious that employment support of all types is essential to dyslexics. This, however, is a worthwhile investment because dyslexics make excellent employees. They are also loyal – dyslexics do not job hop, because they really do hate change.

Do dyslexics make unwise career choices?
Most definitely – and a counsellor can be very helpful in averting this.

Reid and Kirk (2001), for example, were staggered by the number of dyslexic adults who were in employment inappropriate for their skills. This mismatch of dyslexic to job often led to remorseless daily pressure since even the most basic task could trip a dyslexic's processing or literacy weaknesses.

Sometimes a bad choice comes from inaccurate assumptions about what the job will involve, and dyslexics may decide to choose a job that seems to have no need of literacy skills, but find that it is not as easy as it sounds. For example, many dyslexics make fine engineers, architects and artists, but discover on their training course that copious reading and writing is needed for essays and theses. Actors have to study lines, and musicians have to read music. One of the most adaptable career choices was made by a dyslexic counsellor who chose a training course assessed entirely by audio and videotape.

A counsellor may have to explore with a client whether the stress involved in coping with an unsuitable job is worth it. It is no kindness to a dyslexic to encourage him to take a job in which he will suffer in the same way that he did at school. Of course, it is also worth exploring whether it is the stress itself that is significant. Is it a way of avoiding other problems or maintaining a rusty script. Is suffering bringing its own reward?

If, as counsellors, we trust our clients to make the right decision, we also have to establish what is 'right' about a decision that may bring only stress and anxiety to a dyslexic. After all, the dyslexia will not go away. Being dyslexic is a lifelong disorder. The dyslexic adult will have problems in spelling, reading, processing, organization and timekeeping for ever. A counsellor can help by being realistic about possibilities, and encouraging coping and support systems.

Are dyslexic employees bullied at work?

They are – but there is no research on whether they are bullied more than the next person.

Bullying at work is rife (Randall 1997), and it is one of the most common problems encountered by counsellors on employee assistance pro-grammes. One in four people are bullied at work by fellow workers who use a wide variety of methods, including innuendo, sarcasm, intimidatory use of discipline, impossible deadlines, removing responsibility without consul-tation, cold-shouldering, 'death by memo', constant criticism and undermining, encouraging others to bully (which many do for fear of being the next victim) and unreasonable refusal of promotions, leave or training (Douglas 2001).

Dyslexics not only have their own past to disable them, but they can also lack the confidence and verbal skills needed to fight back. A history of iso-lation and abandonment by those in authority also means that they may not know how to ask for help. They are also used to giving away power to stronger, more aggressive people.

As alienated people on the edge of mainstream communities, dyslexics may also not be part of a group that can support and buffer them, and sometimes a counsellor can be the only person to whom the bullied dyslex-ic employee can talk.

Counselling students with dyslexia

What provision is available for dyslexic students?

Higher education has some of the best provision for dyslexic people in this country, and it really shows up the meagre and unhelpful dyslexic support in schools.

I would estimate that around 80% of the published advice and research on dyslexia and counselling involves student support, and the university websites on dyslexia are not only prolific but also sophisticated and informed. Dyslexic students have excellent legal support and onsite provision that is bulwarked by Singleton's report *Dyslexia in Higher Education* (Singleton 1999).

I would like to say that this was just because dyslexic students are as motivated and hard-working as they are: 'dyslexic students who achieve a degree are determined, motivated people who work long hours and make huge efforts. They make extensive use of technology and they take advantage of tutorial support' (Cooke 2001, p. 103).

In reality, another significant reason is economic.

There is a definite financial incentive to attract and support the substantial dyslexic student minority. This is perhaps a good illustration of what dyslexics could achieve if they ever discovered their economic muscle.

What are the recommendations of the *Singleton Report*?

They underline the need to counsel dyslexic students in order to help them deal with their negative experiences, and overcome any problems in their current studies. The report recommends:

- every higher education institution should have at least one student counsellor available who has specific knowledge and/or experience of dyslexic counselling
- all counsellors with students in higher education should have some awareness of the impact of dyslexia on everyday activities as well as educational ones
- counselling for students with dyslexia should be available for immediate crises and long-term problems, an integral part of the support service within the institution, and available as a priority to students recently identified as having dyslexia
- the student's confidentiality must be respected at all times, and information exchange with academic or other staff on the student's dyslexia should only occur with the permission of the student, and always with absolute discretion

How many students are dyslexic?

In the 1990s, there was a substantial rise in the number of dyslexic students in higher education to the extent that, among those with disabilities, students with dyslexia formed the largest group (Smith et al. 1999).

Singleton (1999) estimated that up to 2% of higher education students have dyslexia across all disciplines. In art and design, however, the estimates vary from around 10% to 45% (Kiziewicz 2000). There were about

100 dyslexic students identified in British universities in 1981 and about 5,000 in 1995. Of these, 25% were first diagnosed at university (Morgan and Klein 2000). Five per cent of medical students had their dyslexia diagnosed at course entry.

The provision of access courses has opened up opportunities for dyslexics, particularly those mature students who did not realize they were dyslexic but who now want to give themselves a second chance at education (Pollak 1999).

Some universities pick up at registration if a student is dyslexic. Others do not. Many counselling departments at colleges and universities do not find out if clients are dyslexic, even though establishing this fact might obviate the need for counselling altogether in favour of literacy support.

What problems do dyslexic students face that are different from those faced by non-dyslexic students?

Dyslexic students, more than any other group, will have trouble coping, and not only with the obvious challenges posed by the academic requirements of their chosen course. They can also have a significant number of peer and isolation problems that are a hangover from school.

Dyslexics may also have panic reactions in academic situations, and the additional effort required to cope with studying can make them extremely anxious and tired. Like all dyslexics, they will have bad days when they make more mistakes, misread information, lose things and forget appointments. Dyslexic students will also have problems in lectures – including taking notes while listening, having overheads flashed up and trying to follow the lecturer's lines of thought. Comprehension will continue to be a serious problem (Simmons and Singleton 2000). With all the electronic gadgets and tape recorders in the world, dyslexics still have a struggle on their hands. They must listen hard, sit right at the front and focus for every single second. Dyslexic students also expend much more effort than non-dyslexics on essay writing, and their anxiety at examination time can be disabling. Some students get so disorganized with the additional stress that they have turned up for the wrong exams, on the wrong day, or not at all.

Students with dyslexia are different from adults with dyslexia because they are still in the education system, and are still infected by its many viruses. Morgan and Klein (2000) observe that nearly 60% of academic, counselling and support staff thought dyslexic students showed anxiety and a lack of confidence.

Most of all, dyslexic students need quick support. There is a 'Matthew Effect' at university, too (see Chapter 1), and they can fall faster and harder than other students. Miles and Gilroy (1986) stress the importance of instant support for dyslexic students because, all too quickly, the dyslexic mind can become befuddled and, soon, the various problems will seem insurmountable.

When adult dyslexics opt out of the malign influence of the school system, they develop higher levels of self-esteem (Riddick et al. 1999). Dyslexic students are adults who remain in the learning environment where their literacy skills will continue to be judged. This is a voluntary decision, but it is always worth examining in counselling. Where, for example, is the pressure to use higher education coming from?

Do dyslexic students benefit from counselling services?

What little evidence there is on counselling dyslexic students indicates that they do. Rogan and Harmann (1990) reported that 75% of dyslexic college graduates, and 62% of dyslexic high-school graduates, had experienced some types of psychotherapy or counselling in their lives 'and considered this a significant factor in determining a successful outcome' at college (p. 95).

What about disclosure at university?

The problem is similar to that at work, since many students do not want information about their dyslexia released.

Consequently, the same problems of misinterpreting dyslexic behaviour will also arise. This needs to be discussed, since tutors may not understand the dyslexic's difficulties with reading in class, tests or orals. They also may not have sympathy for late essay submission, or realize how sensitive a dyslexic student may feel. A counsellor can intervene on a student's behalf.

What help is available for study skills?

There are many documents and websites giving a vast amount of information on note-taking, study skills, essay planning and the use of IT (Minton 2002) for dyslexic students. Even a cursory surf on the web yields support sites from a dozen universities all over the world. There are also many useful specialist books on students and dyslexia (Gilroy 1995, Farmer et al. 2002).

There is usually generous one-to-one support from specialist dyslexia tutors in further education, and student-counselling departments are often excellent.

Many colleges and universities provide access to assessment either for visiting, or in-house, psychologists (see below).

Counselling dyslexic children at school

Is there counselling help for dyslexic children at school?

You would think so. Yet, in striking and disgraceful contrast to the quantity of help and understanding for the dyslexic student, dyslexics at school have no coherent counselling support. Where there is the greatest need, there is the least provision.

The requirements of the Children Act (1989) for pastoral provision in schools has encouraged some schools to set up a formalized counselling service, so mentoring and counselling in schools is much more common than it was (Bor et al. 2002), but what is available remains largely ignorant of the special problems of dyslexia.

Things such as Circle Time – a tight discussion group with a teacher – that works fine for non-dyslexic children can be actively harmful for dyslexic children. By its very structure, it is set up to be a nightmare for any dyslexic – speaking in public, lots of people listening, thinking of abstract ideas, face to face with bullies and peer-group derision. This really only works well when all the children in the group are dyslexic, and it is led by someone whose understanding of dyslexia extends beyond some vague idea that they reverse letters.

Are school-based counsellors useful to dyslexics?

Not really. I offer four reasons.

First, many school counsellors are not familiar with dyslexia. They do not know that a child is dyslexic, and they do not know the dyslexic child. They also get little training in dyslexia. Coming unawares upon the dyslexic brain can, however, be like standing on a rake.

Second, school counsellors are not very helpful to dyslexic children for the same reason that they are unable to help many school children; their role is not understood. School counsellors are patronized, underresourced, maligned, ignored and regarded as some human dump for every child problem the teacher cannot deal with. Referral to the counsellor can become a chance of a period without a troublemaker. I have even known teachers who try to 'book out' some children to timetable some peace for the rest of the group.

Good school counsellors are also undermined by the prevailing view that school counselling is little more than a quiet chat – which any teacher can do with half an hour to spare. What commonly happens is that a teacher (or parent, learning-support assistant, dinner lady) creates an ersatz counselling relationship wherein the dyslexic child starts to feel safe. When the adult gets bored, or when some dramatic, new behaviour starts to appear – such as the child becoming overattached – the adult 'counsellor' panics and disappears leaving the child with more serious feelings of abandonment and betrayed trust than they had before. The fallouts from these 'little chats' then add to the school counsellor's case-load.

Third, the problem is already out of control when the school counsellor first sees a dyslexic child. This is because a teacher is creating the dyslexic child's distress in one room faster than the counsellor can extinguish it in another. It is inadequate help with the dyslexic's literacy that is the fundamental handicap, no matter how much counselling they receive. Counselling a dyslexic at school is like sticking your finger in a dam while watching huge cracks radiate out around you. Sometimes, all a school counsellor can do is to give a dyslexic child support, encouragement and – never to be underestimated – a model of someone who can be kind, congruent and respectful to them. She can just hope that this small matchstick of heat can provide some warmth as the dyslexic client steps out again into the vast chiller of school life.

Finally, school counsellors also have profound problems with boundaries. Children identify school counsellors with the school establishment, and it is hard for children to be open in counselling if they imagine that their problems are being discussed over coffee in the staff room.

These problems collide in the situation where all the counselling is left, inappropriately to the overworked special-educational needs coordinator (SENCO) whose case load, from what I have heard, can include all the conduct-disordered children, those with ADHD, Tourette's syndrome, hearing problems and personality disorders, including cases of early psychosis.

Is outside referral a good option?
Yes. Sometimes, the best option is to refer to outside agencies.

Riley and Rustique-Forrester (2002) quote a headmaster's opinion that 'the most successful approach is individual counselling – via external counsellors – not part of the school but personal counselling' (p. 55). Using an independent school-counselling service was found to be more effective, since a proper therapeutic alliance could be formed with an outsider who was on the child's side. Headteachers in this study also liked the idea of a home–school liaison officer; a neutral person who could help build up a positive relationship with both parents and children. Such a counselling provision would also facilitate Ecosystemic counselling which I consider to be very effective for dyslexic children's problems (see Chapter 12).

Outside agencies also sidestep the problem that dyslexic children have with being 'othered' at school. Going to see the school counsellor can join the category of going to the remedial unit, thus adding to the feeling of exclusion. One school described the counselling and remedial unit as the 'support centre', but children are not taken in by such weasel words. The effect of special provision is the same – exclusion from their peers.

Assessment of dyslexia: a counselling tool

What are the practicalities of assessment for a dyslexic client?

If a counsellor suspects that her client is dyslexic, one of the most useful things that she can do is to arrange an assessment. Identifying the problem can provide a major therapeutic boost to a dyslexic client.

Details of what happens in the assessment of dyslexia are given in Appendices A and B. There are also useful texts on this procedure by Thomson (1990, 2001), Fawcett (2001) and Turner (1997).

A full private cognitive assessment with an educational or clinical psychologist costs around £300 for a child and £400 or more for an adult. Lower-level screening tests can be carried out, usually by trained dyslexia teachers. Schools are meant to refer suspected dyslexic children for assessment by the local education authority, but, in practice, this is restricted to the most severe cases. A private communication from the BDA about assessment comments: 'The children who suffer most are those whose parents are unable to afford a private assessment, but whose schools are unable or unwilling to assess the child. In spite of being a neurological inherited condition, specific learning difficulties are sadly neglected by the NHS' (British Dyslexia Association 2003, via email).

When should a dyslexic be assessed?

As early as possible – then there is a chance of real help (see Chapter 1).

This spares children with dyslexia some of the humiliation and trauma that they experience prior to identification. Morgan and Klein (2000) found that late diagnosis led to 'deep scars' in dyslexics. They cite the example of a boy classified as 'borderline mentally retarded' by his school who, at university, was diagnosed as a dyslexic with an IQ of 147 and a 'borderline genius' (p. 50).

Most adults do not have the benefit of childhood diagnosis, and find out late in life that they are dyslexic. They often have an assessment as a matter of practicality (to facilitate a return to education or for employment) or through curiosity (seeing a programme about dyslexia, media people discussing their own dyslexia), and this small act ends up making huge changes to their lives.

Again, it is the universities and colleges who are ahead in helping. They pick up the casualties that the schools leave behind. This is because they often have efficient procedures in place to identify and, therefore, help dyslexics early on in their further education.

The *Singleton Report* on dyslexia in higher education (Singleton 1999) notes that 43% of dyslexic students were identified for the first time while in higher education, and three-fifths of higher-education institutions pay for assessment. About half carry out their own in-house assessments, with others referring on, or expecting students to make their own arrangements. Studies on art and design students showed that over a quarter were diagnosed for the first time at college.

One college in Kent, for example, identifies dyslexic pupils by a tick box on registration that is passed straightaway to the support services. They also have systems for lecturers, and other students, to identify dyslexia in students, and then swiftly arrange for diagnosis. There is optional training for college staff to identify dyslexics.

Some colleges have a dyslexic specialist who diagnoses and supports dyslexic students, often providing more assistance for dyslexic students than the counsellors.

Is counselling useful before or after diagnosis?
Counselling is useful in both instances.

Before the assessment, clients need help with the considerable anxiety about what the test might expose. They are often afraid that the assessment will confirm that they are stupid after all. They know, too, that the test will involve doing things that will re-awaken old school fears, such as reading aloud and spelling.

After assessment, counselling support is needed to deal with the effects of the diagnosis itself. This is because the information can be so destabilizing that some clients can think of nothing else, and have a real identity crisis. Ideally, counselling should follow straight on the confirmation of dyslexia to provide what DePonio (2001) helpfully describes as 'demystifying', including help with the jargon of the report.

McLoughlin et al. (1994) suggest that feedback is the most important part of the assessment process: 'If, following an assessment, clients leave without a greater understanding of the nature of their difficulties and what can be done to overcome them, then it has been a waste of their time' (p. 68). Prins, a dyslexic writing of his own experiences of assessment, insists that the dyslexic client needs time to ask questions so that he 'understands the report's intended meaning and, just as important, what it doesn't mean' (Prins 2002, p. 20). Prins also saw feedback as essential in bringing the assessment process to a close. In the nature of all challenging experiences it needed to be contained.

What are the effects of assessment?
Excellent – for the dyslexic individual.

My experience, which matches that of most professionals in this field, is that diagnosis is beneficial to the dyslexic person, with strikingly positive and immediate effect.

In contrast to diagnosis in other disabilities, where the news can be a source of dismay, the diagnosis of dyslexia can be liberating in the extreme for the sufferer. When it occurs, people report their whole lives being changed for the better. In the study by Riddick (1996) on dyslexic children and their parents, 21 out of 22 children were relieved when they learned that they were dyslexic, and many of the children showed marked improvements in behaviour after assessment and the start of proper teaching. McDougall (2001) found that over 70% of a sample of dyslexic adolescents felt that a diagnosis had had a positive effect on them.

There are other effects of an assessment that are a little more complicated:

Reactions of non-dyslexics

The diagnosis changes the lives of those around the dyslexic client. They, too, will experience change, but against their will and, often, their self-interest.

All significant relationships in the dyslexic's life will need to be revised, and reactions are unpredictable. For example, the response of parents to their child's diagnosis of dyslexia can be that they have gained a disability rather than lost an anxiety. Other parents can be delighted.

This reaction of others plays an absolutely essential part in determining how a dyslexic will cope after the diagnosis, and the counsellor might usefully explore this experience with a dyslexic client.

A thoughtful revision of personal history

Having been motivated by a need to find out – finally – what is wrong, and to extinguish painful childhood labels, the new dyslexic might find that the assessment then acts like a benign computer virus racing and sparking back through his whole life, re-defining almost everything that has happened to him.

To say the least, the effect can be complicated – mostly positive – but with many layers. Some dyslexic clients can experience a form of shock. They have to reconcile their old identity as 'stupid' or 'lazy' with one of 'intelligent' and 'dyslexic'. Just as lottery winners get depressed, so do newly diagnosed dyslexics have problems with the rapid change.

Those who have been diagnosed for longer have integrated the notion of being dyslexic into their identity. Newly hatched dyslexics have a lot of thinking to do. I would compare this process to that of people who have discovered that they are adopted. Dyslexics must find out who they really are, and can spend much time researching dyslexia in their family. When they discover that a parent is also dyslexic, a whole new area of problems can open up.

Dramatic personal change

A counsellor may see her client change dramatically: '[The assessment] is often the starting point of huge changes in self-perception, learning experiences, ambitions, motivation and even personal relations' (Morgan and Klein 2000, p. 21). The client may feel relief that they are not stupid, sadness that they suffered so much unfair criticism, anger at parents and teachers for not helping them. Gold (2002) describes the reaction of a famous dyslexic sculptor who said, with regret, that if he had had some diagnosis 'it would have given me confidence, and it might have stimulated me to be interested in school. I would have had a whole different way of looking at myself'.

When assessment intervenes between two counselling sessions, I can find myself dealing with a different client completely. One university student – charming, 'helpless', adapted – became furious, focused and engaged a solicitor to set about suing his old school. All his old hapless coping strategies were abandoned, and he surged forward psychologically as if he had been spinning his wheels, and now the brake was well and truly off.

Feelings of anger, power and peace

Counselling help is also needed to deal with strong feelings repressed since childhood.

Some clients get very angry, some get vengeful, and others want retribution. *The Times*, for example, reported that 'a man who claimed that his chances in life were ruined because his primary-school teachers did not identify his dyslexia was awarded £52,500 compensation. Robin Johnson, 25, of Stockport said the failure damaged his job prospects and his social and emotional development' (quoted in Parsonage 2002).

Diagnosis of dyslexia can be empowering, and the impetus can take our clients just about anywhere. It is 'the beginning of a process of significant change' (Morgan and Klein 2000, p. 40).

Clients also experience a sense of congruence and peace: a confirmation that something wrong or inappropriate has been laid to rest. The relief of assessment is also a relief from duplicity and distorted perception. It finally provides an explanation for everything that has happened.

It creates a paradox. It is a moment of insight, when light bulbs go on and the way ahead is suddenly bright and clear. It is also a moment of closure, when lights can be turned out and a door very firmly closed behind them.

CHAPTER 11

The counselling process with dyslexic clients

Summary

Over the years of counselling dyslexic clients, I have found that some aspects of the counselling process work and some do not. I offer the following observations in the hope that they might prevent other counsellors from heading off over the fields instead of staying on the road. In these days of brief counselling, limited sessions and evidence-based practice, counsellors have to work fast and effectively.

My objective in this chapter is to enhance the therapeutic relationship with dyslexic clients by facilitating better communication and deeper understanding. To take the official route, the observations to follow are intended to inform practice. My more colloquial objective is to help dyslexic adults and children get more and better counselling. By this, I mean counselling that is based on some intelligent understanding of what the world looks like from their chair; their side of the tissue box.

We do not have a cure for dyslexia. This is because it is a human difference. We might as well look for a cure for blue eyes. We can, however, cure the effects of dyslexia, and counsellors are well placed to do so.

The counselling relationship

What is the single most important aspect of counselling for a dyslexic client?

As always – it is the counselling relationship.

There are hundreds of studies that show that it is the therapeutic bond that makes counselling effective and that 'the therapeutic alliance is vital to both the process and outcome of therapy' (Everall and Paulson 2002, p. 78). This applies to all age groups.

In adolescent and child counselling, for example, 'the perception of the therapist as accepting, supportive and trustworthy' is a central factor in its success (op. cit., p. 78).

Kazdin et al. (1990) also found that 90% of child/adolescent therapists considered the therapeutic relationship to be one of the most important variables influencing change. More recently, a review of over 1,500 studies on child and adolescent therapy concluded not only that it was safe, and had a large treatment effect, but that the relationship emerged as central (Kazdin 2002). The same applies to adult clients. In a study on primary-care adult therapy provision in the NHS, Paley and Lawton (2001) found that the main contribution to patient outcome was the therapeutic relationship, including warmth, expectation of improvement, understanding and encouragement.

In this respect, good dyslexia counselling is no different from good counselling in general. Many dyslexics, however, have problems with relationships. The difficulty can be so profound that they can become socially phobic, defended and distrustful of other people. For this reason, the counselling relationship may not be easy.

There is also good evidence that clients who have difficulty in maintaining social relationships, or who have experienced relatively poor family relationships prior to therapy – all of which can be part of the dyslexic experience – will find it hard to develop strong alliances with their therapist (Horvath and Greenberg 1994).

For dyslexics, however, the counselling relationship may also be the first time that they have experienced an easy, respectful, accepting and supportive relationship with anyone, and herein lies its value. It demonstrates a different model of how relationships could be. It also provides a vehicle for change. As Greenhalgh (1994) points out, children who have experienced emotional abuse 'will only allow themselves to be open to change if they are able to experience acceptance and trust' (p. 84).

On a more practical level, the therapeutic relationship can also be a refuge for a dyslexic client: 'the shielding influence of a good relationship in the midst of discord and disharmony' (Rutter 1985, p. 359).

Do dyslexic clients disclose their dyslexia to a counsellor?

No. If you do not ask, you may never know. Disclosing to a counsellor carries all the same anxieties as disclosing to anyone else.

Even if the client knows that they are dyslexic, they will not give it as a reason for referral. Many are unaware that their dyslexia is the source of the considerable problems that they are facing. I, personally, have no time for issues of whether the matter should disclose itself. I think that this is just sophistry, and of no practical help to a dyslexic client.

While the counsellor is agonizing preciously about whether to raise the issue of possible dyslexia, the client could be out there getting an assessment and receiving some literacy – as well as properly focused counselling help. Appropriate support makes an immediate impact on a dyslexic's well-being, so what are the benefits in waiting?

This may sound like a strong line to take, but, without knowledge of a client's dyslexia, a counsellor is handicapping the counselling process. She might as well try to counsel from behind a curtain, since so much important information can be lost by not establishing this one fact. Not to know is failing the client.

Counselling communication with dyslexic clients

Verbal communication

Do dyslexics have a poor vocabulary?

Sometimes – and this usually comes from literary malnourishment. Dyslexics may have had little access to written text because books and news-papers, even written text on television, are out of their reach. Some undiagnosed or unhelped older dyslexic clients may have never read in their lives. One client in his fifties, a highly successful fishery manager, had only two regrets: that he had never been able to read to his children (this is very common) or share with his friends the content of articles in *The Angling Times*. Some dyslexic clients will be completely illiterate, others will have extremely insecure literacy. Most will appreciate simple vocabulary and short words.

Why does my dyslexic client always sound depressed even when he says that he is not?

Language processing and articulatory problems in dyslexics can lead to rather flat speech and poor intonation. This is not depression, although it sounds like it. Take care, however, that this is not just denial.

Are there problems in expressing language?

Yes – very often. Some dyslexic clients may have cognitive defects in language and speech processing. This gives speech defects that lead dyslexics to clutter speech, stutter or fall over multisyllabic words. All language problems will be contaminated by poor confidence – after all, if you are going to be laughed at for stumbling over the simpler words, you don't attempt the hard ones.

Will a dyslexic client and counsellor understand each other?
Mostly, but not as often as the client will encourage you to believe.

Dyslexic clients often have problems in processing speech – both their own and yours – but can be quite good at concealing this. In fact, many dyslexics go through life having no idea what people are talking about. In this respect, I quote a dyslexic student in the detailed study by Morgan and Klein (2000) who described her loneliness at school. 'I found school particularly difficult, basically because I didn't understand what the teachers were saying.' She had no friends: 'I think a lot of it was because I didn't always understand what people said – even now, as an adult, I sometimes won't understand the words that people say. It was a difficult time. Really sad as well.'

Eventually, any dyslexic client will understand you perfectly. They just need time to get to the information.

Do I need to build a time lag into my responses?
Yes – and there is no harm in checking this out with the client.

Again, this may be due to language-processing problems, but it is much more likely to be due to an information-processing lag – which is very common in dyslexics. In practical terms, dyslexic clients need time to unpack what you have just said, examine it, understand it, work out their response and then reply. In non-dyslexics, this is done in microseconds but, in dyslexics, it can take up to five, or even ten, seconds if there is a profound problem in this area.

Why do we keep talking over each other?
If a counsellor does not build this information-processing lag into her responses with dyslexic clients, she will find herself constantly speaking over the client.

All the responses between counsellor and client will tailback and clash. The solution to all these problems is to talk slowly. Leave gaps between sentences, and try to build in a lag between all utterances. Think of it as speaking on a transatlantic telephone call. Importantly, this will vary by the degree of the client's dyslexia and the particular range of language and articulatory problems that he has.

If you take no account of these problems, the sessions with dyslexic clients can collapse into conversational chaos. Some child clients just get bored and give up. They will simply fill in every gap (your mouth stops moving) with a shrug, 'OK' or, occasionally, 'Dunno' just to offer you some variety. Their mind probably wandered off to more interesting areas some time before you realized there was a problem.

Will my dyslexic client be happy to do CBT homework and keep a diary?
No.

Dyslexic clients – adult or child – will not be ecstatic at therapeutic interventions that require written words, or anything whatsoever that requires organisation and sequencing – whether in homework, diaries or scripts. They may agree to do homework, but you may not see them again. If it is done, you can guarantee that they will have spent hours and hours on it and, far from helping, it has probably exhausted and demoralized them further.

Usually, doing homework between sessions is an effective aspect of CBT, and homework can be much more powerful than work done in the consulting room (Burns and Spangler 2000, Reynolds et al. 2000). This is not the case with dyslexics. All work should be done in the session.

Why do some dyslexic clients talk in a stop-start way?
Dyslexics can be hesitant and often take some time to find the right word. Their speech problems mean that they never get verbally fluent. In a similar way their writing problems mean that they cannot easily get ideas down in words. Thomson and Snow (2002) found, for example, that, compared to non-dyslexics, dyslexic children's writing not only had more spelling errors but was much less fluent and used a less extensive vocabulary. Basic elements of the story were often missing, and they had problems 'with the creative and organisational aspects of narrative story telling' (p. 14).

Do dyslexic clients prefer vague or concrete responses?
Ideally, responses should be communicated in a concrete way.

Counsellors may like to be circumspect – 'I wonder if', 'I'm hearing that' – but dyslexic clients cope better with quite direct and explicit statements. 'This sounds like' and 'When you said that, I had this image of'.

I read with interest the article by Gordon and Toukmanian (2002) on the nature of empathy and attunement in counselling. They found that a measure of good attunement lay in the tentativeness of the counsellor response. This was typified as 'beneficial uncertainty' (p. 90). If a counsellor used 'beneficial uncertainty' with a dyslexic client, he would wonder what the counsellor was talking about.

Crisp, clear, concise and concrete communication really does work best with dyslexic clients, and enables them to feel held. There will be a better chance that you are both communicating well.

Similarly, care is needed about subtle, multilayered phrases. Dyslexics are very concrete thinkers. Morgan and Klein (2000) refer, for example, to a dyslexic student who, on being asked to illustrate an exam question, surrounded her answer with pen drawings. Poor phonological processing also affects the ability of dyslexic individuals to use and manipulate language. Long, multisyllabic words should be avoided.

Should I avoid counselling jargon?
Like the plague.

It is never a good idea to slip into therapy-speak with dyslexics, and long sentences are useless to a client with short-term memory and sequencing problems.

For example, if you were keen on a counselling approach informed by 'beneficial uncertainty' and 'desired not to intrude on the client's self-schema' or were 'feeling your way to a deep empathic understanding of your client's world view in the here and now', and wanted to translate this lot into a response, you might offer your dyslexic client the following: 'I'm wondering what the issue is here with, well, with your – how can I put it? – *unsatisfactory* relationship with your parents, which I feel – (counsellor's hands pressed to chest) as a deep hunger – listen to my stomach rumble – as some fundamental malnourishment, some deep hunger never filled, a life lived constantly at the edge of starvation. What do you think? Hmm?'

At this point, a dyslexic client would be (a) wondering why you are talking about lunch, (b) listening, as instructed, to your stomach rumbling and (c) be gazing with increasing interest at a hovering pigeon because they had tuned out at 'the issue' (which is a meaningless phrase anyway to a visual thinker) and tuned back in at 'Hmm?' because you had stopped talking and were now clearly expecting a response from them.

Alternatively, if, at this point, your dyslexic client is not staring at you like a rabbit in the headlights, they will be wondering if you might use some counselling yourself.

You could have said: 'It sounds like your Mum and Dad's love was a bit like a Chinese meal – you never felt satisfied for long.' That would have made more sense to most clients but, to a dyslexic, it would have been the difference between sense and nonsense, between a counsellor understanding who they were and one who had no idea whatsoever about the reality of being dyslexic.

Why do dyslexic clients often waffle?
Dyslexics can appear unfocused, because they have word-finding or naming difficulties that lead to vague, waffly statements.

Expressive language and communication skills are impaired, but some dyslexics are so good at disguising it by a forbidding articulatory diarrhoea (like the dyslexic who conceals his bad spelling through impenetrable handwriting) that it is only on listening carefully that you realize that the narrative goes nowhere. Your astonishment also gives him breathing space.

At school, this led to problems since dyslexics 'bore or mystify their audience' (Thomson 1995b, p. 37), particularly those who have not the patience to wait, or to find the correct sequence in what they have been told. This is where counselling listening skills come in useful. The counsellor, by giving time, space, patience and respect, can provide a very different form of communication.

Why do dyslexic clients just seem to seize up sometimes?

This is due to a variety of expressive or receptive language problems, such as difficulties with word retrieval.

It manifests in awkwardness of expression or misuse of words, and difficulties in understanding figurative language, words with multiple meanings or grammatical tenses. Some dyslexics will say that something is stuck in their head. 'You know what you want to say, but you can't get it out at all, you're stuck.' I have even known a client to get fixed repetitively on one sound. This is not stuttering. It is almost as if their whole articulatory system seizes up, like a frozen computer, and the stream of sound is the only connection to the outside world.

Are words as important to dyslexics as to counsellors?

Not really. A counsellor and client really are coming from two different worlds.

The meaning of words is important in counselling. Words – written and sometimes spoken – are not only irrelevant to dyslexics but hazardous. Dyslexics associate words with pain, hassle, incomprehension and – often – are so much blahblahblah. Words can be the curtain behind which they have curled themselves away during countless lessons and admonishments from just about everyone.

Therapies that need a client to look at the meaning of words that are subtly different will find a dyslexic client polite but incredulous. Locating the difference between 'can't/won't', 'try/do', 'need/want', 'should/want', 'might/will', as well as phrases such as 'make/feel', and 'maybe/perhaps' is not only not a dyslexic strength, it is also not how they think. Their view of the world is visual and concrete. Bandying words is a waste of time, and disrespectful. You would not ask a blind person to consider gradations in colour.

It is not even as if the dyslexic client gets the same meaning from any word as a non-dyslexic counsellor. One dyslexic client told me that she didn't listen to my individual words but picked out the gist, the general sense, of what I was saying. She was seeing the wood rather than the trees.

How do dyslexics play for time?

Lots of ways – they are absolutely expert at it.

For example, dyslexics use many 'tag questions' such as 'Will it?' or 'Don't you?', or will ask to have questions repeated. I believe these responses serve two functions. First, they reflect the dyslexic's uncertainty and anxiety – their desire to please, and connect with, another person. Second, they give breathing space; a type of verbal semicolon which gives the dyslexic speaker time to catch up by deflecting the listener, however briefly.

Do dyslexic and non-dyslexic clients use 'intention' words in the same way?

Not always. Words such as 'try', 'can't' and 'might be able', which are usually regarded as 'failure' words or expressions of insincere intention, may not mean this to dyslexics.

They can, instead, represent the reality of a dyslexic's lifestyle. They are not cop-out words but a reasonable assessment of predicted success. 'I will *try* to get here on time next week' can mean just that. Dyslexics will often put a huge amount of effort into it. Some of my clients, for example, build an hour into their journeys just to be there waiting. Others load themselves with alarm clocks.

If dyslexics have a bad day, if they get anxious or overwhelmed, then, with the best will in the world, they will lose a grip on time, organization, processing – everything. To say they will 'try' is probably one of the few times in counselling that the word is used in its concrete sense. Also, 'can't' in contexts such as 'I can't get all the reading done for these essays' – is usually an absolutely true statement. The dyslexic can't. He has not the time or the cognitive equipment to do so. Thus, the counsellor's job is not to challenge the meaning of such phrases but to accept them, and look at strategies that might help.

Are words, images and metaphors better for counselling with dyslexics?

Yes. In fact dyslexic counsellors automatically use more visual images, and dyslexic clients instinctively use them in expressing their feelings.

Art therapy is, therefore, an ideal medium for dyslexics (Case and Dalley 1992), but it is time-consuming. Counsellors can, however, make imaginative use of visual images in the more normal person-centred setting. Dainow (1995), for example, has usefully discussed how to uncover a client's script with pictures, mainly cartoons. She notes that such imaging is a very useful approach 'for clients who find it hard to express their feelings in words. The meaning of the image can shine through the tangle of grammar' (p. 291).

Dyslexics think in pictures; they are visual thinkers and learners. Davis (1997) writes that the 'primary thought process of the dyslexic is a non-verbal picture thinking mode which occurs at 32 pictures per second. In a second, a verbal thinker could have between two and five thoughts ... while a picture thinker would have thirty-two' (p. 100). A single picture can show a concept that might require thousands of words to describe. According to Davis (op. cit.), Einstein's theory of relativity came to him in a daydream in which he travelled inside a beam of light. His vision only lasted a second, yet spawned scores of textbooks to describe it. Picture thinking is estimated to be, overall, 400 to 2,000 times faster than verbal thinking.

Davis advises us to encourage a dyslexic to create a personal mental picture that accurately shows the meaning of a concept.

Are dyslexics creative in counselling?

Yes – disconcertingly so, and dyslexic thinking can be hard to follow.

How a dyslexic thinks will be a reflection of his cognitive style. It is on a continuum and will differ in its permutations. A very weak working memory, for example, can result in a random generation of ideas, and some ideas will get lost. There will also be a tendency to go off at tangents.

The gestalt use of 'empty chair' is an excellent counselling tool since it taps into the visuospatial side to dyslexia. Some clients use any objects to hand. No special equipment is needed. Some can create poignant symbols.

One boy, a gifted dyslexic with an IQ of 160, humourless and inarticulate with severe language problems, set his own measure of progress. I had a small Indian birdcage on a shelf. He took a fluffy duck, opened the door and laid the duck inside with its head flopping casually across the cage entrance, but hanging just over the edge of the shelf. He moved the duck out of the cage and onto the shelf over several weeks, as if it were about to take flight. He had to terminate therapy when he left the school to go abroad. The staging of this duck, and its progress from cage to shelf, was a measurable symbol of progress that was far more articulate than words could have conveyed.

I have never moved that duck. It remains a monument for me for all unhappy dyslexic children; their fun and originality lying precariously between two worlds: the cage and the drop from the shelf. Will they fly or will they fall?

How will a dyslexic's sequencing difficulty affect counselling with them?

I once worked with a dyslexic child who had lived in both Greece and Canada before coming to England.

In our session, he would recount, in great detail, events that had happened supposedly that week. Suddenly, he would say – 'Oh no! That was in Cyprus' or 'Sorry – that was Ottawa'. I honestly never knew where anything occurred in space or time, but it was not important. He was chunking events in his head in patterns that made sense to him. Once I got out of a sequential mode of counselling thinking, it made sense to have someone who was coding and filing data into visual, time-independent categories.

Many teachers have problems untangling school altercations when all the dyslexic participants in a fight have different temporal distortions and sequencing problems. You can hear of an incident that happened half an hour or half a year ago. I have a theory that certain events take time to move from short- to long-term memory in a dyslexic. This means that a child can get yelled at suddenly by a friend for something that happened two weeks previously.

I remember a problem with a broken mirror. The child who witnessed the incident named three boys, a certain day and some particular phrase. We put this into the sequence presented and came up with a complete travesty of what had happened. The child had sewn together several boys, several days and several incidents over many weeks and recent hours to create a picture that was coherent for him but which bore no relation to reality. In that instant, I could quite understand how a dyslexic can unwittingly trip himself up in the legal system.

How do short-term memory problems affect dyslexics in counselling?

This makes it hard for some dyslexics to deal with telephone conversations, appointment keeping or long counselling responses, *inter alia.*

Their short-term memory difficulties can also make dyslexics forget what they have said – or are hearing – particularly multiple clause questions, broken sentences, or interpretations that link a number of separate events. Keeping track of what is said is particularly hard if there is a lot of uninterrupted speech thundering towards them.

Dyslexics benefit from breaks and short bursts. It is easier, for example, to fill a bottle in short squirts from the tap than a continuous, fierce stream that leaps back out of the bottle.

Physical factors

Why do my dyslexic clients arrive late, early or sometimes forget to come?

Dyslexia is associated with profound problems in time estimation and organization.

Being late, or not coming are, therefore, rarely to do with acting out, resistance, defence or repressed anger. Problems with time almost always represent problems with dyslexia, not problems with the counsellor or the counselling process. It is best not to waste energy on the reasons for the dyslexic's unpunctuality and unreliability. It is more useful for the counselling, and for the client, to address the practical solutions of how to avoid the problem by laying down some concrete strategies.

I have an agreement with my dyslexic clients that I will wait fifteen minutes, and then I shall go, unless I get a phone call. Being late never leads to a time extension – since good boundaries are also part of work with dyslexia. Most clients quickly find strategies for their appointment and punctuality problems – but a counsellor needs to be unsurprised by what strategies are chosen.

Are dyslexic clients always fidgety and restless?

They can be, but they are as likely to be droopy and languid – depending on the condition associated with their dyslexia (see below).

Some dyslexic clients who have overlap ADHD or ADD will be very fidgety. This is not avoidance behaviour, acting out or boredom; it is a physiological difference. Some will even get up and wander around the room. One such client always had to go to the lavatory halfway through the session. I found out from colleagues outside the room that he would dash out and hare up a staircase and along a corridor then zap back. I did wonder why he was always breathing deeply when he got back, and it gave me cause for much speculation. We built in a stop in the middle of the session, and I recommended a visit to the university medical centre to investigate Ritalin.

Why are dyslexic clients so languid?

Postural control is poor in many dyspraxic clients.

Some dyslexics also have motor-control problems – particularly with posture. Such clients will slouch and droop in the chair, often sliding down through the session. One or two have fallen off their chairs. This slow slide increases markedly as their concentration intensifies and physical control goes in other areas. This can lead to a dramatic and alarming shortening in the space between counsellor and client. In a non-dyslexic client, I would be looking for reasons for this, certainly sharing that I had observed it. With dyslexic clients, it is actually not important and, in fact, a sign that they are really concentrating on what the session holds for them.

Why are dyslexic non-verbal skills so strange?

No one really knows (see Chapter 8) but it is undoubtedly true that some dyslexic clients are truly awful communicators.

This is not intentional. A lot of it has to do with their blank facial expression and eccentric body language. It is significant that non-verbal communication can become more erratic when concentration is on inner processes, and also when the whole process of communication becomes frustrating and difficult. In Chapter 8, there is a detailed account of the ways in which dyslexic non-verbal skills impede communication.

Do dyslexic clients use a lot of comfort and transitional objects?

Yes – dyslexic children and adolescents use transitional objects far more than normal. Adults use symbolic objects such as mobile phones and organizers, and can get quite anxious if they are parted from them.

Winnicott (1974) influentially referred to small coping objects used by children as 'transitional objects'. They help the young child to bridge the gap between self and outer reality, as well as providing a comfort in place of their absent mother. Repetitive sounds or movements can serve the same function. Both objects and sounds are used a lot by dyslexic children and adults, who seem to find them comforting. Dyslexic children carry transitional objects for far longer than non-dyslexic children.

Generally, at five or six years of age, children are saying goodbye to transitional objects. Dyslexic children often start using them at this age, usually as their reading problems start. They can still be deeply attached to them at 12 years or more.

If nothing else, this is a poignant reminder of how stressed many of these children are. Some are still carrying around cuddlies into their teenage years.

Repetitive movements are also common with dyslexics – tapping, clicking, sucking, rocking are all common, and designed to self-soothe as well as to help concentration. Many of these movements are reduced when the children use music as an adjunct to their work, which also improves both standard and output. Music on personal stereos, and played in class while they work, is beneficial to dyslexic children.

Would it be considered tactless to give a dyslexic client forms to fill in?

It depends on how it is done. It is certainly wise to check out whether a particular dyslexic client has problems – and in what areas of literacy. Established in a concrete and neutral way, this is in itself a useful process of acceptance for a dyslexic client. The fact that you are raising the issue as fact, and not through some critical or mickey-taking route, will also be novel and appreciated.

Are dyslexics easily distracted during counselling?

Yes – dyslexic clients are extremely distractible.

The ideal environment would probably be an unfurnished plain white room, with a counsellor dressed from head to toe in taupe. This is unlikely to happen, but any reduction in distractibility is useful so that dyslexic clients can better concentrate on what they are saying and thinking.

Specialist teachers use this reduced-stimulus approach to good effect with severely dyslexic pupils. Knivsberg et al. (1999) specifically recommends that dyslexic children be in a very plain, undecorated room: 'a quiet room with limited stimuli may help them to concentrate' (p. 44).

I worked with one dyslexic male client who would sometimes just stop in the middle of the sentence and waffle aimlessly for a few seconds because he had been distracted by some object that he had caught sight of. A very talented artist, he was highly sensitive to colour and shape and had the dyslexic ability to turn objects around in his head, through dozens of permutations, in a matter of seconds. While he did this, his face would go blank and he could just stare. This had got him into all sorts of trouble at school. When it happened with me, I could see that it must have been challenging for his teachers.

For example, one day, I had laid a pile of books on a shelf and thought nothing of it. In the next session, he was speechless for several minutes – mid-sentence. The colour combinations on the book jackets had totally distracted him. First, they were novel – and dyslexic people are always sensitive to change. Second, the colours – turquoise, orange and pink – had worked visually in an unusual way, and this had fired his creative side. He could not focus on anything else for some minutes. This distractibility can occur with any sensory interruption, and it is random.

Many specialist dyslexia teachers with very dyslexic children (the distractibility tends to increase with the severity of the condition) will encourage the children to look at blank paper for a few minutes before working with them, or give them music over headphones to shut down some of the other distracting sensory channels.

Other distractions during counselling can include traffic noise, cloud movement, a spider on the wall, your new hair colour or an object moved five inches from its place in the last session. I often allow a long, slow period of silence at the beginning of a session so that the dyslexic client can get on with proofreading the counselling room.

Do dyslexic clients get bored?

Yes – particularly if they have to concentrate. There is, for example, a big difference between attention and concentration.

Davis (1997) observes that it is natural and easy for dyslexics to pay attention but difficult for them to concentrate. 'There is a tremendous difference between the two. When people are paying attention, their awareness is spread out; it can encompass the entire immediate environment. When people are concentrating, all or most of their attention is fixed on only one thing in the immediate environment' (p. 56).

A dyslexic can also get bored easily because he has a mind 'working between 400 and 2,000 times faster than the minds of the people around him' (p. 58). A bored dyslexic, of which there are very many, will either use distortion or creative imagination (daydreaming) or shift this attention to something that is interesting (distractibility or inattention). This is not ADD, it is distractibility, and it is a physical part of being a dyslexic – more so the more severely dyslexic they are.

Defences

Are dyslexic clients good at defences?
They are outstanding. Furthermore, the dyslexic child's defences can assume an alarming potency in adults, where aggression, self-deprecation, humour, haplessness and helplessness have achieved a lifetime of refinement and can easily knock the unwary counsellor sideways. Many of these defences were put into place to deflect. When, by adulthood, they have been hardened by many years of sharp survival sense, good intelligence and a highly unusual cognitive style, the defences are about as good as they can get and some of the best that a counsellor may have seen. Adult dyslexic defences are tough, refined and slippery, particularly when combined with the high-class adaptation that comes from years of using a large, invisible radar dish. A counsellor will need all her wits to keep pace, and you certainly never forget a dyslexic client.

With all these types of defence, the subtext is that you get lost in the smoke screen of the dyslexic's behaviours and do not notice the failure and vulnerability beneath.

My view is that this is how it should be – and most of the time these defences get a dyslexic through a difficult life very well indeed. Defences are there, after all, to keep us safe, and dyslexics have learnt the hard way – through a life littered with casual psychological evisceration and the deliberate infliction of physical pain – that safety is a very precious thing indeed.

As counsellors, however, we have to notice when a defence stops being a coping strategy and starts to turn into a 'not coping' signal. We also have to notice when the defences put into place by dyslexics for self-protection start to isolate them from others or distort their ability to lead a normal life. In short, we have to notice when the iron defences turn into iron cages.

What defences are common in dyslexic clients?
Like any human being, a dyslexic will block experience through splitting, denial, projection, repression and distortion. I give below those defences that I have observed to be specifically relevant to dyslexic clients.

Failure as power

It is a tragic fact that sometimes the only power that children have is the spoiling of their own lives.

When the only attention you get is when you fail, why give it up? If failure really aggravates those people you hate and fear, what a wonderful weapon it is. Dwivedi (1993) suggests that 'in a passive-aggressive way, underachievement may become a weapon to punish the persons in authority, i.e. by withholding what they really want' (p. 68).

When masquerading as a sweet mannerism – 'poor me', 'I'm just so awful' – it can also be a useful device for seduction, both sexual and social.

Regressive behaviour

Regression is common in dyslexic children. This is for reasons of infantilization – noted in Chapter 9 – and as a response to acute stress. There are differences to the two presenting forms. The first is usually charming – and elicits maternal transference. The second is distressing – and elicits panic and anxiety in the observer, which is probably a primitive reflex to this earliest and most ancient sign of infant distress.

One interpretation of this regressive behaviour is to see it as the unhappy dyslexic child's retreat back from the latency stage into the earlier oral and anal stages with their narcissistic preoccupations.

Whatever the reason, however, the sudden appearance of these regressive symptoms suggests that the pressure of anxiety is becoming intolerable for the child.

These defences include the sucking of fingers and clothing, curling into balls under desks, bed-wetting and soiling, rocking, holding of genitals and the constant company of furry toys. When these infantile behaviours appear in an older child, they represent a signal that he is no longer coping. We should all be aware that these are not vexatious behaviours but the symptoms of real distress.

Projection

In a judgemental or academically successful family, a dyslexic child may feel that they hold all the losing cards, and seek some way of passing them onto someone else. This can be – through bare-faced lying – onto a younger or older sibling, or it can be onto fantasy figures. Dyslexics are imaginative and think visually, so it can be quite easy for them to imagine some other child in whom they can empty all the hated parts of themselves.

One dyslexic girl talked about a 'sister' who was very 'bad' and, through the session, I formed the opinion that this sister was truly the child from hell. I later found out that my client was an only child. Needless to say, it would have been unwise to challenge this defence since the subsequent rush of perceived 'badness' back into her would have been intolerable, even if she had continued with counselling and not denied my view completely.

Repression and projective identification

This is very common in those dyslexic clients who have long denied their feelings of anger and frustration. This is most marked with highly intelligent dyslexics with profound language problems who are shut off both psychologically and physically. When a good counselling relationship has been established – which can take some time because the communication is handicapped – the atmosphere can become alive with feelings, crackling with an intense energy that I rarely encounter with other clients.

Denial

The most clumsy and dyspraxic child I have ever counselled had a long-running obsession about being a world-class footballer. Other children in a specialist dyslexia school – who, at ten years old, are barely literate – can say that they do not have problem. Others who have just thumped a child in front of 15 witnesses will say that they didn't do it. Being dyslexic is not fun for children, and sometimes they just simply decide that the dyslexia – and its symptoms – does not exist. Success in literacy is the most direct route to this defence collapsing. Counsellors often have to just wait for this to happen.

One variety of denial in adults is covering up. McLoughlin et al. (2002) note that poor handwriting has been used to hide poor spelling, and humour can hide embarrassment.

Humour, extroversion, self-mockery and aggression

This defence puts everything out there and in your face. From classrooms to pubs, such dyslexics are defiant and extrovert. Other such dyslexics can be very funny indeed, or use a charm offensive with such stunning effect that the observer is quite captivated. All these strategies are used principally to deflect attention from any potential failure or criticism.

Getting others to help

Dyslexics can learn to do hapless, hopeless and helpless very well. After all, it has, on occasion, become quite useful to them. The main use of this defence can be that it draws life's rescuers to them. It is one thing, however, to use help and support from others as a coping strategy – that is a positive move – but it is another thing altogether when it becomes a defence against a dyslexic taking responsibility for his life and his dyslexia. Then, it can deflect more independent strategies and become part of a useful 'poor little me' persona. Such dyslexics are, in effect, making their dyslexia into a useful handicap.

This defence can also become an avoidance tactic to prevent such dyslexics from growing up. Children are looked after, is the assumption, but adults are not. Needless to say, a counsellor has to be quite careful with this defence – since it can tug at any counter-transferential rescuer material that she has, and all dyslexics are good at finding our counter-transferential Achilles' heel.

Adaptation

This is a common strategy, particularly among dyslexic girls who can become so over-adapted to the needs of others that they become expert at being exactly what they think you want. Such dyslexics can be so superb and subtle at this that it is easy not to notice their low self-esteem and the lack of any identity of their own.

An adapted dyslexic will quickly become the best client that you have had – ever. Seeing them will be pure pleasure, and they will seem to make astonishing amounts of progress quickly and all – somehow – in the direction of your most deeply held counselling values. They will smile and nod agreeably at anything you say, and you will often wonder why they are there.

Adapted dyslexics are not just 'good' clients, they are super-clients. The problem is that they do not believe that anyone, ever, will like them if they are themselves. The best sign of progress in adapted clients is stroppiness. The best counselling practice is congruence, at every possible opportunity, bolstered by rock-solid acceptance and respect – since being themselves will feel extremely dangerous to deeply adapted clients like these.

The anxiety about the 'bad' part of them can often appear by chance in these clients.

I have known a loose sleeve to drop back, 'accidentally', and reveal the cut marks on a client's arm. In another case, a client had a strong, unwashed smell that was at variance with her pretty, neat, well-dressed exterior. By contrast, another dyslexic client was excessively clean and groomed, filling the room with the smell of aftershave, as if he had sanitized himself – washed and perfumed away any human part of himself – before he came to counselling.

Truculence and aggression

By contrast, there is the aggressive, harmless, 'don't care what you think' defence, which conceals the huge anxiety of someone who cares very much indeed. Sometimes outright aggression is used as a pre-emptive bid against criticism or patronage.

Such dyslexic clients grab attention before someone or something can grab them. Sarcastic, witty and aggressive, such dyslexics can also dress and behave to divert or alarm. I remember some markedly biting, demanding counselling with two fierce and fascinating dyslexic clients – one a huge 19-year-old student, the other a diminutive ten-year-old boy – who were each so covered in chains, leather, studs, their hair in angry hedgehog spikes, that it was obvious that only a brave person would dare to try anything with them, let alone get close.

Academic success: revisiting and fantasy

One complex defence among adult dyslexics is the decision to revisit earlier academic problems and solve them in the safety of adulthood. There are, for example, many dyslexic mature students who decide, with considerable courage, that they can only lay the stressful ghosts of their childhood by going back and facing them. It is as if they want to gain some retrospective control over their childhood misery. They also want to prove finally to themselves and others that 'they can do it'. The ways chosen by these dyslexic adults can be extraordinarily difficult and occasionally unwise. For example, dyslexic students often choose to study such book-infested and language-dominated subjects as English, philosophy, social sciences and psychology.

One dyslexic client, a talented, intelligent artist who was barely literate, insisted on studying psychology at A level. After two weeks of incomprehension and sleeplessness, we were able to look at the issue of choice. Did he need to define himself in this way? Could he lay this fantasy – his father's fantasy – to rest?

Drugs, drink and food

Drugs and alcohol are common solutions to reducing anxiety in dyslexics. Of the dyslexic clients who come to counselling – some as young as 13 – a significant proportion want to beat their addiction to tobacco, cocaine, marijuana, ecstasy and all types of drink. Some dyslexics want to solve the problems that have led to their long-standing use of antidepressants.

Among children, I have, surprisingly, rarely encountered anorexia among dyslexic girls. More common is bulimia, which often represents some need to exert personal control for the sufferer. I have, on the other hand, encountered more undereating problems among male dyslexic children and adult students which – since anorexia is now seen as a function of incongruence in family relationships – may reflect a male dyslexic's need to exert control against family pressure.

Dissociation

This is a defence commonly used by dyslexic children. It is the ability to go deeply inside themselves to a world of fantasy where the distressing outer world is excluded. In these wonderful sanctuaries, dyslexic children are powerful, successful and drive their enemies (teachers, other children, sisters, brothers) to various imaginative forms of destruction. Such children are dissociated, deadened and dreamy in a way comparable to the behaviour presented by victims of child abuse.

In effect, this type of dyslexic has given up on us all and gone away. One young boy I counselled could not even come out of his fantasy world during his counselling session. He just invited me in there – a world of knights, battles and kings where he was always the strongest and bravest. He was happier in there than in a world of people who had done nothing for him.

Boundaries

Are boundaries important in dyslexic counselling?
Essential. The counsellor is faced with a client group that is, on the one hand, in greatest need of good boundaries but, on the other, the best boundary testers imaginable.

Many people with learning disabilities have grown up with people who have kept poor boundaries with them, particularly regarding their self-respect – so their working model is not to respect their own or others' boundaries. This is balanced by the dyslexic's fear of being uncontrolled, unhelped and uncontained – which was their experience at school and often at home.

What types of boundaries are most important?
Strong boundaries help dyslexics to feel safe. I would suggest that there are three important types of boundaries to consider.

First, an essential psychological boundary is maintained by good counsellor congruence. A dyslexic has spent his entire life trying to integrate incongruent reactions (see Chapter 12). The dyslexic is not used to people being straight with him, or trusting him with the truth.

Luckily, this is what a good counsellor is good at, and congruence underpins the best parts of the counselling relationship. Counsellors will find that congruence is essential to deepening, and giving direction to, counselling with a dyslexic client.

Second, boundaries in timekeeping and appointment-setting need to be set in stone with dyslexic clients or the counsellor will soon be more anxious than they are. These are the most difficult boundaries for a dyslexic because of their physiological problems with time estimation and organization.

A counsellor has to be firm about starting and finishing times, and my experience is that if I keep good boundaries – finishing bang on time even if the client arrives late – then even the most time-challenged dyslexic will find ways of learning to arrive and finish within the correct time. If it is a problem, we discuss solutions.

One extremely time-challenged dyslexic client even managed to reach me from a holiday in France, including a tortuous route by boat, train, bus and taxi, and still arrive on time. He had an elaborate system to do it – which I never really grasped – but he did it and never forgot that he did it. This was the model for ever afterwards for any hurdle he faced.

Third, no matter how clear are a counsellor's boundaries, the dyslexic client will test them both consciously and unconsciously. Some of this will simply be their dyslexia – just the way they are. Sometimes, it will be a strategy. Dyslexic children are used to adults giving up on them, being irritated by them and not wanting to be with them. They will think that the counsellor is the same, until proved otherwise, and, like all clients, they will set out to find the proof.

Interestingly, dyslexic clients quickly pick up boundaries as a coping strategy, and the counsellor's model can be carried into the dyslexic's home and work life. I have heard my own boundary principles came bouncing back to me from my client's reported speech to partners, children and employers. One client started to insist on improved boundaries from her two teenage daughters, including a request that her tea be ready when she got in. She used to call it the 'joy of boundaries' and said it was the sexiest concept she had ever learnt.

Challenge and change

How do dyslexic clients respond to challenge?

Not well – and I would give two reasons for this.

First, they can use challenge as another source of direction. The dyslexic experiences of victimization, learned helplessness and overprotection can give them a markedly external attributional style; that is, they will seek to please others and invite them to take control. The thesis of counselling is, however, that the counsellor may work with the client to make things clear but that the choice of how to proceed is ultimately up to him. This degree of choice can be disturbing to people who have comfortably given up control over their lives to others, however much unhappiness this has produced.

Such a client will already have invited the counsellor to give them advice, ask what they 'should' do, what the counsellor thinks. 'Now you can tell me what my problem is.' 'Am I doing the right thing – what do you think?' For such a client, challenge becomes a valuable clue to working out what the counsellor wants from them, not what they want for themselves.

Second, dyslexic clients can see challenge as bullying by the counsellor.

The counsellor will know when the client has taken this stance, because the transference will make a swift turn. Either the counsellor will suddenly feel an urge to overstate the challenge – to harangue and persecute rather than respectfully offer her ideas – or, alternatively, the client will move straight into sad, hurt and hapless child – inviting immediate rescue.

With both responses to challenge it is imperative that the counsellor acts quickly and congruently and that she brings these reactions right out into the room. If not, she might lose the client completely or be faced with the ethical dilemma of working with a client who does not want to change. In such a case, the client may well be using the counsellor and the counselling process to collude with old patterns, such as learned helplessness or an overprotective parent.

I find it useful to use a question favoured by Transactional Analysts – 'Who am I for you right now?'

Do dyslexic clients like change?

No – and this is one of the main problems for a counsellor. For a dyslexic, familiarity breeds content.

Dyslexic clients have enormous problems with all forms of change and transition.

The problem for any therapist is that change is fundamental to the notion of therapeutic growth. Whatever the terminology – whether through reframing, the reunion with the inner self, the shift from child to adult, movement from paranoid-schizoid to a depressive position or the use of the transference to restructure personality, therapeutic change is seen as healthy and organic: a sign of being psychologically alive.

Unfortunately, many dyslexics are not only stuck but feel safe being stuck. If a dyslexic client is utterly opposed, consciously and unconsciously, to change despite all the best therapeutic relationship, supervision and patience in the world – and I have come across this a number of times – the counsellor may need to examine her ethical position in working with them.

CHAPTER 12

Specialist counselling approaches

Summary

I have found some of the ideas in the following counselling therapies to be useful in understanding the dyslexic client. I use these ideas to inform my practice, although my way of being with my client is always person-centred. These are particular points from particular therapeutic perspectives. It is not an exhaustive list but is intended to open discussion on how specific theories can be adapted to the dyslexic client's idiosyncratic needs.

Contributions from the 'inner critic'

What is the 'inner critic'?

The term 'inner critic' was introduced by Gendling (1981) to symbolize the inner voice that people use to lock themselves into ways of behaving.

Other terms for this are 'harsh superego', 'bad parent' and 'negative beliefs'. A strong and punitive 'inner critic' is associated with five client characteristics: a history of rejection, restriction and neglect; negative self-schemas; information-processing deficit and self-protective strategies. All these features are also typically found in the life histories of dyslexic people.

The main feature of the inner critic is that it speaks at the client rather than from the client. It chatters, nags and repeats itself with words such as 'should' and 'ought', and it is nourished by negative introjects.

Does the dyslexic child take in more negative introjects than other children?

Yes.

It is estimated that a dyslexic child will receive up to 25 negative and critical comments a day from school, parents, friends and siblings. It can be far more than this. Over ten years, from the ages of five to 16, this would amount to not far short of 100,000 negative introjects. This will continue, if at a slower pace, as the dyslexic gets older. If there were a balancing fund of positive remarks, that would help, but people do not give praise to dyslexic children unless it is insincere, or in desperation.

Dyslexics grow to neither expect nor attract praise, and can be so allergic to the unfamiliarity of praise that they will cover their ears and furiously shake their heads if it is offered.

Most of the dyslexic's negative introjects will concern their 'stupidity', 'laziness', 'spasticity', 'clumsiness', 'inability to do anything right', 'being thick', 'not talking right' and so on. Being called 'stupid' is the clear winner, followed by 'lazy', 'rubbish', 'a pile of shit' and 'dyslexic cunt'. These are not only expressed verbally and publicly but are also read in the faces, voices, body language and direct statements of parents, siblings, friends, peer group at school, teachers, relatives, work colleagues and employers. These people have also ridiculed and bullied dyslexic people on the basis of their poor reading, writing and spelling, and all the times the dyslexic person has been late or disorganized, lost or forgotten things, and misread or misunderstood instructions. A dyslexic person has internalized this gale of critical information, and often uses it to define both who he is and how he relates to other people.

Not surprisingly, such experiences can contaminate the relationships that dyslexics have throughout their life. They can be suspicious, manipulative, withdrawn, defensive and acutely sensitive to the smallest slight or perceived rejection.

Defences and protective strategies look very sensible in the light of these experiences.

Gerald Ford is reputed to have said: 'Whether you believe you can or whether you believe you can't, you will.' Believing what people say about you is how negative introjects are internalized, and it is how the inner critic gains its clear, subversive voice.

What is the effect of the inner critic?
It discourages change and damages the ability to form relationships by making people feel worthless and inadequate. Casemore (2000) reports: 'As a therapist, I regularly find myself working with clients whose introjected value systems create huge problems for them in their daily lives. As children, they received introjected values which caused them to believe that they must behave in certain ways in order to achieve the strongly conditional love of their parents' (p. 4).

These conditions of worth are transported into adult life so that the adult has the same beliefs about what must be done to achieve others' love and acceptance as he did as a child. This warps the ability of a person to get close to another human being. Individuals with an active inner critic engage in constant and harsh self-scrutiny, and have a chronic fear of being criticized and losing the acceptance and approval of others. They therefore decide that it is altogether easier not to get close to anyone at all, and selectively expose themselves to environments and people that support this view (Zuroff et al. 1995)

How much easier it is for such a dyslexic to stay in a safe orbit way above the world of other human beings. He may just have the company of the old, familiar meteorites that have always pockmarked his self-esteem but this is far, far safer than falling to earth and risking again the pain of human cruelty; of human warmth and connection denied.

In this respect, the counselling relationship is the transitional object, the spaceship, that can bring the dyslexic back into the human fold. Casemore (2000) suggests that a therapist's job is to help the client look at how he has self-imposed his isolation and self-perpetuated his problems. The therapist will help to locate the inner critic introjects and challenge them – often with CBT techniques (see below) – in the safety of the therapeutic relationship. In this way, the counsellor accompanies the client as he re-enters human life with the inner critic silenced by the stronger voice of a new inner advocate who is not only offering new, positive introjects but also not taking any of the old nonsense.

Contributions from cognitive behavioural therapies (CBT)

Why is CBT so useful for dyslexic problems?
As I observed in Chapter 5, the main presenting problems for a dyslexic are related to long-standing anxiety and stress.

While all good therapy will do much to relieve the effects of anxiety through a supportive therapeutic relationship, there is also much excellent research indicating that CBT has the most powerful and long-term effect on anxiety symptoms. Dadds and Barrett (2001), in their extensive review of anxiety disorders in young people, conclude that brief CBT treatments for anxiety disorders in children and adolescents are highly effective, 'with between 60%–90% of those treated showing clinically significant improvements after treatment and at follow-up several years later' (p. 1005). They emphasize that such interventions for anxious children are effective for long-term change.

There are some useful and robust reviews of the CBT technique and its 'numerous strategic options for mood repair' (Terwogt 2002, p. 132). There is, for example, evidence of the successful use of CBT with children

(Spence (1994), childhood depression (Verduyn 2000), post-traumatic stress disorder and anxiety (Smith et al. 1999, Keppel-Benson et al. 2002, Meischenbaum 2000), school refusal (Elliott 1999), depression in adolescence (Fine et al. 1993), social phobia (Spence et al. 2000, Velting and Albano 2001) and children's behavioural problems (Geldard and Geldard 2002).

Barkham (2002) concluded that patients who have received CBT were less likely to relapse than patients receiving medication. The CBT group were also given a long-term protection against subsequent depressive episodes by applying the learned techniques.

Can CBT techniques be integrated into other therapeutic practices?

Yes – easily, but with care.

There are some good CBT and behaviour modification specialists, and these, I believe, are best placed to cope with more extreme and entrenched phobias and anxieties. Techniques such as desensitization and flooding are best left to those trained to use them since there is obvious potential for disaster if such techniques are wrongly applied.

Given this common-sense caveat, I also think that it not necessary to be a specialist CBT therapist to introduce some aspects of its very powerful strategies into other counselling disciplines, including person-centred counselling. Such integration of CBT with humanistic counselling principles is effective and widespread.

As Nelson-Jones (1999) observes: 'Each working day numerous counsellors attempt the task of combining the humanity and whole-person focus of [humanistic counselling] with the clarity and technical precision of [CBT]' (p. 49). He adds: 'Cognitive-humanism stresses the primacy of mind. A basic assumption is that people's minds influence and create their communication, actions, and feelings. People's minds are powerful tools that they always have at their disposal' (p. 49).

My experience is that aspects of CBT are most usefully applied to the negative introjects and anxiety-based thought patterns of dyslexics. In this respect, I note the observation by Hales (1994): 'dyslexia is best understood and located at the cognitive level ... the locus of the learning difficulty lies at the cognitive level where ... an analysis becomes meaningful' (p. 110).

Do I work with cognitive skills or cognitive processes?

Cognitive therapy interventions usually distinguish between those that teach cognitive skills and those that rectify faulty cognitive processes.

The former is based on the assumption that it is inappropriate behaviour that causes the problem, and that the teaching of new skills will solve this; the latter proposes that the inappropriate behaviour is caused by errors or distortions in cognitive processing so the individual is taught how to restructure his thinking. In reality, both approaches overlap.

Cognitive elements can be divided into five domains. These are: *dysfunctional schemas* (general beliefs established at the back of our minds that provide the reference points for choices in our life), *cognitive distortions* (biased interpretations of external events that lead us to catastrophize), *over-generalizations* (taking one event as representative of all others), *personalizing or making internal attributions* (attributing to oneself unwarranted responsibility for all negative events) and *over-abstraction* (focusing on the negative aspects of an event).

What negative thoughts and beliefs are particularly common with dyslexic clients?

These are the most common examples that a counsellor might encounter when working with dyslexic clients:

Oil-slick thoughts

Children and adults who have negative feelings about one aspect of their life can carry them into other parts of their life. This is frequently noted with children who have been victimized (Hawker and Boulton 2000). Dyslexic clients can carry negative attitudes about school failure well into adulthood, still feeling as out of control at 30 as at 13. They have entrenched thoughts about themselves that often bear little resemblance to how they actually live their lives. For example, I have worked with both a ceramic artist and a graphic designer, both dyslexic, who each carried negative thoughts about their 'stupidity' – which depressed them – although both had won awards for innovative design in their respective fields.

With others, these negative thoughts trip them up and mire them in helpless inactivity. There are many intelligent, talented dyslexics, for example, who are steadfastly unblocking drains and digging gardens who have the ability to design the drains and landscape the gardens. The only thing in their way is not their brain but their thought processes.

The habit of beating yourself up

CBT can challenge the punitive self-judgement that is a common reaction in dyslexic children who have blamed themselves for the trouble their disability has caused. Greenhalgh (1994) notes that this is 'a common characteristic of children with emotional and behavioural difficulties who often feel themselves to be worthless, to be unable to complete learning tasks, or who destroy their own work' (p. 76). He places the problem in the concept of the super-ego, and the introjections of parental authority and disapproval. Whatever the origin of the thought, CBT can challenge its manifestation.

Giving power away to other people

Attribution style is the key to how we deal with problems. If we do not feel in control, and we believe that the cause of all our problems is 'out there', then this belief leads us away from a solution: 'Powerlessness is a state of mind, and self talk is the fuel on which it burns' (Steffert 1995, p. 275). Many dyslexic children have experienced failure over which they had no control. They tried hard and it made no difference to the rejection, the academic failure and the parental criticism. They acquired 'learned helplessness', and this led to an external attribution style; that is, they were not in control and could do nothing about their lives. 'The pivot here is one's own attribution; was this negative event my fault or was it due to circumstances beyond my control?' (op. cit., p. 275). CBT teaches clients the art of 'learned mastery', or the ability to take power back to themselves.

Old behaviour that gets in the way

Learnt childhood behaviour that worked as a coping strategy can become obstructive in adulthood. Children may have learnt behaviours that are unhelpful, unnecessarily compliant, aggressive, deceitful or deliberately regressed. Change, however, can be harder in children since the other family members may have a stake in keeping them as they are. In fact, the counsellor may need to include the family as a whole to prevent sabotage. Where there is a change, there is a loss, and the dyslexic's change for the better may be some other family member's change for the worse. This may be a sense of no longer feeling important, needed or clever.

Separating the truth from the lie

There is often a truth behind a destructive belief. It is not always irrational. The important thing is to separate the truthful beliefs from the irrational beliefs. For example, the truth is that a dyslexic child will always be poor at spelling. The irrational belief is that they are the worst speller in the world, and everyone is more skilled than they are. These irrational thoughts can be – may even be intended to be – self-defeating. It may, for example, be easier to think that you will never write a good essay than actually start it.

Which CBT statements and challenges work well with dyslexic clients?
The following ideas have been received well:

'How can I do things differently?'

Dyslexics enjoy the idea of reframing, since inventiveness and creativity are their strengths. The counsellor must be prepared for solutions that will not have occurred to them in their wildest dreams. This notion can also be used to modify process. One university student client asked for three 20-minute sessions three times a week. He had profound problems with concentration and short-term memory and found that he preferred to retain the material from three short sessions than lose most of it from one longer session (and go home with a headache).

'If it doesn't work, stop doing it'

Many dyslexics are good at maintaining and nurturing their anxiety. The Gestalt Therapy question of 'How are you keeping yourself anxious?' is useful here. As O'Connell (2001) observes: 'People under stress may be attached to repetitive behaviour which fails to deliver the desired result' (p. 40).

One useful image to use in this context is that of the 'anxiety weed', an image suggested to me some years ago by a dyslexic child. The 'anxiety weed' describes a disabling worry that chokes off the space in our life that could be more available for fun. These 'anxiety weeds' can be pulled up one by one and the new soil filled with 'growth plants', such as learning a new skill, joining a club or just lying around and watching clouds go by. Since the weed can leave tendrils of root from which a new weed can grow, clients are invited to have a good 'hoe around' every now and then and try to pull out the fragments of 'anxiety root' before they can take hold and grow larger.

'If it works, keep doing it'

If a client does not acknowledge their resources, he cannot draw on them. It comes as a surprise to some dyslexic clients that they have coping strategies already in place, and that a lot of what they have devised for themselves must work or they would not have come this far. 'In the search for solutions, clients will have reported a number of strategies which seem constructive and positive, although this may not be the way in which they are presented. After a period of failure, criticism and blame the client may have come to believe that nothing she does is right' (O'Connell 2001, p. 41). Most dyslexic clients have grown up with people who think that they are stupid, inept, helpless idiots who do not have the resources to solve problems, and that their function in life is to be a problem and to create problems. A therapist who indicates that clients not only can solve problems but also have significant power to do so is an eye-opener.

One of my dyslexic university students was always convinced that he would fail every essay, and became distressed and overwhelmed with anxiety every time one was due. I asked him if he had ever failed an essay. What were his previous marks? There were no failures, and nothing lower than an upper second. With every new essay, he forgot the previous successes. We looked at all the things he had done with his essays that had helped and focused on these. He learnt the strategy of challenging his own disruptive and defeatist thoughts. As O'Connell (2001) notes: 'It is crucial that clients get in touch with the parts of their lives which are healthy and functioning well' (p. 42).

What other CBT approaches can be used?

Most CBT approaches overlap to some extent, and the differences may be subtle. It often depends on what the counsellor finds comfortable and how many sessions are available. The joy of all CBT methods, however, is that they can be adapted to short- or long-term work – from single session to open-ended contracts. The longer work allows more time to establish the history of the client's patterns and script, but even one hour with a dyslexic client can be extremely useful when the counsellor arrives with a wise understanding of the pressures on a dyslexic. The following approaches are flexible:

Neuro-linguistic programming (NLP) and life coaching

This approach is not that different from Solution-focused Brief Therapy (SFBT) in its use of language to challenge client problems (for example, substitute, 'What do I want?' for 'What is my problem?'). This technique is based on the fact that we make a life map from our experiences, and then attend to what we think is relevant to the map and edit out what is not. We make the best choices available to us according to our map, but a new map gives us new choices.

Although NLP is essentially language based, it can be adapted to use visualised symbols. This is particularly so in the NLP concept of 'framing', which is a strategy tailor-made for the dyslexic cognitive style. McDermott and Shircore (1999) explain how you invite a client to 'choose the frame you adopt when you picture a situation, and then change the frame, quite deliberately, when you want to look at it again in a different light' (p. 23). A client can choose 'outcome frames' to identify where they want to go in their lives. There is also the 'as if' frame, which engages the creative imagination of dyslexics and loosens their thinking into visual images.

In this, they are invited to jump ahead to a specific point well beyond the immediate situation and visualize what it looks like and how they are behaving. They look back on the problem as if they had successfully overcome it and work out what they must have done. This is very effective with dyslexics. Fascinatingly, Einstein – arguably one of the most famous dyslexics –

used it a lot as a technique. He used 'thought experiment' so he could 'watch what would happen'. This is not just tinkering. The dyslexic client can really play with different frames, seeing what fits. As a technique 'it always tends to turn you back towards the central truth that it's up to you to make things change for the better' (op. cit., p. 29).

Solution-focused Brief Therapy (SFBT)

This shifts the thinking from problem to solution. It also focuses on any client tendency to choose coping strategies that cause more problems than the problems. The therapy looks at what coping strategies are used, and capitalizes on them in order to find out what the client is doing that works – so he can do more of it. It is therapy based in change, and a belief that even a small change can ripple through a client's system.

This visualization of new solutions works well with the dyslexic client because it 'trusts the client's best instincts and treats him as a resourceful, creative and imaginative person' (O'Connell 2001, p. 16). Using this technique, one dyslexic client decided to leave his cigarettes in the car overnight as a way of getting himself up – he always needed to smoke around 7.30 a.m. There is no better example of the seriousness of the dyslexic's timekeeping problems or the unexpected nature of their solutions.

If you understand the world of the dyslexic, you will also understand why an alarm clock in the morning does not work (but carrying it around in your rucksack during the day does).

Social-skills training (SST)

The dyslexics who have defended themselves through charm, humour and outrageous, delightful, larger-than-life social skills are attractive to others and socially valued. These are the Eddie Izzard, Richard Branson, Felicity Kendall type of dyslexic. They have developed an extremely valuable coping strategy that insulates them from one of the worst aspects of dyslexia – social rejection and isolation. This affliction, which in its extreme form has developed into acute social phobia and abnormal shyness, is like a brick wall between a dyslexic and the warmth of human contact. This is why I constantly emphasize how a good therapeutic relationship is, in itself, so important to dyslexics. Many have simply not been treated with acceptance, warmth, respect, empathy or any form of congruence whatsoever.

There is a point, however, when the counselling relationship, alone, is not enough to help the isolated, socially phobic dyslexic client with poor social skills.

Practical help is justified, if the client is happy to participate, and I have found that additional SST, built on the confidence and support of the counselling relationship, is very useful indeed.

There are three clear objectives of SST.

First, it teaches dyslexic children and adults to behave in a way that stops them appearing so different. Obviously, this objective is irrelevant to those people who are happy that their behaviour is different. They may have already reframed their behaviour as eccentric and distinctive, and may actively enjoy this. There are, however, clients who are lonely because of this difference, and hate the fact that their social skills isolate them. There is a difference between amusing eccentricity and being the rejected butt of others' jokes. Here, as always, I would trust the client's position. For the clients who hate social difference, SST reduces their chance of victimization.

Second, SST models positive skills that enable social interaction. This shows the socially unskilled how to enter groups and make friends, thereby enabling the social support that they have longed for most of their lives.

Much of this is based on straightforward instruction about how to sit, walk, talk, look at people and maintain conversation, including voice modulation and use of different facial expressions. It also teaches non-verbal behaviour, how to manipulate social situations and – joy of joy to dyslexics – how to read the behaviour and speech patterns of others. It is based in group work that provides field-based role play and – as an incidental advantage – creates like-minded friends.

Linked to this is social-perception skills, or social cognitive, training, which teaches how to decode information from others in order to identify feelings. This is implicit in good 'Theory of Mind', a lack of which is associated with bullying and poor peer relationships (see Chapter 4).

Disruptive children are also taught to be sociable, control negative impulses, share and cooperate.

Third, SST teaches dating skills to those young people who feel too anxious and damaged by their peer-group experiences to approach a romantic target. This training is extremely successful, and studies quoted by Argyle (1994) showed that it doubled the number of dates per week among participants. Confidence was increased simply by arranging six practice dates between pairs of clients.

Argyle (1994) is clear that SST is effective: 'It is no longer necessary for a sizeable proportion of the human race to be lonely, isolated, miserable or mentally ill through lack of social skills ... [Learned social skills] raise the whole quality of normal social behaviour so that it is more efficient and enjoyable and results in help, cooperation and trust rather than rejection, misunderstanding and social barriers' (p. 308).

In fact, work on depressive disorders in adolescents shows that SST training is followed by the development of new friendships and marked improvement in depressive affect. A study by Brier (1994), on repeat offenders in the USA, also showed that psychosocial training – along with educational training – can drastically reduce the chances of a relapse. In another study, Spence et al. (2000) found that an integrated CBT programme of social and cognitive training 'produced significant reductions in social anxiety and improvement in social skill among children with social phobia' (p. 722). Treatment effects were maintained at 12-month follow-up. Not only had these children maintained the reduction in social and general anxiety but they had also demonstrated ongoing improvement during the follow-up period.

Training in problem-solving

Clients are encouraged to generate a range of possible solutions to interpersonal or conflict problems.

Self-instructional/self-control/affective training

Children, in particular, are taught to self-monitor and regulate their own behaviour, and emotions through self-talk and relaxing statements, such as 'I am not going to let this annoy/upset me'. They are also taught to use delaying or distracting techniques, such as leaving the scene or counting backwards (the latter absolutely will *not* work with dyslexic children).

Rational Emotive Behavioural Therapy

The identification of the thought associated with a feeling leads to the development of self-talk to challenge irrational reactions to a situation.

Narrative therapy

A client's story about himself is unpicked and rebuilt on new interpretations. Social constructions are challenged. This is useful in post-traumatic stress disorder (Bourne and Oliver 1999).

Relaxation techniques

These are usually based on the idea that a person cannot be anxious and relaxed at the same time. Personally, I find them of little use unless the cognitive biases are also challenged. Otherwise, when the client is no longer relaxed, a single thought can zap them straight back into the old anxiety pattern. Some visualization of walking in quiet places or soothing music can provide respite for dyslexics whose anxiety gives them sleep problems, but it is only a sticking-plaster strategy.

Anxiety management or stress inoculation

This is the most popular form of stress management, and focuses on progressive muscle relaxation, meditation and bio-feedback. It tracks backwards from the physical effects of anxiety (fast to slow breathing, agitation to calm movements, thought management). It works.

Contributions from Transactional Analysis

How can I use the theory of strokes?
It illustrates succinctly, for the counsellor, the types of verbal garbage that are thrown thoughtlessly – and daily – at her dyslexic client.

There are, for example, three particular types of stroke with which dyslexics are familiar. These are 'negative' strokes (in the absence of any positive feedback, criticism is preferable to being ignored), 'counterfeit' strokes (these start off positive but have a sting in the tail, such as 'You draw well – is this because you can't write?') and 'plastic' strokes (which are insincere praise such as 'Wow! John what a marvellous piece of work – well done, well done' to a bored dyslexic child with an IQ of 150 who has written one sentence).

Dyslexics become adept at 'stroke filters'; that is when they get a stroke that doesn't fit in with their preferred script, they ignore or belittle it. Some dyslexics, for example, will not hear anything good about themselves, nor can they make any positive comment about their work or appearance. Some will not look in a mirror, and others destroy their own work.

I have known dyslexic children be unable to say the smallest positive comments, such as 'I have a nice smile'. They can clamp their hands over their mouth and hide their heads to avoid saying such things. Even just trying can distress them. One child would only say a positive affirmation to my dog, another from behind the sofa. Another child told me once that he felt that his reading was improving but later confessed that, while he said this, he was crossing his toes inside his shoes. Some will cover their ears at hearing any good things said to them.

Is the notion of PAC (parent-adult-child) useful?
Yes – and it also gives the counsellor a neat working model of the different dyslexic family dynamics.

For example, many dyslexics have experienced the 'negative nurturing parent' who gives nurturing when it is uninvited or inappropriate. This parent, usually the mother, employs the comments typical of this group, particularly the 'let me do it' instruction, with smothering, engulfing, over-comforting and an abnormally concerned manner.

A common dyslexic experience is also with the 'negative controlling parent' – usually the father – who tries to diminish his child's self-esteem by using harsh, condemnatory phrases combined with a judgemental and distant manner. Teachers who employ the 'controlling parent' will hit, point and shout – sometimes straight into the face of the child.

The dyslexic boy who flinches at any sudden movement is tragically common.

Dyslexics also develop into excellent examples of the 'positive adapted' child who adapts to others in order to get what he wants, or to avoid pain. Dyslexics are also typical of the negative adapted child, who acts purposefully against the expectation of others, often to get attention.

What TA drivers and injunctions are relevant to dyslexic clients?

Most of them. The five Transactional Analysis (TA) drivers, for example, could all have been written for dyslexic adults and children. These – with the balancing counsellor response in brackets are – 'Be perfect' (You are good enough as you are), 'Please others' (Please yourself), 'Be strong' (Be open and express your wants), 'Try hard' (Do it) and 'Hurry up' (Take your time).

Of the 12 injunctions used in TA, the ones most commonly internalized by dyslexics are 'Don't be you', 'Don't think (in the way you are built to)', 'Don't grow up', 'Don't make it' and 'Don't belong'. Dyslexics usually teach themselves the other injunctions – 'Don't be well', 'Don't be important', 'Don't be close' and 'Don't feel'. In my experience, the only one that rarely applies is 'Don't be a child'.

Sometimes, they adopt the worst injunction: 'Don't exist'.

Are notions of 'scripts' unwise for dyslexic clients?

Mostly, yes. This technique is not useful when working with dyslexic clients unless it is translated into visual or cartoon format, when it can work very well. The central notion of scripts as a coherent organization of introjects is useful, but getting a dyslexic to describe a script is probably unwise. Not only do sequencing problems arise but dyslexics just don't think naturally in this way.

What is the main OK/not-OK position for dyslexic clients?

'You're OK – I'm not OK.'

This is the position that exactly typifies a dyslexic child and is, after all, the central message of those thousands of introjects over his lifetime. Harris (1967) summarized the inherent anxiety of the dyslexic in the 'You're OK – I'm not OK' position. This person 'has a magnificent computer ... that can produce brilliant ideas by the thousands if it is not totally involved in working out the problems of "not OK"' (p. 154).

If he does poorly in school, his limitation will be expressed as 'I'm stupid' and his parents' statement will be 'He's not working up to his potential'.

Throughout life, the feelings and techniques for coping with the not-OK position, which the child establishes in the family setting and in school, persist into adulthood and 'deny him the achievements and satisfactions based in a true sense of freedom to direct his own destiny' (op. cit., p. 155).

Harris observes that the primary rule with not-OK is 'when in doubt, stroke' to keep the frightened, anxious child comforted while his adult self learns to take over the realties of the situation. Activating the adult in this model also allows there to be a dialogue to challenge the voice of both the parent and child in the dyslexic. For example, when the parent in the dyslexic says 'Do more', the dyslexic can then respond with the adult voice of 'Do *what* more?'.

Turning on the adult and turning off the frightened child or accusing, critical parent, is the main task. Putting the adult back in control says 'I'm OK and you're OK'.

Interestingly, Harris notes that this model is useful for all children who have been bullied, with their 'catastrophic feelings of terror, fear and hatred' (p. 164). Their need for revenge can switch them in and out of the 'I'm not OK and you're OK' and 'I'm OK – you're not OK' positions, which may, of course, neatly explain the unusual prevalence of the dyslexic bully-victim.

Dyslexic clients enjoy the TA approach because the symbol of PAC (as three little human figures rather than the letters) speaks to them more clearly than more abstract concepts. They can see these three parts and imagine and visualize how they would act.

Contributions from Ecosystemic therapy

What is Ecosystemic therapy?
It is a family therapy that integrates the child's role and behaviour at school.

Of all the family-based therapies, this is the one that works best with dyslexic children since it involves a partnership between counsellor, parents and schools – all working together. When this goes well, it is effective because the child is held in a supportive but well-boundaried circle with everyone communicating. This approach sees the dyslexic child as part of a linked family and school system (for reviews see Cottrell and Boston 2002, and Cooper et al. 1994).

How does it work?
The Ecosystemic approach focuses attention on the school as a factor in family difficulty and vice versa.

Child behavioural problems can then be seen in three ways: a problem in the family that disturbs the school, a problem at school that disturbs the family, a problem at school that does not disturb the family. The theory is that a child's problem behaviour in school can sometimes be related to difficulties in the family, and difficulties in the family to those at school.

For example, a child's disruptive school behaviour can serve 'as a diversion for the family in times of parental disharmony and creates the circumstances in which the parents behave as normal family' (Cooper et al. 1994, p. 94). The problem can be that the parents' dyad is left unacknowledged while attention is focused on the child's school behaviour that is designed to keep the family together. The Ecosystemic approach will, however, integrate it all.

Nonetheless, the counsellor needs to remember that the behavioural problem may actually be vested solely in the school. The family may need to exaggerate those problems for its own end, but the dyslexic child's problems at school will be real enough.

The Ecosystemic approach is also useful in analysing recurring problems, and family situations that maintain the child's symptoms: 'behaviour which functions to maintain an individual's symptomatic condition can often be seen, from a systemic viewpoint, to be serving a goal elsewhere in the system' (op. cit., p. 99). Reframing everyone's position, or just changing one part, can transform the whole.

Contributions from Psychodynamic Theory (transference)

How important is transference in working with a dyslexic client?
It is crucial.

Damaged children transfer onto counsellors and, as we have seen, teachers, their feelings of hurt, anger, frustration, intolerance, anxiety, fear and, most insidious of all, the sense of being useless, deskilled and irrelevant.

As Greenhalgh (1994) observes, one of the most difficult aspects of working with damaged children is 'the problem of what one is made to feel'. These feelings are 'precise and intense' (p. 53). Importantly, countertransference and transference will be strong where there are verbal problems in communication – as there are in dyslexics. Bungener and McCormack (1994) consider that, for impaired-speech clients, transference becomes 'one of the main therapeutic tools' (p. 379).

What aspects of transference are particularly relevant when working with dyslexic clients?

The main transferences from dyslexic clients can include the following broad areas.

Drama triangle

Dyslexics can operate with a strong victim role in which the counsellor can be invited to play a role. This is the classic Transactional Analysis drama triangle, and the counsellor has an almost equal chance of being sucked into persecutor or rescuer roles. Furthermore, the transferences and parallel processes can be both immediate and strong. I have, for example, felt an intense and violent irritation towards a tiny dyslexic child who has done no more than walk into the room and, by contrast, felt fiercely protective of a huge adolescent who just grunts at me.

Implicit in this are a number of parallel processes.

For example, a common school situation involves parents, helplessly stuck in the overprotective rescuer role, who have a child, immersed in victim, who moves, on random select, through the entire school population picking out adults and children as persecutors.

The power of the parallel process is evident when I feel like getting under a desk every time one of these irate, rescuer mothers calls. I am now victim to her persecutor, only to hear the child, moving seamlessly into rescuer, expressing concern at my obvious embattlement.

In a specialist school for dyslexic children, the drama triangle is always present. It whirls through the atmosphere like a gyroscopic Hoover, sucking in every type of adult, child and parent into some permutation of the drama transaction. Some of the most rescuing mothers can ring three or four times a day; many of the worst persecuting parents never offer any comment except criticism of their children, and can even forget to pick up their children at the end of term.

I estimate that the drama-triangle relationship, and the transferences associated with it, represent the predominant feature of working with both dyslexic children and adults.

This is the most obvious transference and the most common. It is also the one that causes most wariness about counter-transference among dyslexic counsellors to whom I have spoken. They are aware of the chance of a powerful amplifying loop being set up between them, in rescuer, and a dyslexic client, in victim.

Disempowerment and deskilling

The second most common transference with dyslexic clients is counsellor disempowerment and deskilling. As I noted in Chapter 3, this is also the main pitfall for teachers working with dyslexic children. The dyslexic child can transfer all his feelings of hopelessness and failure. I have found that this transference emerges about three or four sessions in when I feel, suddenly, that there is no point to the counselling; that I am achieving nothing. For me, this is always the moment when I am most acutely aware of the dyslexic condition. It is clearly transference of the client's feeling that nothing has worked before, this cannot possibly work now and/or they feel like a 'bad' school child again.

When this transference is strongest is also when the client is being faced with a real chance of success, and has no strategy other than giving up, since nothing has worked before. In this sense, it is a sign that we are actually moving forward. I have learnt that an absolutely congruent response at this point is the key. I express my feelings of incompetence; that I am worried about how things will turn out – that maybe he feels the same. By forging empathy from transference we both move forward in partnership.

Disability

The third type of transference revolves around the notion of disability. Segal (1996) refers to the transference of envy from disabled clients to an able-bodied counsellor. With dyslexics, it is their envy of able-literacy and able-communication skills that can be transferred, attitudes brought unconsciously to the therapeutic frame from (old) relationships with parents, siblings and peers.

A dyslexic client, who sees himself as inarticulate, shy and clumsy, meets, every week, with an articulate, socially skilled, relaxed counsellor. In extreme cases, it is not only envy but also ancient and poisonous jealousies towards siblings or a successful father that are transferred to the counsellor.

The other side of this coin is the counsellor's counter-transferential response of graciousness and relief in the face of disability. Segal suggests that both transferences are the product of splitting, and they complement each other.

'The disabled qualities which we dread and the helpless, powerless princess/victim waiting to be rescued are two sides of the same coin' (op. cit., p. 161).

Segal is brutally honest in her focus on this. She suggests that the other side of the counsellor being 'especially kind and considerate to people with disability is the feeling not only that such people are bad but that they actually do not deserve as much of the good things of life as they do get' (p. 161).

Segal also invites us to be careful about the counter-transferential 'think positively' ethos about disability, since this can be a defence against the frightening or depressive aspects of the client's transference. 'Thinking positively can be healthy, but only perhaps after sufficient time to allow negative thoughts and feelings to be brought into the open and made more realistic' (p. 163). Those who retreat into positive thinking may also be placing too much emphasis on the miseries of the condition, and failing to recognize the good bits that are there as well.

Trauma

Casement (1990) wrote of the experience of trauma in the transference. In this, he pointed out that there are often elements of objective reality that function as triggers for transference in the 'here and now' of the counselling relationship. What was experienced in the past can also be enacted in a relationship between two people in the present. Since most dyslexic childhood traumas occurred in relationships with powerful people who were supposed to be caring and protective, it is easy to see how aspects of earlier dyslexic trauma might be remembered in the counselling room with a 'powerful' and 'caring' counsellor.

The problem, as Casement notes, is that this reaction can infect the whole of the therapy. He writes: 'anything associated with a trauma can come to represent the trauma as a whole and may trigger signal anxiety, alerting the unconscious mind as if that trauma were about to be repeated' (p. 76). This may account for why, a few weeks into therapy, dyslexic clients can have apparently random panic attacks during counselling. The client, in response to, say, the counsellor speaking too fast, challenging too hard or even just looking quizzical experiences transference that did not exist when he was not so attached, when the counsellor had not yet established a therapeutic relationship with him.

Furious impotence

Dyslexics are as used to being angry as they are used to not being helped with the cause of their anger. This link of fury and impotence is one of the most marked features of dyslexia.

Fury and impotence are united for dyslexics in a lifetime partnership of thwarted forward motion. They are furious at what has happened to them, but they have no true belief that anything can be done about it, and so are eternally spinning their wheels and permanently stuck in the sand.

What I find fascinating is that this powerful transference is acted out, not only in the counselling room, but also in the writing and lectures of the non-dyslexic people who form the vast majority of activists, researchers and writers in the dyslexia world.

Putting it simply, I believe that inarticulate, illiterate dyslexic people transfer their unexpressed fury and parallel impotence onto the non-dyslexic people who go out and represent them.

How else can we explain the fury and sense of passionate unfairness that roars out of the lectures and writing of the many non-dyslexic people but which never, somehow, gets translated into useful action? It is nearly a hundred years since dyslexia was first identified but I still see abused, illiterate, dyslexic children with almost Dickensian histories of schooling.

I hear a similar transference in the work of people writing about the victims of bullying – that other great unheard, inexpressive, damaged group of adults and children. When Rigby (2002) writes of 'the sound of anguish of people driven to and beyond breaking point, of people striking out in desperation and anger for all they are worth at the sheer injustice of how they are being treated' (p. 264), he is not talking of victims – who do not, in my experience, strike out in anger or anguish – but people who represent them.

Equally, it is not dyslexic people who are striking out in anger, desperation, fury or whatever. It is always other people doing it on their behalf. The issue is that dyslexic feelings are unexpressed consciously and directly.

We can call it lack of political consciousness or learned helplessness or the infantilization of the massive dyslexic minority. It doesn't matter. These feelings are transferred onto non-dyslexic people, like Rigby or me, for us to express them.

Did we, for example, see men act like this in the early feminist movement or whites act like this in the early civil rights movement? Men and whites did not have to because women and blacks were articulate and literate. They could express their anger for themselves.

Another therapeutic interpretation of this phenomenon is to label it as a mass projective identification. This is because one thing I have noted, as a counsellor of dyslexic children and adults, is that they hardly ever get angry.

Dyslexics dress strangely, they act out in sullenness, they get anxious, they get depressed, they overwork, they give up and they shut down. What they do not do is get angry.

It is always a question for me whether it is this unexpressed anger in dyslexics that lies at the bottom of their universal anxiety. Would this be too simple? Or is it one of those facts that is staring us in the face and which we do not recognize?

Contributions from humanistic therapies: empathy and congruence

What problems are there in communicating empathy to a dyslexic client?

Empathy is central to the counselling relationship and, thence, the effectiveness of therapy.

As Mearns and Thorne (2000) summarize, 'If the therapist cannot enter the client's framework, and be at home there, there is no chance that therapy will be effective' (p. 83). The notion of empathy is, however, always integrated with its communication.

The counsellor must pick up accurately the integral feelings of the client and be able to communicate that affective awareness back to the client. Feeling empathy is just self-indulgence if the client does not *experience* that empathy.

With a dyslexic client, hearing is a problem. It must occur at two levels: at the unscrambling level of processing and at the level of decoding words into images that mean something to him. The process from one to the other has to be held in a short-term memory 'suitcase' that may be insecurely fastened or very small. Some of what the dyslexic client hears will fall out of the suitcase of short-term memory and be lost for ever.

Thus, a dyslexic client may hear in the anatomical sense but not in the psychological sense. Even good counsellors will have problems communicating with a dyslexic client if they do not understand the filters that their communication will go through.

One of the problems is how to translate verbal counsellor speak into dyslexic visual speak. There are, in effect, two different languages and receivers in operation.

This can be disastrous since, as May (1989) observes, if client and counsellor do not speak the same language, then no understanding is possible. Common language is the route to rapport. To use the same language allows a 'merging' process (p. 65), and, in good counselling, the participants will 'be automatically employing a common mode of speech' (p. 65).

Unfortunately, a common mode of speech will never come about between a dyslexic and a non-dyslexic. We can offer other things that help a great deal, but the dyslexic's way of being, thinking and communicating may well be something only another dyslexic truly understands.

One client described this translation from dyslexic speak to non-dyslexic speak as a process that sucked out an important essence. The client may have the most wonderful image to communicate but he has to translate it into verbal for you to understand it. To illustrate this, one client asked me if I could describe a rainbow in words. Another compared the translation process of visual to verbal form to capturing a dragonfly. Once caught, it dies and loses all its colours. It becomes black and ugly.

Although the process may be imperfect, a non-dyslexic counsellor must, at least, try to understand the dyslexic client's frame of reference and search for relevant metaphors. If she persists in using verbal and abstract concepts, she is not entering the client's framework and she is not being empathic.

Are words or images more important in communicating empathy to a dyslexic client?

Images, or concrete verbal concepts, are best.

Expressing their felt empathy with a client is very important to counsellors, but they are used to doing this through abstract verbal concepts. Happy, sad, angry, afraid and lost are all abstract concepts, but dyslexics are far more at home with metaphor, visual imagery, symbolism – even eloquent body language. Dyslexic counsellors tell me that they translate the verbal images of non-dyslexic clients into visual images and metaphor before they reflect them back. They tell me that it helps both of them. Certainly, I find that one decent metaphor will communicate more to a dyslexic client than a whole chapter of conventional counsellor responses.

Rennie (2001) agrees. 'Well-placed metaphors succinctly articulate clients' inchoate experience because they compactly gather together many strands of meaning and represent it in shorthand' (p. 85).

This, of course, brings me right up against the arguments of 'whose material is it?' and 'what about counter-transference?' and 'exactly whose image are you working with?' My experience, however, is that dyslexic clients can take your image, wring out the bits that are not relevant to them, reconstruct the rest to take better account of their view then lob it back to you, reformed and relevant to how they are feeling. The more you start doing this, the better you get. This is one area where a really well developed, trusting, warm, respectful therapeutic relationship helps. Also, dyslexics are not good at arguing and challenging. Most are very adapted personalities. So, to say to you that 'the image you offered was crap, but this one is better' is, in itself, a huge leap forward for them.

There is another point, related to this. Empathy involves inhabiting the world of another person. When that other person has problems that you simply do not understand yourself, it will be more difficult, however much you try, to empathize with them. It 'generates a concern about whether there can be a shared reality ... If the surface is very different from the surface we are used to ... the links of coherence we are looking for feel less within reach' (Bungener and McCormack 1994, p. 371). If we voice and share this concern, the dyslexic client will feel trusted, and the breathtaking congruence of such a reply will move both of you forward. They are, after all, on your side. For a dyslexic, for example, 'it is often the first time in their life that they have felt properly understood' (McLoughlin et al. 2002, p. 85).

There is, however, one downside to using visual images. They are far more powerful triggers for physiological anxiety, and much more cognitively available than thought, particularly in stress arousal (Goleman 1995). This may go some way to explaining why the dyslexic anxiety is so trigger-happy. Anxiety is triggered by visual images, and dyslexics are prone to visual images. In short, they are already tuned to the anxiety channel and receiving stress signals neat.

How important is congruence to a dyslexic client?

If I had to choose just one therapeutic skill that is utterly essential to dyslexic counselling, it would be congruence.

This is because it is the one thing that dyslexics trust most and have experienced least. The story of a dyslexic's life is a catalogue of incongruence. It started with those odd, bright smiles and insincere praise in overloud and overhigh voices at school and home. It continued when powerful people insisted that strange shapes on paper made a sound when it was obvious that they did not. It carried on through the constant and inexplicable mismatch of effort and output in their work, the accusations of laziness in the face of hours and hours of work.

It pursued them through those inexplicably failed encounters with people who rejected them despite every effort to please. It was there every night and day in the faces of their parents, and the voices that said 'love' while quietly screaming 'disappointment', 'shame', 'dislike', 'irritation'.

Most of all, the incongruence has lain inside them. It has festered in the irreconcilability between what everyone has called them – 'stupid', 'thick', 'failed' – and what, despite everything, they know they are – bright, clever, creative, imaginative and alive.

This last incongruence will fuel them or destroy them, but it will never quite go away.

So, how important is congruence to a dyslexic client?

It is vital. It is also a gift – and one that all therapists and counsellors know better than anyone how to give.

The individuality of dyslexia

This whole book has been about how to integrate the client's experience of dyslexia into the counselling relationship. At some point, however, our understanding of dyslexia, and our counselling response to it, need to move from conscious competence to unconscious competence. This allows the counselling to get to the rest of a dyslexic client's experience.

It is important when working with this group of clients to move their dyslexic characteristics in and out of focus. Like concentrating on those embedded diagrams that you bring up to your nose so that you can see the image hidden behind the colours, the counsellor will need to stay alert to track a client's dyslexia.

In the therapeutic narrative, the dyslexia will move between foreground and background. Sometimes it will conceal itself; sometimes it will be star-tlingly obvious and spring out at you, but it will always be there somewhere.

Counsellors must take care not to attribute all of a client's problems to dyslexia, but neither can the experience of being dyslexic ever be complete-ly removed from any experience the client has. The client's dyslexia will inform the counselling relationship, and it will inform their worldview and their entire life experiences. Yet, other files lie above and beneath.

The dyslexia is both separate and woven in.

Experience with this client group helps you to disentangle everything. For example, I once worked with a moderately dyslexic man with an obses-sive exercise regime and profound, work-inhibiting anxiety. Much of the dyslexic experience was there, including a withdrawn, hostile, critical non-dyslexic father who had left the client's mother. She was extremely enmeshed with my client. All of this was linked to the dyslexic experience, but his feelings about the enmeshment, his father's absence and the conse-quent need to be a substitute father for his brothers – all these overlay the experience but were not the whole issue. His father might well have left whether my client were dyslexic or not. My client's dyslexic experiences helped to colour the absence, but parts of that absence – the anger, for

287

example – would have been there anyway. It was the dyslexia that made the anger hard to express, but it was the dyslexic's other experience of brutal, rejecting teachers that made it complicated.

My understanding of dyslexic families helped me to get quickly to the fact and relevance of this family set-up, but, from thereon, the issues were also those of a sad and angry human being not just a sad and angry dyslexic human being.

The experiences of dyslexics make them what they are. The feelings that result are as unique and individual as with any client.

In making this point, I am moving in an integrative direction with regard to the dyslexic experience. The literature on dyslexia has concentrated largely on the neurophysiology and cognitive psychology of the condition until, quite recently, when a number of writers have pointed out that the social and behavioural aspects of dyslexia are, in many ways, more important. Their argument is that it is these aspects, and not their brain chemistry, that dyslexics actually have to negotiate on a daily basis.

While it is good to see all the aspects of dyslexia accounted for and included in our understanding of a dyslexic individual, there is still one other indefinable part that is unique to the individual. This is the part that informs and is affected by dyslexia but which takes the dyslexia and weaves it into something original.

We must not lose sight of the fact that dyslexia is important, but how dyslexics integrate and use it, and how they demonstrate it to the world, is a matter of their individuality.

I think a counsellor intuitively understands this, perhaps more so than a pure psychologist, whether cognitive, neurological, genetic, developmental or social. It is the instinct of psychologists to dismember and examine, while the instinct of the counsellor is to understand and integrate.

While psychologists look for the patterns between individuals, the counsellor is looking for the pattern within a single individual.

A counsellor must see that the dyslexia is part of this pattern, might even give major structure to this pattern, but the detail, how it is finally arranged – like a snowflake – is utterly individual.

Signs of dyslexia in children and adults

What are the signs of dyslexia in a child?

- a puzzling gap between written language skills and intelligence
- delayed and poor reading and spelling, often with persistent reversals and disordering of letters, syllables and words (d/b, was/saw, place/palace), bizarre spelling (raul/urchins, kss/snake, tars/trumpet) and others which are more recognizable (wayt/wait, pant/paint, boll/doll)
- confusion of left and right direction
- sequencing difficulties, such as saying months of the year out of order, poor directional scan in reading, weak sequential memory
- poor short-term memory skills (repeating digits, following complex instructions)
- problems in acquiring arithmetical tables
- problems in repeating polysyllabic words (sas'tis'cit'al for statistical, per'im'ery for preliminary)
- difficulties in expressing ideas in written form
- difficulties in dividing words up or recognizing sound-symbol associations

Other associated factors may include late language development and continued pronunciation difficulties, ambidexterity or mixed handedness, similar problems in other members of the family, clumsiness, poor graphic (writing) skills and dyspraxia.

(Copyright: *Dyslexia and Your Child* (2002), booklet produced by East Court School for Dyslexic Children, Ramsgate, Kent.)

What are the signs of dyslexia in an adult?

Positive answers to questions such as:

• Do you find difficulty telling left from right?
• Is map reading or finding your way to a strange place confusing?
• Do you dislike reading aloud?
• Do you take longer than you should to read a page of a book?
• Do you find it difficult to remember the sense of what you have read?
• Do you dislike reading long books?
• Is your spelling poor?
• Is your writing difficult to read?
• Do you get confused if you have to speak in public?
• Do you find it difficult to take messages on the telephone and pass them on correctly?
• When you say a long word, do you sometimes find it difficult to get all the sounds in the right order?
• Do you find it difficult to do sums in your head without using your fingers or paper?
• When using the telephone, do you tend to get the numbers mixed up when you dial?
• Do you find it difficult to say the months of the year forwards in a fluent manner?
• Do you mix up dates and times and miss appointments?
• When writing cheques, do you frequently find yourself making mistakes?
• Do you find forms difficult?

(Adapted from the 'Adult Dyslexia Checklist' (2003) on the British Dyslexia Association website: www.bda-dyslexia.org.uk. Copyright British Dyslexia Association, 1 August 2003.)

APPENDIX B

Dyslexia assessment for children and adults

Children

How do I obtain an assessment for a child?

An assessment has to be carried out by an educational or clinical psychologist. This might include evidence from other sources, such as a doctor, speech therapist, teacher or parent. Crucial evidence comes from a full assessment of intelligence and abilities, attainments in reading, writing and spelling and diagnosis in phonological (sound) coding, memory and other perceptual skills. These are measured by special psychometric tests.

An assessment may be obtained through the local education authority via the Schools Psychological Service or, privately, through an agency specializing in such assessments (e.g. the Dyslexia Institute) or an independent educational psychologist.

What is the assessment process for a child?

The purpose of assessment is to ascertain whether the student is failing and, to what degree, compared with his peers. If he is behind expected levels, it is necessary to establish whether this is due to an overall low ability, physical factors such as hearing or sight difficulty, a repeated absence due to illness, emotional or social factors, such as family problems or bereavement, frequent changes of school or a specific learning difficulty. It is important to remember that more than one factor may be at work in an individual. For example, a failing child who has frequent absences due to asthma attacks may also have a hearing loss or a specific learning difficulty. Differential diagnosis in such cases, as in the case of bilingual children or those for whom English is not their first language, is a delicate and specialized task.

It is necessary when assessing a child to ascertain his strengths as well as his weaknesses. These can then be used in teaching. A distinction must be made between his underlying ability (you may call this intelligence or academic potential) and how he is performing now (i.e. his levels in literacy and numeracy). If there is a discrepancy between these two, the assessment

291

of individual skills and a carefully taken case history will, it is hoped, lead to insights into the areas of skill deficit.

Some of the skills, such as phonological awareness, are essential to the development of literacy. Other skill deficits may be among the effects of literacy failure. Some aspects of development, such as the establishment of laterality, may be useful diagnostic indicators of specific learning difficulty.

Ideally, an educational psychologist will carry out a detailed assessment at a specialist centre or in school. Some tests are, however, available for teachers to use and, although less detailed, they may well be useful as a preliminary to teaching. Wherever a teacher remains concerned about a pupil, a full assessment should be sought from a chartered psychologist.

What tests are used?

Tests of underlying ability

An educational psychologist will normally use either one of the Wechsler battery of IQ tests (Wechsler Intelligence Scale for Children third edition, known as WISC-III, is the most common one) or the British or Differential Ability Scales. Both will yield an overall IQ score and separate IQ scores for verbal and performance (non-verbal) ability, which enable the assessor to compare the subject with his peers. The verbal IQ is recognized as the best predictor of future academic achievement.

These tests are closed to everyone except chartered psychologists; teachers may get some idea of underlying ability by using tests such as Raven's Matrices (published by NFER) or the Matrix Analogies Test (a US publication, available from the Psychological Corporation), supplemented by relevant parts of the Aston Index.

Tests of educational attainment

The assessor will look first at reading ability, and will test both single-word reading and continuous reading. Single-word reading tests include SPAR, Wide-Range Achievement Test, third edition (known as WRAT-3 and published in the USA and available from the Dyslexia Institute), Vernon Single Word Reading Test or an older test, such as Schonell, which is incorporated in the Aston Index – though an equivalent may be substituted. Continuous reading is most often tested using Neale Analysis of Reading Ability (revised), which assesses accuracy, speed and comprehension of prose passages.

Spelling will be assessed in a single-word test, such as WRAT, SPAR, Vernon or Schonell, and within a piece of continuous prose writing. Handwriting can also be looked at in continuous writing. For example, is the size consistent? Is it joined? Are the letters well formed and distinguishable from each other?

Finally, a number test may be administered. There is a useful one within Differential Ability Scales but, for teachers, the Cilham and Hesse Basic Number Screening Test is a valuable tool, as is the Numeracy section of WRAT-3.

For the most reliable results, it is recommended that modern tests be used where possible, as the norms of older tests are likely to be out of date.

Typically, the SpLD student will present with an irregular profile of ability, showing areas of strength and areas of weakness, and there will usually be a discrepancy between his expected levels of attainment on the basis of the IQ test and his actual levels of attainment. Therefore, *something* is preventing him from achieving his potential.

Diagnostic (skills) testing

The student's visual and auditory perceptual skills, including phonological awareness, will also be assessed. The latter is a key factor in the development of literacy, and frequently presents as an area of weakness in the SpLD student. The assessor will wish to measure the skills of auditory and visual memory, speed of information processing and spoken language (receptive and expressive). In addition, the subject's handedness and lateral preference for ear, eye and foot will be looked at; many dyslexic people have mixed laterality (e.g. a preference for the left hand, but a dominant right eye).

Some of the tests used will be norm-referenced. In other words, the scores will relate to age, either as an age score or as a percentile (the sixtieth percentile means that 40% of the same age will do better, and 60% will do less well). Other tests are criterion referenced, which means that success or failure is related to the skill. Some skills cannot be graded as an age continuum; a skill such as rhyming is mastered by most children in the preschool years, but remains a problem to many older SpLD students. Therefore failure can be considered diagnostically useful, and the information of criterion-referenced testing is particularly relevant when planning a teaching programme. For further reading on tests, see Thomson (2001), Turner (1997, 2002).

Adults

How can I obtain an adult assessment?

Assessing an adult for dyslexia requires different psychometric tests than for a child. There are also self-assessment software packages, such as *Quick*

Scan. The British Dyslexia Association (see Appendix C) will supply further contacts. Assessments can be arranged through the Dyslexia Institute (01784 463851) or the British Dyslexia Association (0118 966 2677), who would refer you to an independent, professionally qualified psychologist.

What is the assessment process for an adult?
The assessment procedure would take around two to three hours, including time required to discuss the results of the assessment, for example attainments in basic skills, such as reading, writing, mathematics and spelling. If a specific learning difficulty is present, the following advice should be given:

- extra time should be allowed in examinations
- computer support should be given to help with spelling difficulties
- a learning programme should be set up to address areas of deficiencies in basic skills
- the report will provide evidence of dyslexia, or specific learning difficulty, which can be used, for example, in case of criticism of spelling by an employer or academic tutor

How much will it cost me to have an assessment?
A private assessment can cost between £250 and £500.

Could I be entitled to a free assessment?
You may be entitled to a free assessment under certain conditions.

- a GP may refer you to a clinical psychologist if you believe that having dyslexia is affecting your health adversely
- the Disability Employment Adviser (DEA) at your local Job Centre will be able to tell you what assistance is available. This may include a referral to a psychologist for an assessment
- if you are employed, discuss this with your human resources department
- students at college can ask to be referred to an educational psychologist

What other help can I have?
Specialist tuition is available. While a dyslexic person may have, over the years, developed strategies to cope with reading or writing difficulties, specialist teaching can help and can be arranged through the Dyslexia Institute, or one of their local centres (see Appendix C). The Dyslexia Institute has a program on CD-Rom called *Units of Sound Multimedia* that forms part of the tuition programme.

Examples of methods that can be used by dyslexics include mind-maps, speed reading, mnemonics and visual images.

Can technology help the dyslexic person?
The following are widely used by dyslexic adults and children:

- voice-activated computers
- electronic dictionaries
- dictation machines
- tape recorders
- telephones with memory
- electronic diaries
- spell-checkers
- grammar-checkers
- calculators
- tinted spectacles
- coloured overlays

Minton (2002) provides a comprehensive review of information and computer technology that is helpful to a dyslexic.

What practical help is available for a dyslexic at work?
Dyslexia is a disability and is recognized as such under the relevant legislation. In particular, an employer of a dyslexic person must abide by the terms of the Disability Discrimination Act of 1995.
In day-to-day terms, this means an employer should:

- use multisensory aids, on training courses for example
- highlight any important text when documents are presented or circulated
- ensure that any verbal instructions given should be clear and not lengthy
- give information to a dyslexic person well in advance of a meeting in order for them to assimilate it
- print text on coloured paper; dyslexics find the lowered contrast helps them to read text more easily
- be supportive and make any necessary changes to the job description that will help the dyslexic person to carry out their tasks properly

Bartlett and Moody (2000) provide an excellent, thorough overview of dyslexia in the workplace. But the reader can also contact the British Dyslexia Association at www.bda-dyslexia.org.uk (see Appendix C for more details).

Contact details of useful organizations

For general advice and information

Adult Dyslexia Organisation
336 Brixton Road
London SW9 7AA
Tel: 020 7924 9559

British Dyslexia Association
98 London Road
Reading
Berks RG1 5AU
Tel: 0990 134248 or 0118 668271
Email: info@dyslexiahelp-bda.demon.co.uk
Website: www.bda-dyslexia.org.uk

British Dyslexics
22 Deeside
Enterprise Centre
Deeside
Chester CH5 1PP
Website: www.britishdyslexics.co.uk

Dyslexia Advice and Resource Centre
217 The Custard Factory
Gibb Street
Digbeth
Birmingham B9 4AA
Tel: 0121 694 9944

The Dyspraxia Foundation
8 West Alley
Hitchin
Herts SG5 1EG
Helpline: 01462 454 986
Administration: 01462 455016
Website: www.dyspraxiafoundation.org.uk

Learning to read and write

For a child:

1. Contact the Dyslexia Institute for details of private tutors trained to teach dyslexics.
2. Approach your child's school and discus the problem with the SENCO there.
3. If you consider it appropriate that your child should go to a specialist school for dyslexic children, contact CReSTeD (01242 604852) for details of schools.

For a student at college or university:

1. They should approach their Student Support Unit. Some educational establishments have specialist dyslexic units contained within their student support units or in their disability support units.
2. Students who are resident in the United Kingdom and are either in full-time or part-time study (the latter should be at least 50% of a full-time course) at undergraduate or postgraduate level may be eligible for a Disabled Students' Allowance. This could help towards specialist equipment or other assistance. The Student Support Unit at the university should be able to help obtain the application form. Otherwise, your client should contact their local education authority or the Department for Education and Skills on 0800 731 9133 or text phone 0800 210280.

For an adult:

1. Adult education classes provide basic to advanced literacy skills. The number will be listed in the telephone directory.
2. The Dyslexia Institute (01784 463851) will also provide details of private tutors trained to teach adult dyslexics.

For general advice on assessment and tuition

Dyslexia Institute
133 Gresham Road
Staines TW18 2AJ
Tel: 01784 463851

Helen Arkell Dyslexia Centre
Frensham
Farnham
Surrey GU10 3BW
Tel: 01252 792400

Hornsby International Dyslexia Centre
Glenshee Lodge
261 Trinity Road
London SW18 3SN
Tel: 020 8874 1844

Patoss (RSA tutors)
P.O. Box 10
Evesham
Worcestershire WR11 6ZW

Advice on employment issues

Disability Matters
Berkeley House
West Tytherley
Wiltshire SP5 1NF
Tel: 01264 811120

Employers Forum on Disability (EFD)
Nutmeg House
60 Gainsford Street
London SE1 2NY
Tel: 020 7403 3020

Job Centre: for your local number see the Disability Employment Adviser.

Opportunities for People with Disabilities
1 Bank Buildings
Princes Street
London WC2R 8EU
Tel: 020 7726 4961

Trades Union Congress (TUC)
Congress House
Great Russell Street
London WC1B 3LS
Tel: 020 7636 4030

Disability Advice Organizations

DIAL UK (Local advice centres, telephone helplines and drop-in centres)
Park Lodge
St. Catherine's Hospital
Tickhill Road
Doncaster DN4 8QN
Tel: 01302 310123

Disability on the Agenda
Freepost
Bristol BS38 7DE
Tel: 0345 622633

Disability on the Agenda
Freepost
London SE 99 7EQ
Tel: 0345 622633

Disability Law Service
52–54 High Holborn
London WC1V 6RL
Tel: 020 7831 8031

Equal Opportunities Commission
Tel: 0161 833 9244

Free Representation Unit (for free legal representation to persons on low income)
Tel: 020 7831 0692

Law Centres (for free legal advice and representation)
Law Centre Federation
18-19 Warren Street
London W1P 5DB
Tel: 020 7387 8570

Low Pay Unit
Employment Rights Advice Service
27-29 Amwell Street
London EC1R 1UN
Tel: 020 7713 7616
Helpline: 020 7713 7583

RADAR (The Royal Association for Disability and Rehabilitation)
12 City Forum
250 City Road
London EC1V 8AF
Tel: 020 7250 3222

Specialist dyslexia schools

CReSTeD (Register of schools that help dyslexic children)
The Administrator
Greygarth
Littleworth
Winchcombe
Cheltenham
Gloucestershire GL54 5BT
Tel: 01242 604852
Website: www.crested.org.uk
Email: admin@crested.org.uk

Education appeals

If you need to appeal against a decision that has been made by your LEA
(local education authority) regarding your child's special educational
needs, or need help and advice regarding what the LEA's duties are
towards providing for children who have special educational needs, the following registered charity may be able to help: The Independent Panel for
Special Education Advice (IPSEA) (tel: 01394 382814). They can represent
parents who wish to appeal against a decision made by their LEA. They can
provide independent advice on the duty that the LEA has to provide for
those children who have special educational needs.

Advice regarding computers

Ability Net
P.O. Box 94
Warwick CV34 5WS
Tel: 01926 312847
Helpline: 0800 269545

Computability Centre
P.O. Box 94
Warwick CV34 5WS
Tel: 0800 269 545

Computer Centre for People with Disabilities
University of Westminster
72 Great Portland Street
London W1N 5AL
Tel: 020 7911 5000

Dyslexia Computer Resource Centre
Department of Psychology
University of Hull
Hull HU6 7RX
Tel: 01482 465589

Foundation for Communication for the Disabled
Tel: 01483 727848 or 01684 563684
Iansyst Training Project
The White House
72 Fen Road
Cambridge CB4 1UN
Tel: 01223 420101

Dyspraxia

Dyspraxia Foundation
8 West Alley
Hitchin
Herts SG5 1EG
Tel: 01462 455016
Helpline: 01462 454986
Website: www.dyspraxiafoundation.org.uk
Email: dyspraxia@dyspraxiafoundation.org.uk

Attention deficit/hyperactivity disorder (ADHD) or attention deficit disorder (ADD)?

Contact www.adders.org. This website will provide all sorts of information for those suffering from ADHD or ADD, including information on research, resources and support groups.

Training to be a specialist dyslexia teacher

The Dyslexia Institute
133 Gresham Road
Staines
Middlesex TW18 2AJ
Tel: 01784 463851

Helen Arkell Dyslexia Centre
Frensham
Farnham
Surrey GU10 3BW
Tel: 01252 792400
Email: general_enquiries@arkellcentre.org.uk

Hornsby International Dyslexia Centre
Wye Street
London SW11 2HB
Tel: 020 7223 1144
Email: dyslexia@hornsby.co.uk

APPENDIX D

Help for dyslexics in further education

Colleges of further and higher education have policies for disability aware-ness and support, including dyslexia. Details are usually on college websites. Dyslexics should contact the college disability officer in order to discuss their individual situations with department staff. However, some dyslexics may not have been identified, or may not want to declare their disability, so it is hoped that staff will have some general awareness. Changes to accommodate dyslexic students will improve the learning envi-ronment for them, but dyslexia has not prevented students from achieving excellent results, at all levels.

Indicators of dyslexia in students:

- a marked discrepancy between ability and the standard of work being produced
- a persistent or severe problem with spelling, even with easy or common words
- difficulties with comprehension as a result of slow reading speed
- poor short-term memory, especially for language-based information, which results in inefficient processing into long-term memory
- difficulties with organization, classification and categorization
- note-taking may present problems due to spelling difficulties, poor short-term memory and poor listening skills
- handwriting may be poor and unformed, especially when writing under pressure
- students often show a lack of fluency in expressing their ideas or show difficulties with vocabulary
- some students may have continuing pronunciation or word-finding dif-ficulties, which may inhibit them when talking or discussing in large groups

303

Useful financial resources

The Disabled Students' Allowance (DSA)

A dyslexic student in higher education may be able to get extra funding from a DSA, including finance for the whole of the course, a non-medical helpers' allowance, and a general/other expenditure allowance. The student will have to have had a Study Aids and Study Assessment, which will require proof of your disability or dyslexia (usually a formal assessment is required), as well as agreement of eligibility from the student's LEA. Most colleges can advise on this. University websites have sites with details about this grant and other aspects of disability support, including a helpful site at the University of East London.

Also, try contacting:

- The National Bureau for Students with Disabilities (Tel: 0800 328 5050)
- The Educational Grant Advisory Service (Tel: 020 7249 6636)
- National Federation of Access Centres (Tel: 01752 232278)

The Communication Aids Project

In March 2001, the government announced a commitment of £10 million to provide communication aids for students who have oral or written communication difficulties. This would certainly include dyslexics (who have both). The aim is to provide better access to the curriculum, to increase the ability to interact with others and to help with the transition from school to higher education. It aims to benefit children with speech and language difficulties, hearing-impaired children and those with dyslexia.

The scheme will be managed by the SEN (Special Education Needs) division at the Department for Education and Skills (DfES). It is estimated that up to 1% of the school population will be helped either by augmentative technology or by writing provision for those with severe dyslexia. Further information is on the CAP website: www.becta.org.uk/cap.

Useful websites on disability and dyslexia in education are: www.jiscmail.ac.uk/lists/dis-forum.html (a forum and source site), www.techdis. ac.uk (for a wide range of assistive technologies for students), www.nado. ac.uk (the website for NADA, the National Association for Disability Officers working in Higher and Further Education Institutes).

Legal issues

The Main Acts Affecting Dyslexic Adults and Children

(All publications are available from the Department for Education and Skills (DfES) and obtainable from the HMSO or the DfES website www.dfes.gov.uk.)

The main acts that apply to dyslexic children or adults are:

The **Education Act (1981)** which implemented the Warnock Committee's Report on Special Educational Needs (1978). This decreed that special education would be conceived in terms of need and provision rather than defined categories of handicap. It set out new ways of identifying children who need special help under the education system. In the Act, the term 'specific learning difficulty (dyslexia)' became a recognized educational concept.

The **Education Act (1996)**, which consolidated the law on special needs and further defined 'learning difficulty'. It specified that a disability was something that prevented or hindered a child from making use of educational facilities of a kind generally provided for children in schools. Such a child might also have significantly greater difficulty in learning than the majority of children their age. In such cases, pupils would be eligible for 'special education provision' for children of their age in that particular local education authority (LEA). This Act also required the child's LEA to carry out a statutory assessment if the request were considered to be reasonable. Following this, the LEA must decide if the child, in its opinion, has special educational needs. If the answer is yes, that child's needs can be met from resources generally available. If these resources are not suitable or adequate, the LEA must provide extra resources and write a 'Statement of Educational Needs' for that child.

The **Disability Discrimination Act (1995) (DDA)**, which defines disability. It describes a disabled person as someone with a 'physical or mental impairment that has substantial and long-term adverse effects upon their ability to carry out normal day-to-day activities'. It estimates, on this definition, that there are 8.5 million disabled people in Britain; 1 in 7 of the population. The DDA covers employment practices and applies in any workplace where 15 or more people are employed. (This will also apply to counselling departments and agencies.)

Bartlett and Moody (2000) give a good review of what this Act means for dyslexics. For example, they should not be unfairly disadvantaged (such as in interviews or proficiency tests), and the employer must make 'reasonable adjustment' to reduce or remove any substantial disadvantage caused to a dyslexic person by any of the employment arrangements in force. Adjustment might include modifying equipment, allowing pastel-coloured paper instead of white (the contrast of the latter is difficult for dyslexics) and allocating some of the dyslexic's duties to another person.

Informing an employer of one's dyslexia is not mandatory, unless the employer specifically asks about dyslexic difficulties, such as in an interview. Deliberate concealment of dyslexia may mean the employer does not need to make 'reasonable adjustment'.

The **Special Educational Needs Code of Practice (2001)**, which recommends best practice for the 20% of UK children with learning difficulties who might require, at some point, special educational provision within school, and the 2% of severely afflicted children who warrant support beyond what is available in mainstream schools. This group includes those children with specific learning difficulty (dyslexia). It also includes children with speech and language difficulty, dyscalculia, and emotional and behavioural disturbance – all of which are also associated with dyslexia.

This Code provides practical advice to LEAs and schools on how to carry out their statutory duties to identify, assess and make provision for a child's special educational needs. It particularly supports parental involvement and a good working partnership between parents, children and school.

The **Disability Code of Practice (2002)**, which derives from the Special Educational Needs and Disability Act 1995 (*Disability Rights Commission Code of Practice for Schools*), stipulates that schools, colleges and universities make reasonable adjustments to accommodate disabled students. Disabled pupils cannot be discriminated against in the provision of education and associated services, and in respect of admissions and exclusions. The general consensus is that the Code clearly applies to dyslexics, and that certain practices – such as putting children in lower sets or keeping them in at break to finish work – are discriminatory practices under this Code (see Orton 2002).

The **Quality Assurance Agency Code of Practice for the Assurance of Academic Quality and Standards in Higher Education (Section 3): Students with Disabilities (1999)**, which stipulates that higher-education establishments should provide support and provision for all disabilities, including dyslexia. This reinforces the 'whole institute' approach to dyslexia support. The Disability Discrimination Act was extended to higher education in 2000 to ensure that students with disabilities, such as dyslexia, are not discriminated against.

Many universities now have a Disability Support Officer who arranges for academic and assessment support. Other student counselling departments conduct 'Hidden Disability' workshops, as well as specialist dyslexic groups, which have the advantage of providing a peer group for students, which then continues after the group ends.

The **European Human Rights Act 2000** provides the right of equal opportunity to education irrespective of race, religion, gender or disability.

Disability Service Teams, linked to the Employment Service, provide coherent employment advice and an assessment service, both for employers of, and people with, disabilities. The team consists of a disability employment adviser (DEA), who acts as an intermediary between employers and disabled people, including matching disabled employees with employers. If employers need to make reasonable accommodation for a dyslexic employee, they can apply for a grant through the Access to Work Scheme (below) to cover approved costs, such as computer equipment, which would accommodate the employee's disability.

The Access to Work Scheme provides a service to help assess a dyslexic's difficulties in relation to career goals. Occupational psychologists (OPs) are able to help individuals, including assessing their clients' strengths and weaknesses, and discussing realism about their goals. OPs may also be able to carry out a diagnosis, but there is no legal right to an assessment for dyslexics.

For more on educational and case law see Boyd (1999). For general information on these Acts see Thomson (1990 and 2001) and Fawcett (2001). These matters can get labyrinthine, particularly when LEAs wish to avoid making special provision, or wish to save money.

Also see Alexander (2003) for a very useful review of the current position. Or visit the CAP website: www.becta.org.uk or 'Dyslexia In Adults' – 'A friendly community for adults and students with dyslexia' – on www.dyslexiainadults.com where matters of employment and law are also discussed.

APPENDIX F
Famous dyslexics

Hans Christian Andersen (writer): Danish creator of the fairytales *The Snow Queen* and *The Ugly Duckling*.

Anthony Andrews (actor): 'It's been a painful process and a struggle over the years for me to unjumble words and learn to read. I still find reading a slog, my spelling is atrocious and I often write down telephone numbers wrongly.'

David Bailey (photographer): 'At the age of 59 I have yet to write a letter and still write figures the wrong way round. At school, I was put in the class for the stupid. The British denigrate the visual as something to do at the weekend, not realizing that visual people are luckier than verbal people; they are not limited by their vocabulary. And who's to say what's normal? Maybe dyslexics are the clever ones. Who wants to be an academic, anyway? Most of them are visually illiterate – and art isn't one of those things you can teach. It's natural, and, if you're not careful, you can beat it out of someone.'

Marlon Brando (actor): One of the most celebrated actors of his generation. He won Oscars for his performances in *On The Waterfront* and *The Godfather*.

Richard Branson (entrepreneur): 'At the age of eight I still couldn't read. I was soon being beaten once or twice a week for doing poor classwork or confusing the date of the Battle of Hastings.'

Cher (singer, actress): American singer who made up half of the pop duo Sonny and Cher before turning to acting, starring in films such as *The Witches of Eastwick*, *The Player* and *Moonstruck*, for which she won an Oscar.

Agatha Christie (writer): 'Writing and spelling were always terribly difficult for me. My letters were without originality. I was an extraordinarily bad speller and have remained so until this day.' Agatha Christie is the best-selling and most widely published author of all time; her play *The Mousetrap* is the world's longest-running play.

Winston Churchill (statesman, writer): Possibly the most celebrated war leader of modern times for his conduct as British Prime Minister during the Second World War, Churchill was recently voted the 'Greatest Briton' in a massive television poll conducted by the BBC. His writings include *The World Crisis* and *History of the English-Speaking Peoples*. He won the Nobel Prize for literature in 1953.

Dr Simon Clemmet (scientist): At 28 years old, he analysed the carbon compound found in the meteorite from Mars for Stanford University in California. He was labelled as a slow learner at school until his dyslexia was diagnosed. At the age of 11, he was awarded a grade C for science in a school report, which also said that he showed room for improvement in mathematics. Once he realized he was dyslexic at the age of 12, he flourished and grew in confidence. Even now, he cannot write a letter without the help of his computer spellchecker. He often faxes his scientific papers to his father in England who proofreads them for spelling mistakes. He is about to complete his PhD in physical chemistry.

Brian Conley (comedian, actor, television presenter): 'As I couldn't keep up with the others I was simply written off as being thick. One of the teachers told me – Brian, you'll never get on because you don't concentrate. All you want to do is make the classroom laugh. Now I can read, but my writing's terrible and I spell phonetically.'

Tom Cruise (actor): 'My childhood was extremely lonely. I didn't have many friends. I was dyslexic and a lot of kids made fun of me. That experience made me tough inside because you learn to quietly accept abuse and ridicule'. He was the most commercially viable screen actor of the eighties and early nineties, starring in films such as *Top Gun* and *Mission Impossible*. He received Oscar nominations for *Born on the Fourth of July* and *Jerry Maguire*.

Leonardo da Vinci (painter, sculptor, architect, engineer): As well as painting arguably the most famous painting in the world – 'The Mona Lisa' – his interests ranged from hydraulics to biology. He invented the first armoured tank and anticipated the inventions of the helicopter and the submarine. He is seen by many historians as the leading exponent of the Italian Renaissance.

Ronald Davis (entrepreneur, writer): 'At the age of 12, I was considered uneducably mentally retarded. At the age of 38 I could score 169 on the IQ test but I couldn't read a menu in a restaurant. What the average person could read in five minutes would take me an hour'. He is the author of *Gift of Dyslexia* and a self-made millionaire.

Albert Einstein (scientist): He formulated the special and general theories of relativity and won the Nobel Prize for physics in 1921 for his work on the photoelectric effect.

Whoopi Goldberg (actress): One of the leading comedic actresses of her generation, Goldberg earned an Oscar nomination for her performance in *The Color Purple* and won an Oscar for the film *Ghost*. She was reportedly paid $6,000,000 to write her autobiography.

Duncan Goodhew (Olympic swimmer): 'Being dyslexic does not make life easy, although there are one or two advantages. Dyslexics tend to think laterally because the creative side of the brain is more dominant than the logistical side, which is good for problem-solving.' He was called an 'illiterate moron' at school and became one of the great Olympic athletes for Britain.

Guy Hands (City financier with the Nomura Bank): One of the most powerful and influential men in the City of London, Hands is severely dyslexic and had to take sciences rather than English at school and was examined verbally for his degree finals. He would have liked to have been a writer or even an actor, but his pronunciation is bad too and so instead he decided to make money.

Jack Horner (palaeontologist): Curator of palaeontology at the Museum of the Rockies in Bozeman, Montana and a professor at Montana State University, he is credited with finding more fossils, pioneering more innovative technologies and postulating more theories about dinosaur behaviour than anyone else. He doesn't have a degree, having flunked out of college seven times. He was immortalized as the renegade palaeontologist Allen Grant in the film *Jurassic Park*.

Bob Hoskins (actor): 'The teachers thought I was stupid because I read very slowly. They used to tie one of my hands behind my back because I'd draw pictures with two hands. My brain works both ways, but they didn't notice that. I didn't go home in tears, I just believed I was stupid.' His many film roles include *Who Framed Roger Rabbit* and an Oscar nomination for *Mona Lisa*.

John Irving (writer): 'Bad spelling like mine was considered a psychological problem by the language therapist who evaluated my mysterious case. When the repeated courses of language therapy were judged to have had no discernible influence on me, I was turned over to the school psychiatrist.' An American novelist, he is best-known for his novel *The World According to Garp*.

Felicity Kendall (actress): a highly successful stage actress, she has also starred in several films, but is probably best known for her part in the TV series *The Good Life*. She wrote her autobiography *White Cargo* in 1998.

Lynda La Plante (writer): 'I wasn't diagnosed until I was 12. In those days they thought I was backward. I didn't really feel at home with the written word until somebody gave me a typewriter. But, even today, I never send things out without having them checked by an assistant.' She is one of the most successful writers for television producing such hit series as *Prime Suspect*, *Widows*, *She's Out*, *The Governor* and innumerable best-selling novels.

Simon Menzies (painter): 'We were intelligent, but we were dyslexic. And that toughened us up, made us strive harder. I'm sure we turned to artistic things to prove to other people that we weren't stupid.'

Sarah Miles (actress, writer): 'I was expelled from four schools. Today, I still read with difficulty.' A leading stage actress, she became an overnight star with her screen debut *Term Of Trial*, and won an Oscar nomination for her performance in *Ryan's Daughter*. Her autobiography was published in 1992.

Nicholas Negroponte (founder of the Media Lab at the Massachusetts Institute of Technology): He is described as 'undoubtedly the most venerable of all the new-media gurus'. His company receives millions of dollars of funding each year from top international companies such as BT, Nike and Compaq. They usually want research on technologies that have a quicker payback. Being profoundly dyslexic has, ironically, been something of an aid for him. The digital world rather than the atomic world of paper and print is a godsend. His dyslexia has also made him learn how to stand in front of huge audiences without the need for notes or prompts or any other support.

Steven Redgrave (Olympic rower): At school, he felt as if he were deemed to be lazy and stupid. Now, autography sessions are to be avoided, although he can sign his signature safely, blurring the definition of the letters with a scrawl. Any 'best wishes' message is more of a problem. Dyslexia has left him with a feeling of inadequacy. He has avoided confronting the problem as much as possible and has bolstered his self-esteem elsewhere, proving himself in a boat where he is in control, and wins. He is the winner of five consecutive Olympic Gold medals for Rowing.

Oliver Reed (actor): One of the great British screen actors of his generation and rumoured to have turned down the role of James Bond, Oliver Reed starred in films such as the *The Three Musketeers*, *The Jokers* and *Women In Love*. He died while making his final film *Gladiator*.

Anita Roddick (entrepreneur): She is the founder of the Body Shop – the internationally recognized chain of health and beauty products that introduced environmental awareness to the High Street.

Auguste Rodin (sculptor): His most famous works are 'The Kiss' and 'The Thinker'.

Lord Richard Rogers (architect): He achieved international recognition as a postmodernist architect for his designs of the Lloyd's Building in London and the Pompidou Centre in Paris.

Ben Way (entrepreneur): At the age of nine, his teachers wrote him off as 'unteachable'. By the age of 17, he was the head of a £60,000 computer business. He is now a self-made millionaire.

Toyah Wilcox (singer, television presenter): 'I am dyslexic and have to have special help with spelling and elocution. I didn't pass a single GCE. I think anyone can do anything if there is a will and enough self-esteem.' One of the icons of the pop scene of the late seventies and early eighties, she is now a presenter on Sunday morning television.

Mark Wilkinson (furniture designer and maker): He left school at 15 with no qualifications. He helped to set up Smallbone high-quality kitchens, sold out and set up the highly successful Mark Wilkinson kitchens. He still feels a failure.

William Butler Yeats (poet): When he was a child, he did so poorly in school that his father decided to teach him at home. In his memoirs, Yeats wrote that his father got so impatient with him that he 'flung the reading book at my head'. His handwriting and spelling were atrocious, and he had difficulty with pronunciation and pacing when he tried to read his own poetry out loud. His poem *The Lake Isle of Innisfree* was recently voted one of Britain's favourite poems of all time. He won the Nobel Prize for literature in 1923.

Murray Lachlan Young (poet): 'I was dyslexic and failed all my exams.' He is now a self-made millionaire.

(This appendix is based on a BDA list, copyright British Dyslexia Association, 1 January 2000, X07.)

References

Abramson L, Seligman M, Teasdale J (1978) Learned helplessness in humour: Critical reformulation. Journal of Abnormal Psychology 87: 49-74.

Ackerman P, Dykman R (1996) The speed factor and learning disabilities: The toll of slowness in adolescents. Dyslexia 2(1): 1-21.

Ackerman P, Anhalt J, Dykman R, Holcomb P (1986) Effortful processing deficits in children with reading and/or attention disorders. Brain and Cognition 5: 22-40.

Adams J, Snowling M, Hennessy S, Kind P (1999) Problems of behaviour, reading and arithmetic: Assessments of co-morbidity using the strengths and difficulties questionnaire. British Journal of Educational Psychology 69: 571-585.

Alexander S (2003) Disability and employment. Dyslexia Contact 22(2): 19-21.

Alm J, Anderson J (1997) A study of Prisons in Uppsala. Dyslexia 3(4): 245-246.

Anderson K (1997) Gender bias and special education referrals. Annals of Dyslexia 47: 151-162.

Apiafi J (2001) The PALS project – Positive action through learning support. Dyslexia Review 12(2): 10-12.

Appleyard B (2002) Get a life. The Sunday Times, 18 October 2002.

Argyle M (1994) The Psychology of Interpersonal Behaviour (5th edn). London: Penguin.

Asendorpf J (1993) Abnormal shyness in children. Journal of Child Psychology and Psychiatry 34(7): 1069-1081.

Babinski L, Hartsough C, Lambert N (1999) Childhood conduct problems, hyperactivity-impulsivity and inattention as predictors of adult criminal activity. Journal of Child Psychology and Psychiatry 40(3): 347-355.

Banerjee, R (2000) The development of an understanding of modesty. British Journal of Developmental Psychology 18(4): 499-517.

Barkham, M (2002) Methods, Outcomes and Processes in the Psychological Therapies across Four Successive Research Generations. In Dryden W (ed.) Handbook of Individual Therapy (4th edn). London: Sage.

Barkham M (1992) Research on Integrative and Eclectic Therapy. In Dryden W (ed.) Integrative and Eclectic Therapy: A Handbook. Buckingham: Open University Press.

Barrett P, Shortt A, Healy L (2002) Do parent and child behaviours differentiate families whose children have obsessive-compulsive disorder from other clinic and non-clinic families? Journal of Child Psychology and Psychiatry 43(5): 597-607.

Barrett H, Jones D (1996) The Inner Life of Children with Moderate Learning Difficulties. In Varma V (ed.) The Inner Life of Children with Special Needs. London: Whurr.

Bartlett D, Moody S (2000) Dyslexia in the Workplace. London: Whurr.

Beresford B (1994) Resources and strategies: How parents cope with the care of a disabled child. Journal of Child Psychology and Psychiatry 35(1): 171-209.

Berndt T (1981) The effects of friendship of prosocial intentions and behaviour between friends. Developmental Psychology 17: 408-416.

Biddulph S (1998) Manhood. London: Hawthorn.

Bifulco A, Moran P, Ball C, Jacobs C, Baines R, Bunn A, Cavagin J (2002) Childhood adversity, parental vulnerability and disorder: Examining inter-generational transmission of risk. Journal of Child Psychology and Psychiatry 43(8): 1075-1086.

Bishop E (2001) Writing speed and extra time in examinations. Dyslexia Review 12(3): 13-16.

Blagg N (1992) School Phobia. In Lane D, Miller A (eds.) Child and Adolescent Therapy: A Handbook. Buckingham: Open University Press.

Boetch E, Green P, Pennington B (1996) Psychosocial correlates of dyslexia across the lifespan. Development and Psychopathology 8: 539-562.

Bor R, Ebner-Landy J, Gill S, Brace C (2002) Counselling in Schools. London: Sage.

Boulton M, Smith P (1994) Bully/victim problems in middle school children: Stability, self-perceived competence, peer perceptions, and peer acceptance. British Journal of Developmental Psychology 10(2): 315-330.

Bourne I, Oliver B (1999) The telling of terror: Helping trauma survivors construct a therapeutic narrative. Counselling 10(2): 135-138.

Bowlby J (1991) Loss: Sadness and Depression (Vol. 3). London: Penguin.

Boyd R (1999) Independent Schools – Law, Custom and Practice. London: Jordan.

Brand V (2000) Music and dyslexia. Perspectives 26(1): 36-37.

Bray A, Skelton E, Ballard K, Clarkson J (1995) Fathers of children with disabilities: Some experiences and reflections. New Zealand Journal of Disability Studies 1(1): 164-176.

Brier N (1994) Targeted treatment for adjudicated youth with learning disabilities: Effects on recidivism. Journal of Learning Disabilities 27: 215-222.

Brigden A (2000) Results of the Surrey Institute HEFCE Dyslexia Project. In Brigden A, McFall C (eds.) Dyslexia in Higher Education Art and Design (Conference Report). Farnham: The Surrey Institute of Art and Design, University College.

BDA (1996) British Dyslexia Association: Guide for the Medical and Health Care Profession. Reading: British Dyslexia Association.

BDA (2003) Website: www.bda-dyslexia.org.uk.

BPS (1999) British Psychological Society Report by the Working Party of the Division of Educational and Child Psychology of The British Psychological Society. Dyslexia, Literacy and Psychological Assessment. Leicester: The British Psychological Society.

Brody L, Mills C (1997) Gifted children with learning disabilities. Journal of Learning Disabilities 30(3): 282-286.

Brooks G, Giles K, Harman J, Kendall S, Rees F, Whittaker S (2001) Assembling the Fragments: A Review of Research in Adult Basic Skill. Department for Education and Skills (DfES) Research Report RR220.

Bruce E, Schultz C (2002) Non-finite loss and challenges to communication between parents and professionals. British Journal of Special Education 29(1): 9-13.

Bryan T, Burstein K (2000) Don't worry, be happy: The effect of positive mood on learning. Thalamus 18(2): 34-42.

Bryant P, Nunes T, Bindman M (1998) Awareness of language in children who have reading difficulties: Historical comparison in a longitudinal study. Journal of Child Psychology and Psychiatry 39(4): 501-510.

Bungener J, McCormack B (1994) Psychotherapy and Learning Disability. In Clarkson P, Pokorny M (eds.) The Handbook of Psychotherapy. London: Routledge.

Burns D, Spangler D (2000) Does psychotherapy homework lead to improvements in depression in cognitive-behavioural therapy or does improvement lead to increased homework compliance? Journal of Consulting and Clinical Psychology 68: 46-56.

Burns RB (1979) The Self Concept: Theory, Measurement, Development and Behaviour. London: Longman.

Butkowsky I, Willows D (1980) Cognitive-motivational characteristics of children varying in reading ability: Evidence for learned helplessness in poor readers. Journal of Educational Psychology 72(3): 408-422.

Butler R (1996) Effects of age and achievement goals on children's motives for attending to peers' work. British Journal of Developmental Psychology 14(1): 1-18.

Calhoun L, Tedeschi R (1999) Facilitating Posttraumatic Growth: A Clinician's Guide. Mahwah, New Jersey: Lawrence Erlbaum.

Carpenter B (2000) Sustaining the family: Meeting the needs of families of children with disabilities. British Journal of Special Education 27(3): 135-144.

Case C, Dalley T (1992) The Handbook of Art Therapy. London: Routledge.

Casement P (1990) Further Learning from the Patient: The Analytic Space and Process. London: Tavistock/Routledge.

Casemore R (2000) Should we challenge a client's prejudices? Counselling 11(1): 4-6.

Chadwick O, Taylor E, Taylor A, Heptinstall E, Danckaerts M (1999) Hyperactivity and reading disability: A longitudinal study of the nature of the association. Journal of Child Psychology and Psychiatry 40(7): 1039-1050.

Chamberlain K, Zika S (1990) The minor events approach to stress: Support for the use of daily hassles. British Journal of Psychology 8(4): 469-481.

Chavira V, Lopez S, Blacher J, Shapiro J (2000) Latina mothers' attributions, emotions and reactions to the problem behaviours of their children with developmental disabilities. Journal of Child Psychology and Psychiatry 41(2): 245-252.

Childline Annual Review (2001) London: Childline.

Chinn S, McDonagh D, van Elswijk R, Harmsen-Kay J, McPhillips T, Power A, Skidmore L (2001) Classroom studies into cognitive style in mathematics for pupils with dyslexia in special education in the Netherlands, Ireland and the UK. British Journal of Special Education 28(2): 80-85.

Chivers M (2001) Practical Strategies for Living with Dyslexia. London: Jessica Kingsley.

Clark C, Prior M, Kinsella G (2002) The relationship between executive function abilities, adaptive behaviour and academic achievement in children with externalising behaviour problems. Journal of Child Psychology and Psychiatry 43(6): 785-796.

Clayton P (2001) Some thoughts on maths and dyslexia. Dyslexia Review 13(1): 19-21.

Cline T (2000) Multilingualism and dyslexia: Challenges for research and practice. Dyslexia 6(1): 3-12.

Cline T, Ganschow L, Reason R (2000) Editorial: Multilingualism and dyslexia, including the teaching of modern foreign languages. Dyslexia 6(1): 1-2.

Cohen N, Menna R, Vallance D, Barwick M, Im N, Horodezky N (1998) Language, social cognitive processing and behavioural characteristics of psychiatrically disturbed children with previously identified and unsuspected language impairments. Journal of Child Psychology and Psychiatry 39(6): 853-864.

Coleby M (1995) The school-aged siblings of children with disabilities. Developmental Medicine and Child Neurology 37: 415-426.

Congdon P (1995) Stress Factors in Gifted Dyslexics. In Miles T, Varma V (eds.) Dyslexia and Stress. London: Whurr.

Cooke A (2001) Critical response to dyslexia, literacy and psychological assessment: A view from the chalk-face. Dyslexia 7(1): 47-52.

Cooke A (2002) Case study: A virtual non-reader achieves a degree. Dyslexia 8(2): 102-115.

Cooper P (1996) The Inner Life of Children with Emotional and Behavioural Difficulties. In Varma V (ed.) The Inner Life of Children with Special Needs. London: Whurr.

Cooper P (ed.) (1999) Understanding and Supporting Children with Emotional and Behavioural Difficulties. London: Jessica Kingsley.

Cooper P, Smith C, Upton G (1994) Emotional and Behavioural Difficulties: Theory to Practice. London: Routledge.

Coopersmith S (1967) The Antecedents of Self-esteem. San Francisco, CA: Freeman.

Cottrell D, Boston P (2002) Practitioner review: The effectiveness of systemic family therapy for children and adolescents. Journal of Child Psychology and Psychiatry 43(5): 573-586.

Couchman A (2003) Member's Communication from the British Association of Counselling and Psychotherapy Research Department, January 2003.

Cowie H, Dawkins J (2002) Proven Benefits of Psychotherapeutic Interventions with Children and Adolescents. In Feltham C (ed.) What's the Good of Counselling and Psychotherapy? London: Sage.

Craib I (1994) The Importance of Disappointment. London: Routledge.

Crombie M (2000) Dyslexia and the learning of a foreign language in school: Where are we going? Dyslexia 6(2): 112-123.

Crozier W (2002) Shyness. The Psychologist 15(9): 460-463.

Crozier W, Rees V, Morris-Beattie A, Bellin W (1999) Streaming, self-esteem and friendships within a comprehensive school. Educational Psychology in Practice 15(2): 128-134.

Cutting A, Dunn J (2002) The cost of understanding other people: social cognition predicts young children's sensitivity to criticism. Journal of Child Psychology and Psychiatry 43(7): 849-860.

Czeschlik T, Rost D (1995) Sociometric types and children's intelligence. British Journal of Developmental Psychology 13(2): 177-189.

Dadds M, Barrett P (2001) Practitioner review: Psychological management of anxiety disorders in childhood. Journal of Child Psychology and Psychiatry 42(8): 999-1011.

Dainow S (1995) Uncovering a TA script with pictures. Counselling 6(2): 291-293.

Davis R (1997) The Gift of Dyslexia. London: Souvenir.

Davis S, Howell P, Cooke F (2002) Sociodynamic relationships between children who stutter and their non-stuttering classmates. Journal of Child Psychology and Psychiatry 43(7): 939-947.

Deary I, Peter A, Austin E, Gibson G (1998) Personality traits and personality disorders. British Journal of Psychology 89(4): 647-661.

Deater-Deckard K (2001) Annotation: Recent research examining the role of peer relationships in the development of psychopathology. Journal of Child Psychology and Psychiatry 42(5): 565-579.

DePonio P (2001) Dyslexia and Self-Awareness: Issues for Secondary Schools. Proceedings of the 5th BDA International Conference, York (website: www.bdainternationalconference.org)

Dockrell J (2001) Assessing language skills in pre-school children. Child Psychology and Psychiatry Review 6(2): 74-85.

Donaldson M (1978) Children's Minds. London: Fontana.

Douglas E (2001) Beating the workplace bullies. Special (Autumn): 22-23.

Duane D (1991) Dyslexia: Neurobiological and behavioural correlates. Psychiatric Annals 21: 703-708.

Duck S (1988) Relating to Others. Milton Keynes: Open University Press.

Dummer-Smoch L (1998) Dyslexia in Germany – An educational policy for meeting dyslexic children's needs in the German school system. Dyslexia 4(2): 63-72.

Dunn J, Brown J, Slomkowski C, Tesla C, Youngblade L (1991) Young children's understanding of other people's feelings and beliefs: Individual differences and their antecedents. Child Development 62: 1352-1366.

Durham M (2003) Fighting fathers breed a better adjusted child, The Sunday Times, 23 March 2003.

Dwivedi K (1993) Confusion and Underfunctioning in Children. In Varma V (ed.) How and Why Children Fail. London: Jessica Kingsley.

Dyslexia Institute (2002) Recognising the Dyslexic Child. Learning in the Classroom. www.dyslexia-inst.org.uk/articles/recog.htm

Eaude T (1999) Learning difficulties: Dyslexia, bullying and other issues. London: Letts Educational.

Edwards J (1994) The Scars of Dyslexia. London: Continuum.

Elliott J (1999) Practitioner review: School refusal: Issues of conceptualisation, assessment and treatment. Journal of Child Psychology and Psychiatry 40(7): 1001-1012.

Elliott J, Thomas Z (2003) Ten-year-old self is the key to adult success, The Sunday Times, 29 June 2003.

Emery E (1982) Interpersonal conflict and the children of discord and divorce. Psychological Bulletin 92: 310-330.

Engfer A (1988) The Interrelatedness of Marriage and the Mother-child Relationship. In Hinde R, Stevenson-Hinde S (eds.) Relationship within Families: Mutual Influences, 104-118. London: Clarendon.

Erikson E (1968) Identity: Youth and Crisis. New York: Norton.

Etkin H (1993) Fear and Underachievement. In Varma V (ed.) How and Why Children Fail. London: Jessica Kingsley.

Everall R, Paulson B (2002) The therapeutic alliance: adolescent perspectives. Counselling and Psychotherapy Research 2(2): 78-87.

Everatt J, Steffert B, Smythe I (1999) An eye for the unusual: Creative thinking in dyslexics. Dyslexia 5(1): 28-46.

Everatt J, Brannan P (1996) The effects of a spelling task on the subsequent performance of dyslexics. Dyslexia 2(1): 22-30.

Ezpelata L, Granero R, de la Osa N, Guillamon N (2000) Predictors of functional impairment in children and adolescents. Journal of Child Psychology and Psychiatry 41(6): 793-801.

Fairhurst P, Pumphrey P (1992) Secondary school organisation and the self-concepts of pupils with relative reading difficulties. Research in Education 47(May): 19-28.

Farmer M, Riddick B, Sterling C (2002) Dyslexia and Inclusion: Assessment and Support in Higher Education. London: Whurr.

Farrell P (1999) The limitations of current theories in understanding bereavement and grief. Counselling 10(2): 143-146.

Farrell P, Critchley C, Mills C (1999) The educational attainments of pupils with emotional and behavioural difficulties. British Journal of Special Education 26(1): 50-53.

Fawcett A (1995) Case Studies and Some Recent Research. In Miles T, Varma V (eds.) Dyslexia and Stress. London: Whurr.

Fawcett A (ed.) (2001) Dyslexia Theory and Good Practice. London: Whurr.

Fawcett A (2003) The international adult literacy survey in britain: impact on policy and practice. Dyslexia 9(2): 99-121.

Fine S, Haley G, Gilbert M, Forth A (1993) Self-image as a predictor of outcome in adolescent major depressive disorder. Journal of Child Psychology and Psychiatry 34(8): 1399-1407.

Fink R (1995) Literacy development in successful men and women with dyslexia. Annals of Dyslexia 48: 311-334.

Firman C, Francica C, Grech K (2001) Paired reading and the dyslexic child – How effective? Dyslexia Review 13(1): 15-18.

Fisher B, Rhiannon R, Rose G (1996) The relationship between anxiety and problem solving skills in children with and without learning difficulties. Journal of Learning Disabilities 29: 439-446.

Fiske S, Taylor S (1984) Social Cognition (1st edn). Reading, MA: Addison-Wesley.

Flory S (2003) Dyslexia and dyspraxia. In Thomson M (ed.) Dyslexia Included. London: Fulton.

Flouri E, Buchanan A (2003) What predicts fathers' involvement with their children? A prospective study of intact families. British Journal of Developmental Psychology 21(1): 81-98.

Foote R, Holmes-Lonergan H (2003) Sibling conflict and theory of mind. British Journal of Developmental Psychology 21(1): 45-58.

Francis-Smythe J, Robertson I (1999) On the relationship between time management and time estimation. British Journal of Psychology 90(3): 333-347.

Freinkel E (2000) Dyslexia in South Africa. Perspectives 26(1): 24-25.

Freud A (1981) Psychoanalytic Psychology of Normal Development. London: Hogarth.

Freud S (1905) Three Essays on the Theory of Sexuality. Hogarth: London.

Frith U (1999) Paradoxes in the definition of dyslexia. Dyslexia 5(4): 192-214.

Fromm (2000) The Art of Loving. New York: Harper Collins.

Galaburda A (1983) Developmental dyslexia: Current anatomical research. Annals of Dyslexia 33: 41-53.

Gallagher A, Frith U, Snowling M (2000) Precursors of literacy delay among children at genetic risk of dyslexia. Journal of Child Psychology and Psychiatry 41(2): 203-213.

Ganschow L, Sparks R, Schneider E (1995) Learning a foreign language: Challenge for students with language learning difficulties. Dyslexia 1: 75-95.

Ganschow L, Sparks R, Javorsky J (1998) Foreign language learning problems: An historical perspective. Journal of Learning Disabilities 31: 248-258.

Garralda M, Bailey D (1986) Children with psychiatric disorders in primary care. Journal of Child Psychology and Psychiatry 27(5): 611-624.

Gathercole S, Pickering, S (2001) Working memory deficits in children with special educational needs. British Journal of Special Education 28(2): 89-97.

Geldard K, Geldard D (2002) Counselling Children: A Practical Introduction. London: Sage.

Gendling E (1981) Focussing. New York: Bantam.

Gilroy D (1995) Stress Factors in the College Student. In Miles T, Varma V (eds.) Dyslexia and Stress. London: Whurr.

Glaser D (1995) Emotionally Abusive Experiences. In Reder P, Lucey C (eds) Assessment of Parenting: Psychiatric and Psychological Contributions. London: Routledge.

Glaser D (2000) Child abuse and neglect and the brain – A review. Journal of Child Psychology and Psychiatry 41(1): 97-116.

Gold K (2002) The pupils with a hidden intelligence, The Sunday Times, 29 September 2002.

Goldup W, Ostler C (2000) The Dyslexic Child at School and at Home. In Townend J, Turner, M (eds.) Dyslexia in Practice: A Guide for Teachers, New York: Kluwer Academic/Plenum.

Goleman D (1995) Emotional Intelligence. London: Bloomsbury.

Gomez J (1991) Psychological and Psychiatric Problems in Men. London: Routledge.

Gordon K, Toukmanian S (2002) Is how it is said important? The association between quality of therapist interventions and client processing. Counselling and Psychotherapy Research 2(2): 88-98.

Goulandris N (ed.) (2003) Dyslexia in Different Languages. London: Whurr.

Grant D (2001) 'That's the way I think – Dyslexia and creativity'. Proceedings of the 5th BDA International Conference, York (website: www.bdainternational conference.org).

Greenbaum B, Graham S, Scales W (1996) Adults with learning disabilities: occupational and social status after college. Journal of Learning Disabilities 29: 167-173.

Greenhalgh P (1994) Emotional Growth and Learning. London: Routledge.

Grigorenko E (2001) Developmental dyslexia: An update on genes, brains and environments. Journal of Child Psychology and Psychiatry 42(1): 91-125.

Grossman A, Churchill J, McKinney B, Kodish I, Otte S, Greenough W (2003) Experience effects on brain development: Possible contributions to psychopathology. Journal of Child Psychology and Psychiatry 44(1): 33-63.

Gurney P (1988) Self-esteem in Children with Special Educational Needs. London: Routledge.

Gyarmathy E (2000) Holistic Learners: Identifying gifted children with learning disabilities – an experimental perspective. In Montgomery D (ed.) Able Underachievers. London: Whurr.

Hales G (1994) The Human Aspects of Dyslexia. In Hales G (ed.) Dyslexia Matters: A Celebratory Contributed Volume to Honour Professor TR Miles. London: Whurr.

Hales G (1995) Stress Factors in the Workplace. In Miles T, Varma V Dyslexia and Stress. London: Whurr.

Hales G (2001a) How we felt and how we tackled it! – The experiences of dyslexic people and their parents. Proceedings of the 5th BDA International Conference, York (website: www.bdainternationalconference.org).

Hales G (2001b) The Pattern of Personality in Dyslexic Children and Adults: The invisible symptoms and the effects they produce. Proceedings of the 5th BDA International Conference, York (website: www.bdainternationalconference.org).

Hardy L, Mullen R, Jones G (1996) Knowledge and conscious control of motor actions under stress. British Journal of Psychology 87(4): 621-636.

Hargie O, Saunders C, Dickson D (1994) Social Skills in Interpersonal Communication. London: Routledge.

Harrington R (1995) Depressive Disorder in Childhood and Adolescence. Chichester: Wiley.

Harrington R, Bredenkamp D, Groothues C, Rutter M, Fudge H, Pickles A (1994) Adult outcomes of childhood and adolescent depression. III, Links with suicidal behaviours. Journal of Child Psychology and Psychiatry 35(7): 1309-1319.

Harris P (1994) The child's understanding of emotion: Developmental change and the family environment. Journal of Child Psychology and Psychiatry 35(1): 3-28.

Harris T (1967) I'm OK – You're OK. London: Pan.

Hawker D, Boulton M (2000) Twenty years' research on peer victimisation and psychosocial maladjustment: A meta-analytic review of cross-sectional studies. Journal of Child Psychology and Psychiatry 41(4): 441-455.

Hay D, Vespo J, Zahn-Waxler C (1998) Young children's quarrels with their siblings and mothers: Links with maternal depression and bipolar illness. British Journal of Developmental Psychology 16(4): 519-538.

Hay I (2000) Gender self-concept profiles of adolescents suspended from high school. Journal of Child Psychology and Psychiatry 41(3): 345-352.

Heath N (2001) Learning disabilities and depression. Thalamus 19(1): 2-10.

Hellendoorn J, Ruijsenaars W (2000) Personal experiences and adjustment of dutch adults with dyslexia. Remedial and Special Education 21: 227-239.

Henderson M (2003) Social skills trap the artist within, The Times, 28 May 2003.

Hermann K (1959) Reading Disability. Copenhagen: Munsksgaard.

Heyman I (1997) Children with obsessive compulsive disorder. British Medical Journal 315: 444.

Hiebert E, Winograd P, Danner F (1984) Children's attributions for failure and success in different aspects of reading. Journal of Educational Psychology 76(16): 1139-1148.

Hill J (2002) Biological, psychological and social processes in the conduct disorders. Journal of Child Psychology and Psychiatry 43(1): 133-164.

Hiscock N (1995) We dyslexics need to communicate. Dyslexia 1(2): 128-129.

Hodges E, Parry D (1996) Victims of peer abuse: An overview. Journal of Emotional and Behavioural Problems 5: 23-28.

Hollin C (1993) The Lack of Proper Social Relationships in Childhood Failure. In Varma V (ed.) How and Why Children Fail. London: Jessica Kingsley.

Honess T, Charman E, Zani B, Cicognani E, Xerri M, Jackson A, Bosma H (1997) Conflict between parents and adolescents: Variation by family constitution. British Journal of Developmental Psychology 15(3): 367-385.

Horvath A, Greenberg L (1994) The Working Alliance: Theory Research and Practice. New York: Wiley.

Huges W, Dawson R (1995) Memories of school: Adult dyslexics recall their school days. Support for Learning 10: 181-184.

Hughes C, Dunn J (2002) When I say a naughty word. A longitudinal study of young children's accounts of anger and sadness in themselves and close others. British Journal of Developmental Psychology 20(4): 515-535.

Humfress H, O'Connor T, Slaughter J, Target M, Fonagy P (2002) General and relationship-specific models of social cognition: explaining the overlap and discrepancies. Journal of Child Psychology and Psychiatry 43(7): 873-883.

Hummel S (2000) Developing comprehension skills of secondary students with specific learning difficulties. Australian Journal of Learning Disabilities 5(4): 22-27.

Humphrey N (2002) Teacher and pupil ratings of self-esteem in developmental dyslexia. British Journal of Special Education 29(1): 29-34.

Humphrey N, Mullins P (2002) Personal constructs and attribution for academic success and failure in dyslexia. British Journal of Special Education 29 (4): 196-203.

Hurry J (1999) Annotation: Children's reading levels. Journal of Child Psychology and Psychiatry 40(2): 143-150.

Jackson M, Tisak M (2001) Is prosocial behaviour a good thing? Developmental changes in children's evaluations of helping, sharing, cooperating and comforting. British Journal of Developmental Psychology 19(3): 349-367.

Jacobs M (1986) The Presenting Past: An introduction to practical psychodynamic counselling. Buckingham: Open University Press.

Jenkins G (2002) Good Money after Bad? The Justification for the Expansion of Counselling Services in Primary Health Care. In Feltham C (ed.) What's the Good of Counselling and Psychotherapy: The benefits explained. Sage: London.

Kappers E, Veerman J (1995) The family environment of young adolescents with dyslexia. Dyslexia 1(2): 108-119.

Kavale K, Forness S (1994) Social skills deficits and learning disabilities: A meta-analysis. Journal of Learning Disabilities 29: 226-237.

Kazdin A (2002) The state of child and adolescent psychotherapy research. Child and Adolescent Mental Health 7(2): 53-59.

Kazdin A, Siegal T, Bass D (1990) Drawing on clinical practice to inform research on child and adolescent psychotherapy: Survey of practitioners. Professional Psychology: Research and Practice 21: 189-198.

Keane T (2002) Violent siblings let cat out of the bag, The Sunday Times, 20 October 2002.

Kemp-Wheeler S, Hill A (1987) Anxiety responses to subliminal experience of mild stress. British Journal of Psychology 78(3): 365-374.

Kennedy E, Spence S, Hensley R (1989) An examination of the relationship between childhood depression and social competence amongst primary school children. Journal of Child Psychology and Psychiatry 30(4): 561-573.

Keppel-Benson J, Ollendick T, Benson M (2002) Post-traumatic stress in children following motor vehicle accidents. Journal of Child Psychology and Psychiatry 43(2): 203-212.

Kirk J, Reid G (2001) An examination of the relationship between dyslexia and offending in young people and the implications for the training system. Dyslexia 7(2): 77-84.

Kirkby R (1995) Dyslexia and car driving. Dyslexia 1(2): 130-131.

Kiziewicz M (2000) Ourselves in Place. In Brigden A, McFall C (eds.) Dyslexia in Higher Education Art and Design (Conference Report). Farnham: The Surrey Institute of Art and Design, University College.

Kline C, Kline C (1973) Severe reading disabilities: The family's dilemma. Bulletin of the Orton Society XXIII: 146-160.

Knivsberg A, Reichelt K, Nodland M (1999) Co-morbidity or co-existence between dyslexia and attention deficit hyperactivity disorder. British Journal of Special Education 26(1): 42-47.

La Fontaine J (1991) Bullying: The Child's View. London: Calouste Gulbenkian Foundation.

Lane B (2001) Personality and Academic Achievement in Dyslexic Children. Unpublished paper, University of Sunderland.

Lane D (1992) Bullying. In Lane D, Miller A (eds.) Child and Adolescent Therapy: A Handbook. Buckingham: Open University Press.

Lawrence D (1971) The effects of counselling on retarded readers. Educational Research 13: 119-124.

Lawrence D (1996) Enhancing Self-esteem in the Classroom. London: Paul Chapman.

Lazarus R (1984) Puzzles in the study of daily hassles. Journal of Behavioral Medicine 7: 375-380.

Leach R (1994) Children First: What Society Must Do – and Is Not Doing – for Children Today. London: Penguin.

Legrand L, McGue M, Iacono W (1999) A twin study of state and trait anxiety in childhood and adolescence. Journal of Child Psychology and Psychiatry 40(6): 953-958.

Lewis C, Hitch G, Walker P (1994) The prevalence of specific arithmetic difficulties and specific reading difficulties in 9- to 10-year-old boys and girls. Journal of Child Psychology and Psychiatry 35(2): 283-292.

Leymann H, Gustaffson A (1996) Mobbing at work and the development of post-traumatic stress disorder. European Journal of Work and Organisational Psychology 5: 251-275.

Lightfoot L (2003) Special needs pupils make majority suffer, Daily Telegraph, 17 April 2003.

Linley P, Joseph S (2002) Post-traumatic growth. Counselling and Psychotherapy Journal 13(1): 14-17.

Lu L (1991) Daily hassles and mental health: A longitudinal study. British Journal of Psychology 82(4): 441-447.

Lundberg I (1995) Trends in dyslexia research in Sweden. Dyslexia 1(1): 46-53.

Maccoby E (1980) Social Development: Psychological growth and the parent–child relationship. Orlando, FLA: Harcourt Brace Jovanovich Inc.

Mackay M (2002) From cure to prevention. Counselling at Work 31: 1-2.

Mackinnon D (1962) The Personality Correlates of Creativity. A study of American Architects. In Vernon P (ed.) Creativity. Harmondsworth: Penguin.

Macrae C, Bodenhausen G (2001) Social cognition: Categorical person perception. British Journal of Psychology 92(1): 239-255.

Magiste E (1986) Processing in bilinguals: psycholinguistic and neuropsychological perspective. In Magiste E (ed.) Selected Issues in Second and Third Language Learning. Hillsdale, NJ: Erlbaum.

Malofeev N, Kukushkina O (2000) Advances in diagnosis and treatment of dyslexia in Russia. Perspectives 26(1): 14.

Mannoni M (1973) The Retarded Child and the Mother. London: Tavistock.

Marchington-Yeoman C, Cooper C (2002) The Benefits of Counselling and Employee Assistance Programmes to British Industry. In Feltham C (ed.) What's the Good of Counselling and Psychotherapy: The Benefits Explained. London: Sage.

Mardell-Czudnowski C (2001) The top-ten predictors for identifying young children at risk. Thalamus 19(1): 34-40.

Margalit M, Heiman T (1986) Family climate and anxiety in families with learning disabled boys. Journal of the American Academy of Child and Adolescent Psychiatry 25: 841-846.

Martin P (2001) The therapist as a person. Counselling and Psychotherapy Journal 12(10): 10-12.

Martlew M, Hodson J (1991) Children with mild learning difficulties in a special school: Components of behaviour, teasing and teachers' attitudes. British Journal of Educational Psychology 61: 355-372.

Maslow A (1954) Motivation and Personality (3rd edn.). New York: Harper.

Masten A, Garmezy N, Tellegen A, Pellegrini D, Larkin K, Larsen A (1988) Competence and stress in school children: The moderating effects of individual and family qualities. Journal of Child Psychology and Psychiatry 29(6): 745-764.

Mathijssen J, Koot H, Verhulst F, De Bruyn E, Oud J (1998) The relationship between mutual family relations and child psychopathology. Journal of Child Psychology and Psychiatry 39(4): 477-487.

Mattison R (2001) Learning disabilities in special education students referred for psychiatric consultation. Thalamus 19(1): 11-19.

Matty J (1997), Dyslexia and Society in the 4th BDA International Conference Supplement. Dyslexia Contact 16(2): 7-9.

Maughan B (1995) Annotation: Long-term outcomes of developmental reading problems. Journal of Child Psychology and Psychiatry 36(3): 357-371.

May R (1989) The Art of Counselling. New York: Gardner.

McArthur G, Hogben J, Edwards V, Heath S, Mengler E (2000) On the 'specifics' of specific reading disability and specific language impairment. Journal of Child Psychology and Psychiatry 41(7): 869-874.

McCormick M (2003) Continents and Valves: An evidence-based approach to dyslexia. In Thomson M (ed.) Dyslexia Included. London: Fulton.

McDermott I, Shircore I (1999) Manage Yourself, Manage Your Life. London: Piatkus.

McDougall S (2001) Experiences of dyslexia: Social and emotional factors associated with living with dyslexia. Dyslexia Review 12(2): 7-9.

McFarlane A, Bellisimo A, Norman G (1995) Family structure, family functioning and adolescent well-being: the transcendent influence of parental style. Journal of Child Psychology and Psychiatry 36(5): 847-864.

McGee R, Prior M, Williams S, Smart D, Sanson A (2002) The long-term significance of teacher-rated hyperactivity and reading ability in childhood: Findings from two longitudinal studies. Journal of Child Psychology and Psychiatry 43(8): 1004-1017.

McKinney J, Feagans L (1987) Current issues in research and services for learning disabled children in the United States. Paedoperisse 1(1): 91-107.

McLoughlin D, Fitzgibbon G, Young V (1994) Adult Dyslexia: Assessment, Counselling and Training. London: Whurr.

McLoughlin D, Leather C, Stringer P (2002) The Adult Dyslexic: Interventions and Outcomes. London: Whurr.

McNamara S (2000) Stress in Young People: What's new and what can we do? London: Continuum.

Meade J, Lumley M, Casey R (2001) Stress, emotional skill and illness in children: The importance of distinguishing between children's and parents' reports of illness. Journal of Child Psychology and Psychiatry 42(3): 405-412.

Mearns D (1999) Person-centred Therapy with Configurations of Self. Counselling 10(2): 125-130.

Mearns D, Thorne B (2000) Person-centred Therapy Today. London: Sage.

Meijer S, Sinnema G, Bijstra J, Mellenbergh G, Wolters W (2000) Social functioning in children with a chronic illness. Journal of Child Psychology and Psychiatry 41(3): 309-317.

Meischenbaum D (2000) What Can Be Done to Help Clients with PTSD and DES? In Scott M, Palmer S (eds.) Trauma and Post-traumatic Stress Disorder. London: Cassell.

Mellor-Clark J (2000) Counselling in Primary Care in the Context of the NHS Quality Agenda: The Facts. Rugby: British Association for Counselling and Psychotherapy.

Meridian (2002) Meridian Broadcasting On Line. That's Esther Factsheet. Programme 4, 12 October 2002 (www.meridian.tv.co.uk).

Miles E (1995) Can there be a single definition of dyslexia? Dyslexia 1(1): 37-45.

Miles E (2000) Dyslexia may show a different face in different languages. Dyslexia 6(3): 193-201.

Miles T (1993) Dyslexia: The Pattern of Difficulties (2nd edn.). London: Whurr.

Miles T (2001) Editorial: A chain of editorial reflections (Crime and Dyslexia). Dyslexia 7(2): 57-61.

Miles T, Gilroy D (1986) Dyslexia at College. London: Methuen.

Miles T, Varma V (eds.) (1995) Dyslexia and Stress. London: Whurr.

Miles T, Westcombe J (eds.) (2001) Music and Dyslexia. London: Whurr.

Milton M (2000) How do schools provide for children with difficulties in numeracy? Australian Journal of Learning Disabilities 5(2): 23-27.

Minton P (2002) Using information and communication technology (ICT) to help dyslexics and others learn spelling. Australian Journal of Learning Disabilities 7(3): 26-31.

Minuchin S (1974) Families and Family Therapy. Cambridge, MA: Harvard University Press.

Mittler H (1995) Families Speak Out: international perspectives on families. In Mittler P (ed.) Families Speak Out: international perspectives in families' experiences of disability. Cambridge, MA: Brookline.

Moody S (2001) Dyslexia in the dock: How the disability discrimination act is being applied. Dyslexia Review 13(1): 8-10.

Moradi A, Doost H, Taghavi M, Yule W, Dalgleish T (1999) Everyday memory deficits in children and adolescents with PTSD: Performance on the Rivermead behavioural memory test. Journal of Child Psychology and Psychiatry 40(3): 357-361.

Morgan E, Klein C (2000) The Dyslexic Adult in a Non-Dyslexic World. London: Whurr.

Morgan W (1997) Dyslexia and crime. Dyslexia 3(4): 247-248.

Morris L (2001) Emotional literacy for kids. Counselling and Psychotherapy Journal 12(8): 15-18.

Nabuzoka D, Smith P (1993) Sociometric status and social behaviour of children with and without learning difficulties. Journal of Child Psychology and Psychiatry 34(8): 1435-1448.

National Children's Bureau (1996) Factsheet No. 144 (Highlight: Suicidal Behaviour in Children and Young People). NCB: London (www.ncb.org.uk).

Nelson-Jones R (1999) Towards cognitive-humanistic counselling. Counselling 10(1): 49-54.

Newman M, Black D, Harris-Hendriks J (1997) Victims of disaster, war, violence or homicide: Psychological effects on siblings. Child Psychology and Psychiatry Review 2(4): 140-149.

Nicholson R (2000) Dyslexia and dyspraxia: Commentary. Dyslexia 6(3): 203-204.

Ochse R (1990) Before the Gates of Excellence: The determinants of creative genius. Cambridge: Cambridge University Press.

O'Connell B (2001) Solution-focused Stress Counselling. London: Continuum.

Ofsted Report (1999) Pupils with specific learning difficulties in mainstream schools (HMI 208) and the SEN Code of Practice: Three years on (HMI 211). London: Ofsted Publications Centre.

Oglethorpe S (1996) Instrumental Music for Dyslexics: A Teaching Handbook. London: Whurr.

O'Leary V, Alday C, Ickovics J (1998) Models of Life Change and Posttraumatic Growth. In Tedeschi R, Park C, Calhoun L (eds.) Posttraumatic Growth: Positive changes in the aftermath of crisis. Mahwah, NJ: Lawrence Erlbaum.

Ollendick T, King N, Muris P (2002) Fears and phobias in children: Phenomenology, epidemiology, and aetiology. Child and Adolescent Mental Health 7(3): 98-106.

Olson R (2002) Dyslexia: Nature and nurture. Dyslexia 8(3): 143-159.

O'Moore A, Hillery B (1992) What do Teachers Need to Know? In Elliott M (ed.) Bullying: A practical guide to coping for schools. Harlow: Longman.

O'Moore M (2000) Critical issues for teacher training to counter bullying and victimisation in Ireland. Aggressive Behaviour 26(1): 99-111.

Orton C (2002) The new SEN code of practice. Dyslexia Contact 21(1): 13.

Orton S (1937) Reading, Writing and Speech Problems in Children. London: Chapman and Hall.

Paley G, Lawton D (2001) Evidence-based practice: Accounting for the importance of the therapeutic relationship in UK National Health Service therapy provision. Counselling and Psychotherapy Research 1(1): 12-17.

Park J (1995) Sons, Mothers and Other Lovers. London: Little, Brown.

Parsonage M (2002) The Social Effects of Dyslexia. Unpublished master's thesis (private communication to the author).

Patton J, Holloway E (1992) Learning disabilities: The challenge of adulthood. Journal of Learning Disabilities 25: 410-415.

de Pear S (1997) Excluded pupil's views of their educational needs and experiences. Support for Learning 12(1): 19-22.

Pearson, W (2001) Is dyslexia a gift? Dyslexia Contact 20(3): 33.

Peer L (2002) Dyslexia – Not a condition to die for. Special Children (September): 31-33.

Pellegrini A, Long J (2002) A longitudinal study of bullying, dominance and victimisation during the transition from primary school through secondary school. British Journal of Developmental Psychology 20(2): 259-280.

Pepler D, Craig W (1998) Assessing children's peer relationships. Child Psychology and Psychiatry Review 3(4): 176-182.

Perin D (1997) Workplace literacy assessment. Dyslexia 3(3): 190-200.

Perrin S, Smith P, Yule W (2000) Practitioner review: The assessment and treatment of post-traumatic stress disorder in children and adolescents. Journal of Child Psychology and Psychiatry 41(3): 277-289.

Piaget J (1932) The Moral Judgment of the Child. London: Routledge.

Pine D, Cohen E, Cohen P, Brook J (2000) School phobia and the persistence of conduct problems. Journal of Child Psychology and Psychiatry 41(5): 657-665.

Pollak D (ed.) (1999) Dyslexic Learners: A Holistic Approach to Support. Leicester: De Montfort University.

Pollock J, Walker E (1994) Day-to-day Dyslexia in the Classroom. London: Routledge.

Porter J, Rourke B (1985) Socio-emotional Functioning of Learning-disabled Children. A subtype analysis of personality patterns. In Rourke B (ed.) Neuropsychology of Learning Disabilities: Essentials of Subtype Analysis. New York: Guildford.

Povey R, Todd J (1993) The Dyslexic Child. In Varma V (ed.) How and Why Children Fail. London: Jessica Kingsley.

Prins E (2002) Psychological assessment and the importance of feedback. Dyslexia Review 13(3): 20-21.

Prior M (1996) Understanding Specific Learning Difficulties. Hove, East Sussex: Psychology Press.

Prior M, Sanson A, Smart D, Oberklaid F (1995) Reading disability in an Australian community sample. Australian Journal of Psychology 47(1): 32-37.

Pumphrey P (1979) Improved Reading Through Counselling – Royal Road or Cul-de-sac? In Thackeray D (ed.) Growth in Reading. London: Ward Lock.

Pumphrey P, Reason R (1991) Specific Learning Difficulties (Dyslexia). London: Whurr.

Purves L (1996) The voices of children, The Sunday Times, 19 March 1996.

Puura K, Almquist F, Tamminen T, Piha J, Kumpulainen K, Rasanen E, Moilanen I, Koivisto A (1998) Children with symptoms of depression – What do adults see? Journal of Child Psychology and Psychiatry 39(4): 577-585.

Qualter P, Munn P (2002) The separateness of social and emotional loneliness in childhood. Journal of Child Psychology and Psychiatry 43(2): 233-244.

Quinn P (1996) Bullying in schools: Detection in an adolescent psychiatric clinic practice compared with questionnaire survey. Child Psychology and Psychiatry Review 1(4): 139-145.

Rack J, Hatcher J (2001) The characteristics of pupils with specific literacy difficulties: evidence from SPELL IT. Dyslexia Review 13(1): 11-14.

Rachman S (1977) The conditioning theory of fear acquisition: A critical examination. Behaviour Research and Therapy 15: 375-387.

Ramaa S, Kurian N (2000) Two views on dyslexia in India. Perspectives 26(1): 16.

Ramus F, Rosen S, Dakin S, Day B, Castellote J, White S, Frith U (2002) Theories of Developmental Dyslexia: Insights from a multiple case study of dyslexic adults on Cogprints. Website: www.cogprints.soton.ac.uk.

Randall P (1997) Adult Bullying: Perpetrators and Victims. London: Routledge.

Rawson M (1996) Dyslexia over the Lifespan: A fifty-five-year Longitudinal Study. Cambridge: Educators Publishing Service.

Reid G, Kirk J (2001) Dyslexia in Adults: education and employment. Chichester: Wiley.

Reid M (2001) Evaluating the effectiveness of counselling in primary care: Taking a fresh look. Counselling and Psychotherapy Research 1(1): 24-28.

Rennie D (2001) The client as a self-aware agent in counselling and psychotherapy. Counselling and Psychotherapy Research 1(2): 82-89.

Reynolds A, Gregg, N (2002) Do Learning Difficulties Impact on the Emotional Profile of College Students? Proceedings of the 5th BDA International Conference, York (website: www.bdainternationalconference.org).

Reynolds M, Brewin C, Saxton M (2000) Emotional disclosure in school children. Journal of Child Psychology and Psychiatry 41(2): 151-159.

Riddick B (1996) Living with Dyslexia: The social and emotional consequences of specific learning difficulties. London: Routledge.

Riddick B, Sterling C, Farmer M, Morgan S (1999) Self-esteem and anxiety in the educational histories of adult dyslexic students. Dyslexia 5(4): 227-248.

Rigby K (2002) New Perspectives on Bullying. London: Jessica Kingsley.

Riley K, Rustique-Forrester E (2002) Working with Disaffected Students: Why students lose interest in school and what we can do about it. London: Paul Chapman.

Rivers I (2001) Retrospective reports of school bullying: Stability of recall and its implications for research. British Journal of Developmental Psychology 19(1): 129-142.

Roberts C, Smith P (1999) Attitudes and behaviour of children towards peers with disabilities. International Journal of Disability, Development and Education 46(1): 35-50.

Robinson G, Whiting P (2001) The Interpretation of Emotion from Facial Expression for Children with Visual Sub-Type of Dyslexia. Proceedings of the 5th BDA International Conference, York (website: www.bdainternational conference.org).

Rogan L, Harmann L (1990) Adult outcomes of learning disabled students ten years after initial follow-up. Learning Disabilities Focus 5: 91-102.

Rolland J (1987) Chronic illness and the life-cycle: A conceptual framework. Family Process 26: 203-221.

Rose S (2002) Theoretical approaches to psychological trauma: Implications for research and practice. Counselling and Psychotherapy Research 2(1): 61-72.

Rourke B (1988) Socioemotional disturbances of learning disabled children. Journal of Consulting and Clinical Psychology 56: 801-810.

Rourke B, Fuerst D (1996) Psychosocial dimensions of learning disabilities Subtypes. Assessment 3: 277-290.

Rowan J (1990) Subpersonalities. London: Routledge.

Rowe D (1996) Depression and Happiness. In Palmer S, Dainow S, Milner S (eds.) Counselling: The BAC Reader. London: Sage.

Rucklidge J, Tannock R (2002) Neuropsychological profiles of adolescents with ADHD: Effects of reading difficulties and gender. Journal of Child Psychology and Psychiatry 43(8): 988-1003.

Russell G (1982) Writing and dyslexia – An historical analysis. Journal of Child Psychology and Psychiatry 23(4): 383-400.

Rutter M (1975) Helping Troubled Children. London: Penguin.

Rutter M (1985) Family and school influences on behavioural development. Journal of Child Psychology and Psychiatry 26(3): 349-368.

Rutter M, Tizard J, Whitemore K (1970) Education, Health and Behaviour. London: Longman.

Salmon G, Kemp A (2002) ADHD: A survey of psychiatric and paediatric practice. Child and Adolescent Mental Health 7(2): 73-78.

Sandberg S, Rutter M, Pickles A, McGuiness D, Angold A (2001) Do high-threat life events really provoke the onset of psychiatric disorder in children? Journal of Child Psychology and Psychiatry 42(4): 523-532.

Saunders R (1995) Stress Factors within the Family. In Miles T, Varma V (eds.) Dyslexia and Stress. London: Whurr.

Saunders S (2000) Examining the relationship between the therapeutic bond and the phases of treatment outcome. Psychotherapy 37: 206-218.

Scarborough H (1984) Continuity between childhood dyslexia and adult reading. British Journal of Psychology 75(4): 329-348.

Schafer M, Werner N, Crick N (2002) A comparison of two approaches to the study of negative peer treatment: General victimisation and bully/victim problems among German schoolchildren. British Journal of Developmental Psychology 20(2): 281-306.

Schlichte-Hiersemenzel B (2000) The Psychodynamics of Psychological and Behavioural Difficulties of Highly Able Children: Experiences from a Therapeutic Practice. In Montgomery D (ed.) Able Underachievers. London: Whurr.

Scott C (2003) Out for justice (Special needs provision review), The Sunday Times, 23 February 2003.

Scott M, Palmer S (eds.) (2000) Trauma and Post-traumatic Stress Disorder. London: Cassell.

Scott M, Stradlin S (2000) Brief group counselling and post-traumatic stress disorder. In Scott M, Palmer S (eds.) Trauma and Post-traumatic Stress Disorder. London: Cassell.

Seeman L (2002) The Sociological Implications of Untreated Dyslexia: Linkage of dyslexia with crime. Available: seeman@netvision.net.il.

Segal J (1996) Whose disability? Counter transference in work with people with disabilities. Psychodynamic Counselling 2(2): 155-166.

Seligman M (1975) Helplessness: On Depression, Development and Death. San Francisco, CA: Freeman.

Selye S (1956) Stress of Life. New York: McGraw-Hill.

Shafran R (2001) Obsessive-compulsive disorder in children and adolescents. Child Psychology and Psychiatry Review 6(2): 50-58.

Shaw R (2000) The status of dyslexia in Chile. Perspectives 26(1): 32.

Shaywitz S, Shaywitz B, Fletcher J, Escobar M (1990) Prevalence of reading disability in boys and girls. Journal of the American Medical Association 264(3): 998-1002.

Simmons F, Singleton C (2000) The reading comprehension abilities of dyslexic students in higher education. Dyslexia 6(3): 178-192.

Sinason V (1993) Understanding Your Handicapped Child. London: Rosendale.

Singleton C (1999) Dyslexia in Higher Education Policy, Provision and Practice. Report of the National Working Party. Hull: University of Hull.

Skuse D (2003) Fear recognition and the neural basis of social cognition. Child and Adolescent Mental Health 8(2): 50-60.

Slaughter V, Dennis M, Pritchard M (2002) Theory of mind and peer acceptance in pre-school children. British Journal of Developmental Psychology 20(4): 545-564.

Smith P, Perrin S, Yule W (1999) Cognitive behaviour therapy for post-traumatic stress disorder. Child Psychology and Psychiatry Review 4(4): 177-182.

Smith P (1991) The silent nightmare: Bullying and victimisation in school peer groups. Bulletin of the British Psychological Society 4: 243-248.

Smith S, Carroll A, Elkins J (1999) University students with learning disabilities: Results of a national survey. Australian Journal of Learning Disabilities 4(1): 18-30.

Smyth M, Anderson H (2000) Coping with clumsiness in the school playground: Social and physical play in children with co-ordination impairments. British Journal of Developmental Psychology 18(3): 389-413.

Smyth M, Anderson H (2001) Football participation in the primary school playground: The role of coordination impairments. British Journal of Developmental Psychology 19(3): 369-379.

Snowling M (2000) Dyslexia (2nd edn). Oxford: Blackwell.

Snowling M (1998) Dyslexia as a phonological deficit: Evidence and implications. Child Psychology and Psychiatry Review 3(1): 4-11.

Snowling M, Bishop D, Stothard S (2000) Is preschool language impairment a risk factor for dyslexia in adolescence? Journal of Child Psychology and Psychiatry 41(5): 587-600.

Snowling M, Nation K (1997) Development and dyslexia: Further comments on Ellis, McDougall and Monk. Dyslexia 3(1): 9-11.

Speece D, McKinney J, Appelbaum M (1985) Classification and validation of behavioural subtypes of learning disabled children. Journal of Educational Psychology 77: 67-77.

Spence S (1987) The relationship between social-cognitive skills and peer sociometric status. British Journal of Developmental Psychology 5(4): 347-356.

Spence S (1994) Practitioner review: Cognitive therapy with children and adolescents: From theory to practice. Journal of Child Psychology and Psychiatry 35(7): 1191-1228.

Spence S, Donovan C, Brechman-Toussaint M (2000) The treatment of childhood social phobia: The effectiveness of a social skills training-based, cognitive-behavioural intervention, with and without parental involvement. Journal of Child Psychology and Psychiatry 41(6): 713-726.

Stallard P, Velleman R, Baldwin S (1999) Psychological screening of children for post-traumatic stress disorder. Journal of Child Psychology and Psychiatry 40(7): 1075-1082.

Stanovich K (1986) Matthew Effects in reading: Some consequences of individual differences in the acquisition of literacy. Reading Research Quarterly 21: 360-407.

Stanovich K (1994) Does dyslexia exist? 35(4): 579-595.

Staudacher C (1987) Beyond Grief: A Guide for Recovering from the Death of a Loved One. London: Souvenir.

Steffert B (1995) You are what you think. Counselling (November): 275.

Sterling C, Farmer M, Riddick B, Morgan S, Matthews C (1998) Adult dyslexic writing. Dyslexia 4(1): 1-15.

Stevenson J, Pennington B, Gilger J, De Fries J, Gillis J (1993) Hyperactivity and spelling disability: Testing for shared genetic aetiology. Journal of Child Psychology and Psychiatry 34(7): 1137-1152.

Sutton J (2001) Bullies: Thugs or thinkers? The Psychologist 14(10): 530-534.

Sutton J, Smith P, Swettenham J (1999) Social cognition and bullying: Social inadequacy or skilled manipulation? British Journal of Developmental Psychology 17(3): 435-450.

Svensson I, Lundberg I, Jacobson C (2001) The prevalence of reading and spelling difficulties among inmates of institutions for compulsory care of juvenile delinquents. Dyslexia 7(2): 62-76.

Sylva K (1994) School influences on children's development. Journal of Child Psychology and Psychiatry 35(1): 135-170.

Tattum D (1993) Understanding and Managing Bullying. London: Heinemann.

Taylor S (2001) Gifted and Talented Children: A Planning Guide. London: Jessica Kingsley.

Terwogt M (2002) Emotional states in self and others as motives for helping in 10-year-old children. British Journal of Developmental Psychology 20(1): 131-147.

Thompson B, Snow P (2002) The written expression of children with reading disabilities: A comparison of written and dictated narratives. Australian Journal of Learning Disabilities 7(4): 13-19.

Thompson C, Rudolph L (1996) Counselling Children (4th edn). Pacific Grove, CA: Brooks/Cole.

Thomson M (1990) Developmental Dyslexia (3rd edn). London: Whurr.

Thomson M (1995a) Sport and dyslexia. Dyslexia 1(1): 54.

Thomson P (1995b) Stress Factors in Early Education. In Miles T, Varma V (eds.) Dyslexia and Stress. London: Whurr.

Thomson M (2001) The Psychology of Dyslexia: A Handbook for Teachers. London: Whurr.

Thomson M (2003) Monitoring dyslexics, intelligence and attainments: A follow-up study. Dyslexia 9(1): 3-17.

Thomson M, Hartley G (1980) Self-concept in children with dyslexia. Academic Therapy 26: 19-36.

Tillich P (1952) The Courage to Be. Newhaven and London: Yale University Press.

Tolan J (2001) The fallacy of the real self. Counselling and Psychotherapy Journal 12(2): 18-22.

Torrance D (2000) Qualitative studies into bullying within special schools. British Journal of Special Education 27(1): 16-21.

Townend J, Turner, M (eds.) (2000) Dyslexia in Practice: A Guide for Teachers. New York: Kluwer Academic/Plenum.

Trower P, Casey A, Dryden W (1988) Cognitive-Behavioural Counselling in Action. London: Sage.

Tsui E (1990) Effects of a Disaster on Children's Academic Attainment. Unpublished master's thesis, University of London.

Tunali B, Power T (1993) Creating satisfaction: A psychological perspective on stress and coping in families of handicapped children. Journal of Child Psychology and Psychiatry 34(6): 945-957.

Tur-Kaspa M, Weisel A, Segev L (1998) Attributions for feelings of loneliness of students with learning disabilities. Learning Disabilities Research and Practice 13(2): 89-94.

Turner M (1990) Sponsored reading failure. An object lesson. Warlingham, UK: IPSET Education Unit.

Turner M (1997) Psychological Assessment of Dyslexia. London: Whurr.

Turner M (2000a) Dyslexia and Crime. Dyslexia Review 12(1): 4-5.

Turner M (2000b) Special arrangements in standard assessment tasks (SATs). Dyslexia Review 11(4): 8-9.

Turner M (2002) A round up of new tests. Dyslexia Review 13(3): 14-19.

Underdown T (1999) Dyspraxia: One-to-one support. Special (Spring): 16-19.

Van den Oord E, Rispens J (1999) Differences between school classes in preschoolers' psychosocial adjustment: Evidence for the importance of children's interpersonal relations. Journal of Child Psychology and Psychiatry 40(3): 417-430.

Van der Wissel A, Zegers F (1985) Reading retardation revisited. British Journal of Developmental Psychology 3(1): 3-9.

Vanzetti N, Duck S (1996) A Lifetime of Relationships. Pacific Grove, CA: Brooks/Cole.

Veerman J (1995) Family stress, family functioning and emotional/behavioural problems following child psychiatric treatment. European Child and Adolescent Psychiatry 4: 21-31.

Velting O, Albano A (2001) Current trends in the understanding and treatment of social phobia in youth. Journal of Child Psychology and Psychiatry 42(1): 127-140.

Verduyn C (2000) Cognitive behaviour therapy in childhood depression. Child Psychology and Psychiatry Review 5(4): 176-180.

Viall J (2000) Shhh... don't talk about it. Perspectives 26(1): 3.

Vogel S (1990) Gender differences in intelligence, language, visual-motor abilities and academic achievement in students with learning disabilities: A review of the literature. Journal of Learning Difficulties 23: 44-52.

Vogel S, Adelman, P (1999) Teachers with learning disabilities: How do they fare? Thalamus 17: 72-74.

Von Gontard A (1998) Annotation: Day and night wetting in children – A paediatric and child psychiatric perspective 39(4): 439-451.

Vostanis P, Nicholls J, Harrington R (1994) Maternal expressed emotion in conduct and emotional disorders of childhood. Journal of Child Psychology and Psychiatry 35(2): 365-376.

Wagner R, Garon T (1999) Learning Disabilities in Perspective. In Sternberg R, Spear-Swerling L (eds.) Perspective in Learning Disabilities. Boulder, Colorado: Westview.

Walker A, Harris G, Baker A, Kelly D, Houghton J (1999) Post-traumatic stress responses following liver transplantation in older children. Journal of Child Psychology and Psychiatry 40(3): 363-374.

Wallander J, Varni J (1998) Effects of paediatric chronic physical disorders on child and family adjustment. Journal of Child Psychology and Psychiatry 39(1): 29-46.

Waring S, Prior M, Sanson A, Smart D (1996) Predictors of recovery from reading disability. Australian Journal of Psychology 48(3): 160-166.

Warr P, Downing J (2000) Learning strategies, learning anxiety and knowledge acquisition. British Journal of Psychology 91(3): 311-333.

Watson J (1999) Working in groups: social and cognitive effects in a special class. British Journal of Special Education 26(2): 87-95.

Wearmouth J (1999) Another one flew over: 'Maladjusted' Jack's perception of his label. British Journal of Special Education 26(1): 15-22.

Weavers, J (2003) Dyslexia and Mathematics. In Thomson M (ed.) Dyslexia Included: A Whole School Approach. London: Fulton.

Weekes S (1997) Book reviews. Dyslexia 3(1): 58.

West T (1997) In the Mind's Eye: Visual Thinkers, Gifted People with Dyslexia and Other Learning Difficulties, Computer Images and the Ironies of Creativity. Amherst, New York: Prometheus.

Whitney I, Smith P, Thompson D (1994) Bullying and Children with Special Educational Needs. In Smith P, Sharp S (eds.) School Bullying: Insights and Perspectives. London: Routledge.

Willcutt E, Pennington B (2000) Psychiatric comorbidity in children and adolescents with reading disability. Journal of Child Psychology and Psychiatry 41(8): 1039-1048.

Winkley L (1996) Emotional Problems in Children and Young People. London: Cassell.

Winnicott D (1965) The Family and Individual Development. London: Tavistock.

Winnicott D (1974) Playing and Reality. London: Pelican.

Wolke D, Woods S, Bloomfield L, Karstadt L (2000) The association between direct and relational bullying and behaviour problems among primary school children. Journal of Child Psychology and Psychiatry 41(8): 989-1002.

Wood G (1983) The Myth of Neurosis: A Case for Moral Therapy. London: Macmillan.

Woodward L, Ferguson D (2000) Children's peer relationship problems and later risks of educational under-achievement and unemployment. Journal of Child Psychology and Psychiatry 41(2): 191-201.

Woodward L, Taylor E, Dowdney L (1998) The parenting and family functioning of children with hyperactivity. Journal of Child Psychology and Psychiatry 39(2): 161-169.

The World Factbook (CIA) (2002) Available: www.odci.gov/cia/publications/factbook/ geos/uk.html.

Yamada J (2000) The myth of absence of dyslexia in Japan. Perspectives 26(1): 22.

Zuroff D, Stotland S, Sweetman E, Craig J, Koestner R (1995) Dependency, self-criticism and social interaction. British Journal of Clinical Psychology 34(4): 543-553.

Index

Ability Net, 301
abstract concepts
   diagnosis of dyslexia, 23
   phonological deficit, 15
academic success
   idealization of, 62
   revisiting and fantasy, 261
acceptance of dyslexics
   by family members, 121
   by teachers, 84–86
access courses for higher education, 236
Access to Work Scheme, 307
adaptation, 260
ADD, *see* attention deficit disorder
ADHD, *see* attention deficit hyperactivity
   disorder
adjustment phase of family adaptation,
   111
Adult Dyslexia Centre, 293
Adult Dyslexia Organisation, 296
adult dyslexics, counselling
   bullying, 234
   career choices, 232–234
   disclosure of dyslexia, 231
   employment problems, 230–234
   issues, 229
   literacy problems, 230
   practical support, 231–232
adult education classes, 297
advantages
   of dyslexia, 10–11
   of dyslexics' experiences, 219–220
adversity, strengthening power of,
   217–218
affective training, 275

age factors
   academic problems, 63–64
   bullying, help against, 93
   psychological and social effects of
   dyslexia, 156
   sibling conflicts, 112, 113
aggression and violence
   as defence strategy, 259, 260–261
   between siblings, 111–113
   see also anger; bullying
alcoholism and alcohol abuse
   and anxiety, 169, 261
   parents with dyslexia, 135
alienation, *see* isolation, social
Allen, Rick (Def Leppard), 36
alphabet, history of, 4–5
ambidexterity, 36
ambiguity
   and social isolation, 190
   tolerance of, 42
ambitious parents, 132–133
amygdala, 160, 161
Andersen, Hans Christian, 308
Andrews, Anthony, 308
anger
   diagnosis as trigger, 243
   furious impotence, 282–283
   and maladaptive behaviour, 63
   at school, 63
   see also aggression and violence
anorexia nervosa, 261
antisocial behaviour, *see* conduct
   disorders
anxiety, 157
   bed-wetting, 171–172

causes in childhood, 169–170
cognitive behavioural therapy, 271
defence strategies, 258, 261
effects of, 60–61
evidence, 168–169
excessive, 170–171
gender factors, 157
and intelligence, relationship
    between, 171
isolation, social, 191
management, 275–276
normal, 169
obsessive-compulsive disorder,
    172–173
overprotective parenting, 148
parental, 131–132
physical and psychosomatic
    symptoms, 171
as protective factor, 174
regressive behaviour, 258
research critique, 221
school phobia, 68, 69–70
and self-esteem, relationship between,
    208
separation
    mothers', 144
    school phobia, 67, 68, 69
students, 236
and visual images, 285–286
see also stress
anxiety management, 275–276
appeals, education, 300
appearance of dyslexics
    childlike, 149
    eccentricity, 44
    unattractive, 57, 193
    untidiness, 23
architects, 39
Army careers, 233
artistic talents, see creativity
art therapy, 251
    post-traumatic stress disorder, 163
assessment of dyslexics
    adults
        cost, 294
        free assessment, entitlement to,
            294
        help, 294–295
        obtaining an assessment, 293–294

practical help at work, 295
process, 294
technological help, 295
children
    obtaining an assessment, 291
    process, 291–292
    tests, 292–293
contact details, 298
counselling combined with, 226, 241
counselling as extension of, 225
as counselling tool, 240–243
effects, 241–243
importance, 25
practicalities, 240
students, 304
timing of, 240–241
associated conditions, 26–27
    see also attention deficit disorder;
    attention deficit/hyperactivity
    disorder; dyscalculia; dysphasia;
    dyspraxia and clumsiness
Aston Index, 292
attention, vs. concentration, 256–257
attention deficit disorder (ADD), 26, 28,
    178
    contact details, 302
    counselling, 254
attention deficit hyperactivity disorder
    (ADHD), 26, 28
    conduct disorder, 175, 178–179
    contact details, 302
    counselling, 179–180, 254
    crime, 179
    depression, 166
    family life
        effects on, 108–109, 118, 120
        organization of home, 105
    isolation, social
        gestures, inappropriate use of, 191
        peer problems, 186
        routes to, 184
    special schools, 67
attitudes to dyslexia, 7–8, 33
attractiveness, lack of, 57, 193
auditory memory, 293
auditory perceptual skills, 293
automaticity difficulties
    brain differences in dyslexia, 11–12
    diagnosis of dyslexia, 23

and reading comprehension
    problems, 21
avoidance techniques, 63

Bailey, David, 308
bed-wetting, 171–172
behavioural treatment for school phobia,
    70–71
benefits
    of dyslexia, 10–11
    of dyslexics' experiences, 219–220
bereavement, 123
    counselling, 124
    grief for a 'normal' child, 123–124
    pathological mourning, 125–126
    signs and stages, 125
bewilderment, parental, 129
bisexuality, 214
bonding between teacher and child, 85
boredom
    in counselling, 256–257
    and maladaptive behaviour, 63
boundaries, counselling, 262–263
    school counselling, 239
brain differences in dyslexics, 11–12
    handedness, 36
    post-traumatic stress disorder,
        160–161, 162
Brando, Marlon, 308
Branson, Richard, 209, 273, 308
British Ability Scales, 292
British Association of Counselling and
    Psychotherapy (BACP), 227
British Dyslexia Association (BDA)
    assessment of dyslexia, 294
    befrienders, 232
    contact details, 296
    employment issues, 232
    founding, 5
    specialist tuition, 21
British Dyslexics, 296
bulimia nervosa, 261
bullying
    eccentricity as defence mechanism, 44
    and overprotective parenting,
        relationship between, 143
    paternal horseplay as protection
        against, 142
    post-traumatic stress disorder, 163

relational, 95
research, 96
at school, 56
    action against, 96–100
    background, 88–91
    context, 94–95
    by dyslexics, 89, 100
    effects, 91, 186
    extent, 88–89
    help against, 91–94
    mainstream vs. special schools, 66,
        89–90
    by teachers, 83
    transition, 58
and self-esteem, relationship between,
    205
by siblings, 109, 112
social, 95
types, 95
at work, 234
see also aggression and violence

car driving, 34
career choices, 232–234
castration fears, 210
CBT, see cognitive behavioural therapy
cerebellar dysfunction, 11
challenge, response to, 263–264
change
    cognitive behavioural therapy, 270
    dislike of, 264
cheque writing, 37
Cher, 308
chess, 35
Children Act (1989), 238
Chile, 7
chiropractors, 39
Christie, Agatha, 40, 308–309
chromosomes associated with dyslexia,
    10
    see also inheritance
Chronically Sick and Disabled Persons
    Act (1970), 5
chronic phase of family adjustment, 111
Churchill, Winston, 40, 309
Cilham and Hesse Basic Number
    Screening Test, 293
Circle Time, 97, 238
class environment, 73–74, 87–88

Clemmet, Simon, 309
clumsiness, *see* dyspraxia and clumsiness
cognitive behavioural therapy (CBT)
    application to dyslexic problems,
        267–268
    approaches, 272–276
    cognitive skills vs. cognitive processes,
        268–269
    common negative thoughts and
        beliefs, 269–270
    effective statements, 270–272
    homework, 248
    integration into other therapeutic
        practices, 268
    obsessive-compulsive disorder, 173
    post-traumatic stress disorder, 163
    self-esteem, 207
cognitive style, distinctive dyslexia, 38–39
colleges and universities, 297, 303
    assessment of dyslexia, 226, 240–241
    counselling
        and assessment, combination of,
            226
        benefits, 237
        disclosure issues, 237
        prevalence of dyslexia, 235–236
        problems, 236–237
        provision, 234–235
        Singleton Report, 235
        study skills, 237
        voluntary projects, 2s6–227
    financial resources, 304
    help for dyslexics, 65
    hope unreleased during schooldays,
        74
    prevalence of dyslexia, 235–236
    transition to, 59
    see also education
comfort objects, 255
communication
    in counselling, 246–253
        empathy, 283–286
    and isolation, 184
        language problems, 193–196
        non-verbal skills, 187–193
    siblings of dyslexic children, 110
Communication Aids Project (CAP),
    304
co-morbidity, *see* associated conditions

compensated dyslexics, 219
    see also coping strategies
competition between siblings, 111
complexity of dyslexia, 9
Complex post-traumatic stress disorder,
    159, 160
comprehension difficulties, 21
Computability Centre, 301
Computer Centre for People with
    Disabilities, 301
computers, *see* technology
concentration
    attention vs., 256–257
    diagnosis of dyslexia, 23–24
conduct disorders, 174–175
    anxiety, 174
    attention deficit hyperactivity
        disorder, 178–179
    depression, 166
configurations, and self-esteem, 206
conflict, *see* aggression and violence;
    anger; bullying
confusion, 36, 38
    of date, 47–49
    directional, 46–47
    of left and right, 46–47
        driving, 34
    of time, 47–49
congruence, counsellor, 262, 263, 286
Conley, Brian, 309
contagion of dampening reactions, 190
contextual style, 39
continuous reading tests, 292
continuous spelling tests, 292–293
control
    as coping strategy, 217–218
    of ego, 217–218
    lack of, at school, 62–63
    perceived, 218
    sense of
        parental, 115
        and time management, 48–49
conversation problems
    reasons for, 194
    types of, 195
coordination problems, *see* dyspraxia and
    clumsiness
coping strategies, 204
    academic work, 219

adults' reading abilities, 22
anxiety, 171
benefits of dyslexia experiences,
    219–220
boundaries as, 263
career choice, 232
cognitive behavioural therapy, 271
creativity, 41, 42–43
crime, 178
development, 215–216
eccentricity, 44
infantilization, 208–214
intergenerational, 131–132
learned helplessness and, 37
maternal, 138
parents', 115–116
post-traumatic growth, 219–220
research, critique of, 220–222
self-esteem, 204–208
self-sufficiency, 38
sequencing problems, 46
siblings' 110–111
survival of negative experiences, 214
types, 216–219
unacknowledged, 214–215
see also defence strategies
counselling relationship, 244–246
counsellors and counselling, 223, 225,
    244
adult dyslexics, 229–234
anxiety, 169
assessment of dyslexia, 240–243
attention deficit hyperactivity
    disorder, 179–180
boundaries, 262–263
    school counselling, 239
bullying
    action against, 97–100
    effects, 94
challenge and change, 263–264
communication, 246–253
counselling relationship, 244–246
defences, 257–262
dyslexic counsellors, 227
effective counselling systems, 225–227
families
    bereavement, 124
    disability notion, 122–123
    mothers, 117

overprotective parenting, 148–149
    parents, 109, 121–123, 128
    sibling dynamics, 110
infantilized dyslexics, 208–209
isolation, misinterpretation of, 202
jargon, 249
language difficulties, 194
obsessive-compulsive disorder, 173
physical factors, 253–257
post-traumatic growth, 220
post-traumatic stress disorder, 163
primary care, 228–229
self-esteem, 207
social cognition, 198
specialist approaches, 265
    Ecosystemic therapy, 239, 278–279
    humanistic therapies, 283–286
    inner critic, 265–267
    Psychodynamic Theory, 279–283
    see also cognitive behavioural
        therapy; Transactional Analysis
students with dyslexia, 234–237
suicidal clients, 182
and teachers
    dyslexics' similar expectations of,
        75
    transferential issues, comparison,
        77–78
transference and counter-
    transference, 77–78
see also school counsellors/counselling
counter-transference
    between counsellor and client, 260
    Psychodynamic Theory, 281
    between teacher and child, 77, 78–80
creative writing, 43, 63
creativity, 39–43
    as coping process and defence, 42–43
    in counselling, 252
    creative process, 41–42
    infantilized dyslexics, 213
    musical ability, 35
    and severity of dyslexia, relationship
        between, 40–41
    solitary dyslexics, 203
    and work effort, relationship between,
        42
CReSTeD, 297, 300
cricket, 32

crime
    and dyslexia, relationship between,
        176, 177–178
        attention deficit hyperactivity
            disorder, 179
        prisoners with dyslexia, help for, 177
    and reading disability, relationship
        between, 175–176
crisis phase of family adjustment, 110
criterion-referenced tests, 293
criticism
    hypersensitivity to, 59–60
    inner critic, 265–267
    at school, 83–84
cross-dressing, 213
Cruise, Tom, 309
cultural issues, 33
cuneiform, 4
Czech language, 8

daily hassle stress, 164
    causes, 165
    'final straw', 165
    generality vs. particularity, 165
    theory, 164
dampening reactions, contagion of, 190
Danish language, 8
dates, confusion of, 47–49
da Vinci, Leonardo, 40, 309
Davis, Ronald, 309–310
death wish, 122
    see also suicide and suicidal tendencies
defence strategies
    adeptness, 257
    common, 257–262
    creativity, 42–43
    eccentricity, 44
    at school, 63
    see also coping strategies
Def Leppard, 36
delinquency, see conduct disorders
denial, 259
Department for Education and Skills
    (DfES), 297, 304
depression
    correlation vs. cause, 167
    definition, 167
    evidence, 166–168
    false indications, 246

friends, lack of, 56
gender factors, 157
isolation, 184, 190
maternal, 118, 139
    and favouritism towards dyslexic
        sons, 113
parents with dyslexia, 134
school phobia, 68, 69–70
social-skills training, 274
suicide, 181
desensitization, 268
desexualization of dyslexics, 210, 213–214
deskilling, 280–281
determination, 217
developmental nature of dyslexia, 25–26
diagnosis of dyslexia, 23–30
    effects, 241–243
        on family relationships, 103–104,
            114–115
    laterality, 36
    parents' reactions to, 128, 130
    at university, 236
    at work, 230
diagnostic skills, 293
DIAL UK, 299
diaries, 47–48, 248
difference, 43–44
    and isolation, 184
    at school, 79–80
Differential Ability Scales, 292, 293
directional confusion, 46–47
disability
    family and home life, see family and
        home life, disability
    Psychodynamic Theory, 281–282
disability advice organizations, 299–300
Disability Code of Practice
    1995: 231
    2002: 306
Disability Discrimination Act (DDA)
    1995: 305–306
        employment, 295
    2000: 307
Disability Employment Advisers (DEAs),
    298, 307
    assessment of dyslexia, 294
Disability Law Service, 299
Disability Matters, 298
Disability on the Agenda, 299

*Disability Rights Commission Code of
    Practice for Schools*, 306
Disability Service Teams, 307
Disability Support Officers, 307
Disabled Students' Allowance (DSA), 297,
    304
disclosure of dyslexia
    to counsellors, 245–246
    to employers, 231
    by parents with dyslexia, 129–130
    to universities, 237
disempowerment, 280–281
disorientation, 36
dissociation, 262
distractibility during counselling,
    255–256, 257
distress, parents', 122
dominance and submission, mixed
    signals, 191–192
drama triangle, 280
driving, 34
drug abuse, 169, 261
Dutch language, 8
dyscalculia, 26, 28–29
Dyslexia Advice and Resource Centre, 296
Dyslexia Computer Resource Centre, 301
Dyslexia Institute, The
    assessment of dyslexia, 291
        tests, 292, 294
    contact details, 294, 298, 302
    specialist tuition, 21, 294, 297
    Units of Sound Multimedia, 294
Dyspel Pilot Project, 177
dysphasia, 26–27
dyspraxia and clumsiness, 26, 27
    contact details, 297, 301
    counselling, 254
    diagnosis of dyslexia, 23
    family life
        effects on, 120
        organization of home, 105
        play, parents' abandonment of, 118
        public problems, 118
    isolation
        mixed dominance and submission
    signals, 191
        peer relationships, 186
        poor social synchrony, 189
    posture, 254

speech therapy, 22
sport, 57–58
    bullying, 89
    peer relationships, 87, 186
    unattractiveness, 57
Dyspraxia Foundation, The, 297, 301

early intervention, 24–25
    advantages of, 18
    effects of lack of, 18–19
eating disorders, 261
eating habits, 22
eccentricity, 43–44
Ecosystemic therapy, 239, 278–279
education
    appeals, 300
    legal issues, 305, 306, 307
    see also colleges and universities;
        specialist tuition and schools; teachers
        and schools
Education Act
    1981: 305
    1996: 64, 306
educational attainment, tests of, 292–293
Educational Grant Advisory Service, 304
educational psychologists, 291, 292, 294
    see also school counsellors/counselling
Education Otherwise, 70
effects, *see* psychological and social
    effects of dyslexia
effort, *see* work effort of dyslexics
ego-control, 217–218
Einstein, Albert, 29, 40, 252, 272–273, 310
emasculation fears, 210
embarrassment, *see* shame
emotional abuse by parents, 132
emotional and behavioural difficulties
    (EBD), 175
    near absence in rigid family
        structures, 106
    and reading disability, relationship
        between, 156
    teacher and dyslexic child,
        relationship between, 85
empathy, in counselling, 283–286
    see also social cognition
Employee Assistance Programmes
    (EAPs), 232
    bullying, 234

Employers Forum on Disability (EFD), 298
employment issues, 229–234
    assessment of dyslexia, 294
    bullying, 234
    career choices, 232–234
    contact details, 298–299
    disclosure of dyslexia, 231
    legal aspects, 306, 307
    literacy problems, 230
    practical help, 231–232, 295
Employment Service, 307
empty chair technique, 252
encouragement
    as coping strategy, 216
    by family, 150–151
English language, 8
    as foreign language, 32–33
enuresis, 171–172
Equal Opportunities Commission, 299
erratic behaviour, 188
ethnic issues, 33
European Human Rights Act (2000), 307
examinations
    help, 84
    and suicide, 181
excluded pupils
    bullies, 97–98
    hope for teachers' approval, 74
exclusion, see isolation, social
existence of dyslexia, 3
expectations
    dyslexics', 74
    parents', 133
    teachers', 75–76, 83–84, 85
externalizing effects of dyslexia, 157
    attention deficit hyperactivity disorder, 178–180
    conduct disorder, 174–175
    crime, 175–178
    suicide, 180–182
extroversion, 218, 259
eye contact, 198
    see also gaze

facial expressions
    contagion of dampening reactions, 190
    conversation problems, 194

difficulty in reading and conveying, 192
    mixed signals, 191–192
    see also gaze
failure
    as power, 258
    transference and counter-transference between teacher and child, 78–79
family and home life, 101–102, 103, 127
    ambitious parents, 132–133
    anxiety, parental, 131–132
    attention deficit hyperactivity disorder, associated problems, 108–109
    bereavement, 123
        counselling, 124
        grief for a 'normal' child, 123–124
        pathological mourning, 125–126
        signs and stages, 125
    bewilderment, parental, 129
    diagnosis of dyslexia, 103–104, 128–130
    disability
        counselling, 122–123
        cure, desire for, 121
        feelings of parents, 121–122
        help for mother, 116–117
        impact on home, 119, 120
        information for parents, 117
        isolation of parents, 119
        normal family life, 120–121
        parents' reactions to, 114–116
        and play, 118
        public problems, 118–119
        self-image, parents' impact on dyslexic's, 116
        sex life of parents, 120
        siblings' reactions to, 110–111
        transference issues, 117–118
    drama triangle, 280
    dyslexic parents
        ambitious, 133
        anxiety, 131
        'coming out', 129–130
        damaged, 134
        emotional abuse by, 132
        fathers, 141, 146
        guilty feelings, 128
        homework, child's, 108

hostility and jealousy towards child,
    146
infantilization, 212
inheritance, 9
mothers, 138–139
organization of home, 106
overprotectiveness, 144
parented by dyslexic children,
    134–135
pathological mourning, 125
reactions to child's dyslexia,
    128–129
Ecosystemic therapy, 278–279
emotionally abusive parents, 132
encouragement of dyslexic child,
    150–151
guilt, parental, 128, 131
infantilized dyslexics, 211
influences on dyslexic children, 104
inheritance issues, 131
isolation of dyslexic child, 184–185
marital difficulty, 119–120, 130
optimism, 115, 116, 151
organization of home, 105–106
overprotective parenting
    counselling issues, 148–149
    effects, 148
    parent-child alliance, 147–148
    prevalence, 143
    reasons for, 146–147
    relevance to dyslexia, 142–143
    repressed and denied dislike of
child, 143
post-traumatic stress disorder,
    protection against, 162
realization that a child is dyslexic,
    104–105
rigidity vs. flexibility, 106–107
and schools, relationship between,
    130
    homework, 108
    LEAs' attitudes, 64–65
    school phobia, 68, 69, 70
    special needs tribunals, 64–65
    transference between teacher and
child, 79
siblings
    coping with dyslexic child's
        disability, 110–111

favouritism issues for parents, 114
    importance, 109–110
    isolation, 185
    long-lasting effects of sibling
        relationships, 113–114
    relationship with dyslexic child,
        111–114
    violent/aggressive behaviour,
        111–113
support/lack of support for dyslexic
    child, 107, 150–151
teaching reading at home, 107–108
training for parents, 109
unambitious parents, 133–134
warmth towards dyslexic child, 138,
    150
see also fathers; mothers
famous dyslexics, 40, 43, 308–312
fathers
    critical, 142
    engagement with dyslexic children,
        141
    grief, 124
    horseplay, 142
    hostility and jealousy, 145–146
    infantilized dyslexics, 211–212
    marital problems, 119–120
    and mothers, relationships with
        dyslexic children compared,
        139–140
    protection, 142
    reintegration of absent, 140–141
    as role models, 141
    sexual problems, 120
    support for wife, 141
    transforming, 141
    triadic relationships, 112
    unconditional, 141
    see also family and home life
favouritism, parental, 113, 114
fear, 168–174
    of bullies, 93
    excessive, 170–171
    normal, 169
    overprotectiveness caused by, 146–147
    and school phobia, 69–70
    see also anxiety
Feliciano, Jose, 36
fidgety behaviour, 254

financial issues
    assessment of dyslexia, 240, 294
    Communication Aids Project, 304
    Disabled Students' Allowance, 297,
        304
Finnish language, 8
flexibility of teachers, 84
flicker-motion detection, 12
flooding, 268
Ford, Gerald, 266
foreign language, 33–34
    English as, 32–33
forgetfulness, 23
    see also memory
Foundation for Communication for the
    Disabled, 301
framing, 272–273
France, Anatole, 40
Free Representation Unit, 299
French language, 8
friends, 72
    failure to make friends, 56
    help against bullying, 92–94, 100
    see also peers
frustration, 63
further education, see colleges and
    universities

gaze, 192–193
    mixed signals, 191
    see also eye contact; facial expressions
gender factors
    bullying
        help against, 93
        types, 95
    dyslexia, 29–30
    dyspraxia, 27
    eating disorders, 261
    infantilization of dyslexics, 210, 213–214
    modesty, 202
    psychological and social effects of
        dyslexia, 157
    sexuality, 213–214
    siblings of dyslexic children
        maternal favouritism towards
    dyslexic sons, 113
        psychological disturbance, 110
    suicide and parasuicide, 181
general practitioners, 228–229

genetic factors
    attention deficit hyperactivity
        disorder, 28
    dyspraxia, 27
    see also inheritance
German language, 8
Germany
    English language, 33
    history of dyslexia, 5
gestures, inappropriate use of, 191
giftedness, 44–46
    and infantilization, 213
    and maladaptive behaviour, 63
    and non-verbal behaviour,
        interpretation, 187
Glennie, Evelyn, 36
glucocorticoid, 161
Goldberg, Whoopi, 310
Goodhew, Duncan, 32, 310
GPs, 228–229
grammar, 21
Greek language, 8
grief
    life-span, 124
    at loss of a 'normal' child, 123–124
    pathological mourning, 125–126
    see also bereavement
group work, 163
Guaranteed Interview Scheme, 232
guilt
    counter-transference between teacher
        and child, 79
    parental, 128

handedness, 36, 293
hand-eye coordination, 32
Hands, Guy, 310
handwriting
    assessment, 292–293
    diagnosis of dyslexia, 23
Harris City Technology College, 226
Hatcher, Peter, 20
Hebrew language, 8
Helen Arkell Dyslexia Centre, 298, 302
helplessness, learned, 37
    nature of, 200
    at school, 62–63
heritability issues, see genetic factors;
    inheritance

hesitant speech, 194–195, 248
'Hidden Disability' workshops, 307
hieroglyphs, 4
higher education, *see* colleges and
    universities
hippocampus, 160–161
historical perspective on dyslexia, 3–8
home life, *see* family and home life
home–school liaison officers, 239
homework
    cognitive behavioural therapy, 248
    parents with dyslexia, 108
homosexuality, 213
Hong Kong, 5
hope, expectation of, 74
hopelessness, 78–79
Horner, Jack, 310
Hornsby International Dyslexia Centre,
    298, 302
Hoskins, Bob, 310
humanistic therapies
    congruence, 286
    empathy, 283–286
humiliation
    and maladaptive behaviour, 63
    at school, 63, 64
        transference between teacher and
            child, 81
humour, 218, 259
Hungarian language, 8
hyperactivity, *see* attention deficit
    hyperactivity disorder

idealization of academic ability, 62
ideograms, 4
ignorance of dyslexia, 82
illiteracy, *see* literacy
imagery, written, 43
images in counselling, 251–252, 285–286
incidence of dyslexia, 3–4
Independent Panel for Special Education
    Advice (IPSEA), 300
India
    attitudes to dyslexia, 7
    English language, 33
    history of dyslexia, 5
indicators, *see* signs of dyslexia
individual difference, dyslexia as, 3
    diagnosis of dyslexia, 23–30

literacy, 14–23
    physical factors, 8–14
    social and historical perspective, 3–8
individuality of dyslexia, 287–288
infantilization of dyslexics, 43, 49, 156,
    208–209
    internalization, 209–214
    regressive behaviour, 258
    in research, 221
information
    about disability, 117
    for parents, 117
    for siblings, 110
information processing problems
    reasons for, 194
    time lags, 247
information processing speed, 293
inheritance
    dyslexia, 9
        diagnosis of dyslexia, 25
        genetic evidence, 10
        genetic point of dyslexia, 10–11
        parents' feelings, 131
        reading difficulty, 10
    see also genetic factors
inner critic, 265–266
    effects, 266–267
insensitivity, teachers', 83–84
insincerity, teachers', 84
insula, 11
intelligence
    and anxiety, relationship between, 171
    dyslexia's independence from, 24,
        44–46
    and literacy, relationship between, 23,
        24
    non-verbal skills, independence from,
        187
    and reading, relationship between, 24
    see also IQ
intelligence quotient, *see* IQ
intention words, 251
internalizing effects of dyslexia
    anxiety and fear, 168–174
    depression, 166–168
    stress, 158–165
International Dyslexia Association (IDA),
    7
international perspective on dyslexia, 6–7

attitudes to dyslexia, 7–8
history of dyslexia, 5
literacy standards, 6
Invalid Children's Aid Association, 5
IQ
    and anxiety, relationship between, 171
    assessment, 292
    dyslexia's independence from, 24,
        45
    non-verbal, 292
    underperformance in tests, 61
    verbal, 292
    see also intelligence
irrational beliefs, 270
Irving, John, 310
isolation, social, 37–38, 183
    attention deficit hyperactivity
        disorder, 67, 109
    depression, 167–168
    through kinaesthetics, 196–197
    through lack of social cognition,
        197–198
    through language problems, 193–196
    through latency stage, 200–202
    misinterpreting, 202–203
    through non-verbal skills, 187–193
    parents', 119
        attention deficit hyperactivity
            disorder's effects, 109
    and parents, relationship between,
        184–185
    routes to, 184–185
    school life, 64, 87
        bullying, 90, 93
        class environment, 87–88
        peer problems, 185–186
        special schools, 67–67
        transference between teacher and
            child, 79–80
    and siblings, relationship between, 185
    vehicle for, 186
    through victim behaviour, 198–200
Israel, 33
Italian language, 8
Italy, 68
Izzard, Eddie, 273

Japan
    attitudes to dyslexia, 8

denial of dyslexia's existence, 5
    Kanji, 8
jargon, counselling, 249
Job Centre, 298
    see also Disability Employment
        Advisers

Kanji, 8
Kendall, Felicity, 273, 311
'Kevin' syndrome, 217
kinaesthetics, isolation through, 196–197

labels for dyslexia, 31–32
    at school, 81–82
language aspects of dyslexia, 8
language difficulties, 26–27
    counselling communication, 246
    isolation through, 193–196
    nature of, 193
    reasons for, 194
    types of, 194–196
language processing, 10
languor, 254
La Plante, Lynda, 311
latency stage
    effects of problems, 201–202
    importance in social relationships,
        201
    infantilized dyslexics, 212
    relevance to relationship problems,
        200
laterality, 36
    assessment, 293
Law Centres, 299
leakage, 191
learned helplessness, 37
    nature of, 200
    at school, 62–63
learning difficulties loop, 19
    see also Matthew Effect
learning style, distinctive dyslexic, 38–39
left and right, confusion of, 46–47
    driving, 34
left-handedness, 36, 293
legal issues, 305–307
life coaching, 232, 272–273
Link into Learning, 226
listening skills
    counsellors', 250

and isolation, 193, 196
literacy, 14–23
    diagnosing dyslexia, 23, 24
    employment problems, 230, 231–232
    failure in, 56–57
    historical perspective, 4, 6
    inheritance aspects, 10
    and intelligence, discrepancy between,
        23, 24
    parents with dyslexia, 130
    prisoners' help with, 177
    and self-esteem, relationship between,
        62, 207–208
    see also phonological deficit; reading;
        writing
local education authorities (LEAs)
    appeals, 300
    assessment of dyslexia, 291
    legal issues, 305, 306, 307
    organization of schools, 64–65
loneliness, see isolation, social
long-term memory, 12, 14
Low Pay Unit, 300
loyalty to employer, 233

magnocellular deficits, 11–12
    directional confusion and sequencing
        difficulties, 46
maladaptive behaviours, 63
    see also defence strategies
Mandelbrot, Benoi, 40
maps, 32
marginalization, see isolation, social
mathematics, problems with, 26, 28–29
Matrix Analogies Test, 292
Matthew Effect, 19
    elimination, 20
    at university, 236
memory
    forgetfulness, 23
    long-term, 12, 14
    post-traumatic stress disorder, 161,
        163
    short-term, 12–14
        brain differences in dyslexia, 11
        counselling, 253
        dyscalculia, 29
        phonological deficit, 16
        problem-solving ability, 41–42

school life, 58
speech problems, 195
mentoring services, 232, 238
Menzies, Simon, 311
metaphors in counselling, 251–252, 285
Miles, Sarah, 311
mirror writing, 36
mnemonics, 46–47
modelling, parental, 138, 140, 141, 216
modesty, 202
mothers
    actions to solve dyslexia, 136
    detection of dyslexia, 136
    dyslexic, 138–139
    effects of dyslexia, 137
    emotional support for children,
        137–138
    and fathers, relationships with
        dyslexic children compared, 139–140
    grief, 124
    help for, 116–117
    husband's support, 141
    infantilization of dyslexics, 210, 211
    as main carers, 136
    marital problems, 119–120
    overprotectiveness
        embodiment of female 'tiger' role,
            145
        mother's mother, importance of,
            144–145
        prevalence, 143
        as reaction against a hostile, jeal-
            ous father, 145–146
        relevance to dyslexia, 142–143
        separation anxiety, 144
    positive effects on children, 138
    post-traumatic stress disorder, 124
        protection against, 162
    practical support for children, 137
    sexual problems, 120
    triadic relationships, 112–113
    unhappiness, and favouritism towards
        dyslexic sons, 113
    warmth, 138
    see also family and home life
motor coordination problems,
    see dyspraxia and clumsiness
mourning, see bereavement; grief
mouth sensitivity, 22

multisensory learning, 19, 20
musical ability, 35–36
    see also creativity
music as soothing factor, 255

narrative therapy, 275
    post-traumatic stress disorder, 163,
        275
National Association for Disability
    Officers (NADA), 304
National Bureau for Students with
    Disabilities, 304
National Federation of Access Centres,
    304
Neale Analysis of Reading Ability
    (revised), 292
neglect of non-dyslexic siblings, 112
Negroponte, Nicholas, 311
neurolinguistic programming (NLP),
    272–273
neuroticism, 201–202
NFER, 292
Nietzsche, Friedrich, 40
non-conforming behaviour, 188–189
non-medical nature of dyslexia, 8–9
non-verbal IQ, 292
non-verbal skills
    counselling, 254–255
    importance, 187
    isolation, social, 187–193
'normality', and family life, 111, 120–121
norm-referenced tests, 293
Norway, 8
Norwegian language, 8
numbers, problems with, 26, 28–29
number tests, 293

obsessive-compulsive disorder (OCD),
    172–173
occupational psychologists, 307
Oedipal stage, 140, 211
oil-slick thoughts, 269
Opportunities for People with
    Disabilities, 299
optimism
    counsellors', 281–282
    parental, 115, 116, 151
oral problems, see speech problems
over learning, 19, 20

overprotectiveness, see family and home
    life, overprotective parenting

PALS Project, 177, 226
panic attacks, 168, 170
parasuicide, 181
parent-adult-child (PAC) notion,
    Transactional Analysis, 276–277
parental modelling, 138, 140, 141, 216
parents, see family and home life; fathers;
    mothers
pathological mourning, 125–126
Patoss, 298
peace following diagnosis, 243
peers, 72
    effects of problems with, 88
    importance, 86
    isolation, 185–186
    relationship with dyslexic children,
        86–88
    social bullying, 95
    see also bullying; friends
Pentonville Prison, 177
perfectionism, 45
performance anxiety, 37
persistence, 217
personal history, revision after diagnosis,
    242
personality factors
    bullies and victims, 94–95
    post-traumatic stress disorder, 162
    teachers, 76–77
personal space, 196–197
phobias, 170
    school, see school phobia
phonemes, 14
phonetic writing, 4–5
phonics
    decline in teaching, 6
    structured, 19–20
phonography, 4
phonological awareness, 14, 293
phonological deficit, 14
    brain differences in dyslexia, 12
    dyslexic's perspective on, 15
    early identification of dyslexia, 24–25
    effect on reading, 16
    help, 18
        lack of, 18–19

historical perspective, 4, 5
importance, 14–15
inheritance, 10
Matthew Effect, 19
spelling, 22
unignorability, 16
varying severity, 16–18
phonological training, 18, 20
physical appearance, *see* appearance of
    dyslexics
physical differences associated with
    dyslexia, 8–14
Picasso, Pablo, 40
picture script, 4
picture thinking, 251–252
plana temporale, 12
play, 118, 142
poetry, 43
Polish language, 8
political issues, 49, 210
Portuguese language, 8
positive attitudes, *see* optimism
post-traumatic growth (PTG), 219–220
post-traumatic stress disorder (PTSD)
    acquisition, 158–158
    behavioural effects, 159
    bullying as cause, 91
    Complex (Type II), 159, 160
    counselling response, 163
    cure, lack of, 162
    maternal, 124
    narrative therapy, 163, 275
    physical effects, 160–161
    protective factors, 162–163
    psychological effects, 159–160
    vulnerability to, 161–162
posture, 254
power
    cognitive behavioural therapy, 270
    failure as, 258
    teaching as, 74–75
practical help for dyslexics
    by mothers, 137
    at school, 84
    at work, 231–232
pregnancy, 120
prevalence of dyslexia, 3–4
primary care, 227–229
printed work by dyslexics, 214

prisoners, dyslexic, 176
    help for, 177
problem-solving
    creative process, 41–42
    training, 275
projection, 258–259
projective identification, 283
    anger at school, 63
    and repression, 259
promotion, avoidance of, 230
pronunciation problems, 38
protest mechanisms, 209–210
Psychodynamic Theory, 279–283
Psychological Corporation Matrix
    Analogies Test, 292
psychological and social effects of
    dyslexia, 153–154, 155
    externalizing effects, 157
        attention deficit hyperactivity dis
            order, 178–180
        conduct disorder, 174–175
        crime, 175–178
        suicide, 180–182
    internalizing effects, 157
        anxiety and fear, 168–174
        depression, 166–168
        stress, 158–165
    reading problems, 155–157
    research, critique, 220–222
psychologists, assessment of dyslexia,
    292, 294
    see also educational psychologists;
        occupational psychologists
psychosocial training, 274–275
    prisoners, 177
PTSD, *see* post-traumatic stress disorder
public behaviour of dyslexics, 118–119
published work by dyslexics, 214

Quality Assurance Agency Code of
    Practice for the Assurance of
    Academic Quality and Standards in
    Higher Education (Section 3):
    Students with Disabilities (1999), 307
Quick Scan, 294

RADAR, 300
Rational Emotive Behavioural Therapy,
    275

Raven's Matrices, 292
Redgrave, Steven, 32, 311
reading
  ability
    assessment, 292
    attention deficit hyperactivity dis-
      order, 28
    decline in, 6
    historical perspective, 6
    and inheritance, 10
    and intelligence, relationship
      between, 24
    unhelped adult dyslexics, 22
  comprehension difficulties, 21
  developmental nature of dyslexia, 26
  effects of problems, 155–157
    conduct disorder, 174–175
    crime, 175–176
  idealization by dyslexics, 62
  learning, 297
  process, 16
  teaching, 19–20
    parents' attempts at, 107–108
  see also literacy
Reed, Oliver, 311
referrals of dyslexics, 228, 239
regressive behaviour, 258
relational bullying, 95
relaxation techniques, 275
'remedial' classes, 65–66
repetitive movements, 255
repression, 259
repulsion hypothesis, 189
resilience literature, 150
restlessness, 254
reversal errors, 38, 46–47
rhyming, 43, 293
right and left, confusion of, 46–47
  driving, 34
right-handedness, 36, 293
rigidity of family structure, 106–107
rivalry, sibling, 111
road signs, 34
Roddick, Anita, 312
Rodin, Auguste, 312
Rogers, Lord Richard, 312
role models, parental, 216
  fathers, 140, 141
  mothers, 138

romantic relationships, see sexual
  relationships and dating
rowing, 32
Royal Association for Disability and
  Rehabilitation (RADAR), 300
rugby, 32
Russia
  attitudes to dyslexia, 7
  history of dyslexia, 5, 82

Schonell test, 292
school counsellors/counselling
  lack of provision, 238
  outside referral, 239
  teachers' need for counselling, 78
  usefulness, 238–239
school phobia, 67–69
  fear and anxiety about school,
    importance of, 69–70
  as rational learning response, 70
  and separation anxiety, relationship
    between, 69
  treatment, 70–71
school refusal, 67, 68–69
  as rational learning response, 70
  treatment, 70–71
  see also school phobia
schools, see specialist tuition; teachers
  and schools
Schools Psychological Service, 291
secondary school, transition to, 59
second language, see foreign language
self-assessment software packages, 294
self-confidence
  and criticism, 60
  school life, 83
  students', 236
self-control training, 275
self-deprecation
  as defence strategy, 259
  and hesitant speech, 195
  and isolation, 202
self-esteem
  and academic failure, relationship
    between, 61–62
  associated bodies of evidence, 205
  career choice, 232
  defence against bullying, 100
  dyslexics vs. non-dyslexics, 204–205

effects of bullying, 91
encouragement from adults, 216
improving, 207–208
insensitivity and criticism by teachers,
    83
judging, 206–207
and literacy, relationship between, 62,
    207–208
multi-facetedness, 205–206
nature of, 204
respect for dyslexia, 208
at special schools, 66, 205
strategic choice of poor self-esteem, 207
teachers', 76–77
    and acceptance, 86
    high expectations, 85
    and transference, 81
self-harm, 181
self-image
    diagnosis of dyslexia, 242
    influences on, 116
self-instructional training, 275
self-sufficiency, 38
separation anxiety
    mothers', 144
    school phobia, 67, 68, 69
sequencing problems, 46
    cognitive behavioural therapy, 163
    counselling, 252–253
    diagnosis of dyslexia, 23
    narrative therapy, 163
    school life, 57
    in speech, 195
severity of dyslexia
    and creativity, relationship between,
        40–41
    and distractibility, relationship
        between, 256
    and social deficits, relationship
        between, 41
    variations, 16–18
sexual relationships and dating
    bullying's effects on, 91
    infantilized dyslexics, 213–214
    parents of dyslexic children, 120, 145
    social-skills training, 274
shame
    parents', 121
        with dyslexia, 129

school life, 81
    see also humiliation
Shaw, George Bernard, 55
short-term memory, see memory, short-
    term
    visual, 293
siblings, see family and home life
signification, 82
signs of dyslexia, 23–24
    in adults, 23, 290
    in children, 23, 24–25, 289
    in students, 303
Singleton Report, 235, 240
single-word reading tests, 292
single-word spelling tests, 292
situationally accessible memories (SAMs),
    163
smiling, 191–192
social bullying, 95
social cognition
    bullies and victims, 94–95
    and isolation, 184, 186, 197–198
    nature of, 197
    sibling relationships, 114
    training, 198, 274
social deficits
    depression, 167–168
    isolation, routes to, 184, 186
    psychosocial training for prisoners,
        177
    school
        bullying, 94–95
        friends, lack of, 56, 86–87
        phobia, 70
    and severity of dyslexia, relationship
        between, 41
    teachers', 76
social effects, see psychological and social
    effects of dyslexia
social isolation, see isolation, social
social perspectives on dyslexia, 31
    cheque writing, 37
    chess, 35
    cognitive and learning style, 38–39
    confusion, 36, 47–49
    creativity, 39–43
    cultural issues, 33
    date confusion, 47–49
    driving, 34

eccentricity, 43–44
English as foreign language, 32–33
ethnicity issues, 33
famous dyslexics, 43, 308–312
foreign languages, 32–34
giftedness, 44–46
handedness, 36
individual differences, 3–8
intelligence, 44–46
isolation, 37–38
labels for dyslexia, 31–32
musical ability, 35–36
political issues, 49
pronunciation and vocabulary
    problems, 38
reversal errors, 38, 46–47
sequencing problems, 46–47
sport, 32
time confusion, 47–49
visuospatial ability, 32
work effort, 36–37
written imagery, 43
social-skills training (SST), 273–275
effectiveness, 198
for prisoners, 177
social support, as coping strategy, 216
social synchrony, 189
software, 294
solitary vs. lonely people, 203
Solution-focused Brief Therapy (SFBT),
    272, 273
sound coding, 20
Sound Linkage, 20
South Africa, 8
Spanish language, 8
SPAR, 292
spatial intelligence, 196–197
    see also visuospatial skills
Special Educational Needs and Disability
    Act (1995), 306
Special Educational Needs Code of
    Practice (2001), 306
Special Educational Needs CoOrdinators
    (SENCOs), 239, 297
specialist tuition, 20–21, 66–67, 294–295,
    297
bullying, 89–90
contact details, 298, 300, 302
self-esteem, 205

special classes in mainstream schools,
    65–66
structured phonics, 19–20
special needs tribunals, 64–65
specific learning difficulties, 5–6
speech problems, 38
assessment, 293
counselling communication, 246
implying depression, 246
patterns of speech, 196, 248
types of, 194–196
speech therapy, 22
spelling
assessment, 292–293
difficulties, 21–22
and grammar, 21
teaching, 19–20
spoken language, see speech problems
sport, 32
parental context, 118
at school, 87
Springboard For Children, 226
Statements of Educational Needs, 305
stereotypes, 188
Stewart, Jackie, 34
stigma associated with dyslexia, 33
stress, 157, 158
and career choice, 233–234
daily hassles, 164–165
inoculation, 275–276
regressive behaviour, 258
at school, 63, 64
    transference between teacher and
        child, 80
see also anxiety; post-traumatic stress
    disorder
strokes, theory of, 276
structured phonics, 19–20
students, see colleges and universities
Student Support Units, 297
Study Aids and Study Assessment, 304
stuttering, 195
submission and dominance, mixed
    signals, 191–192
suicide and suicidal tendencies
counselling, 182
dyslexia as cause, 180–181
facts, 181
obsessive-compulsive disorder, 173

signs of suicidal tendency, 181
survival strategies, *see* coping strategies;
    defence strategies
Swedish language, 8
swimming, 32
symmetry of brain hemispheres, 12
synchrony, social, 189

tag questions, 251
teachers and schools, 51–52, 53, 72
    assessment of dyslexia, 291
        process, 292
        tests, 292, 293
    bullying
        action against, 96–100
        background, 88–91
        context, 94–95
        help against, 91–94
    class environment, 73–74, 87–88
    developmental nature of dyslexia,
        26
    drama triangle, 280
    dyslexic teachers, 219, 232–233
    effects of school, 54–56
    failures of dyslexics, 56–58
    and family, relationship between, 107,
        130
        fathers, 136
        mothers, 136
        parents with dyslexia, 108, 136
    helpful teachers, 84–86
    importance
        of schools, 53–54
        of teachers, 72–73
    infantilization of dyslexics, 210
    isolation, 185–186
        misinterpretation, 202
    organization of school, 64–67
    peer relationships, 86–88
    personality of teachers, 76–77
    phobia, school, 67–71
    power of teachers, 73–76
    reaction of dyslexics to school,
        59–64
    self-image of dyslexic child, 116
    structured phonics, 19–20
    transference and counter-
        transference, 77–84
    transition, 58–59

see also colleges and universities;
    education; school counsellors/
    counselling; specialist tuition and
    schools
teaching, *see* colleges and universities;
    specialist tuition and schools; teachers
    and schools
technology, 295
    advice on, 301
    software, 294
    timekeeping, 47–48
tests
    of diagnostic skills, 293
    of educational attainment, 292–293
    of underlying ability, 292
theory of mind, *see* social cognition
therapeutic alliance, 244–246
threat, perception of, 216–217
three-dimensional style, 38–39
    see also visuospatial skills
time estimation, 11
timekeeping problems, 47–49
    counselling, 253–254, 262–263
    diagnosis of dyslexia, 23
time lags in counselling communication,
    247
Tizard Report, 5–6
touch
    inappropriate, 197
    lack of, 189–190
Trades Union Congress (TUC), 299
trade unions, 232
Transactional Analysis (TA)
    drivers and injunctions, 277
    infantilized dyslexics, 209
    OK/not-OK position, 277–278
    PAC (parent-adult-child) notion, 276–277
    scripts, 277
    strokes, theory of, 276
transference
    between counsellor and client, 77–78
        aspects of, 280–283
        bullying's challenges, 94
        challenges, 264
        importance, 279
        overprotective parenting, 149
        post-traumatic stress disorder, 163
    between employer and dyslexic
        employee, 230

between parent and child
  attention deficit hyperactivity
    disorder, 109
  disability, 117–118
  dyslexic parents, 129
  overprotectiveness, 147
between teacher and child, 77–78
  actions of teacher, 81–84
  types, 78–80
  unacknowledgement, 78
  see also counter-transference
transition, school or class, 58–59
transitional objects, 255
transvestism, 213
trauma, 282
triadic family relationships, 147–148
  effect on siblings, 112–113
tribunals, special needs, 64–65
truancy, 68
truculence, 260–261
trust, 94
tuition, specialist, *see* specialist tuition
  and schools
Type I post-traumatic stress disorder, *see*
  post-traumatic stress disorder
Type II post-traumatic stress disorder,
  159, 160

unambitious parents, 133–134
unattractiveness, physical, 57, 193
underlying ability, tests of, 292
understanding in counselling
  communication, 247
unfamiliarity, and social isolation, 189
UNISON, 232
United States of America
  attitudes to dyslexia, 7–8
  crime, 176
  employment issues, 231, 232
  history of dyslexia, 5
  sibling relationships, 109
  special schools, 66
Units of Sound, 20
universities, *see* colleges and universities
University of East London, 304
University of Wales, 226
USDAW, 232

variation in dyslexia, 16–18

verbal IQ, 292
verbally accessible memories (VAMs), 163
verbal reasoning, 21
Vernon Single Word Reading Test, 292
victim behaviour, 37
  bullying, 98, 99–100
  family life, 113
  prevalence, 198–199
  reasons for, 199–200
  see also learned helplessness
victimization, *see* bullying
violence and aggression
  as defence strategy, 259, 260–261
  between siblings, 111–113
  see also anger; bullying
visibility, and risk of being bullied, 90
visual images in counselling, 251–252,
  285–286
visual memory, 293
visual perceptual skills, 293
visuospatial skills, 32, 45–46
  distinctive cognitive learning style,
    38–39
  genetic point of dyslexia, 11
vocabulary
  counselling communication, 246
  problems, 38
  teaching, 19–20
voice problems, *see* speech problems
voluntary counselling projects, 226–227

waffle, in counselling, 249–250
warmth towards dyslexics
  from family, 150
    mothers, 138
  from teachers, 84–85
Warnock Committee, 305
watches, 47
Way, Ben, 312
Wechsler Intelligence Scale for Children
  third edition (WISC-III), 292
Wide-Range Achievement Test (WRAT),
  292, 293
Wilcox, Toyah, 312
Wilkinson, Mark, 312
wiring of dyslexic brain, 12
Wonder, Stevie, 36
work effort of dyslexics, 36–37
  as coping strategy, 216

and creativity, 42
students, 236
working memory, *see* memory, short-term
writing
adults' skills, 23
assessment, 292–293
cheques, 37
creative, 43, 63

history, 4–5
learning, 297
mirror, 36
see also handwriting; literacy
written imagery, 43

Yeats, William Butler, 40, 43, 312
Young, Murray Lachlan, 312